Cold, hard steel

Manchester University Press

SOCIAL HISTORIES OF MEDICINE

Series editors: David Cantor, Anne Hanley and Elaine Leong

Social Histories of Medicine is concerned with all aspects of health, illness and medicine, from prehistory to the present, in every part of the world. The series covers the circumstances that promote health or illness, the ways in which people experience and explain such conditions, and what, practically, they do about them. Practitioners of all approaches to health and healing come within its scope, as do their ideas, beliefs and practices, and the social, economic and cultural contexts in which they operate. Methodologically, the series welcomes relevant studies in social, economic, cultural and intellectual history, as well as approaches derived from other disciplines in the arts, sciences, social sciences and humanities. The series is a collaboration between Manchester University Press and the Society for the Social History of Medicine.

To buy or to find out more about the books currently available in this series, please go to: https://manchesteruniversitypress.co.uk/series/social-histories-of-medicine/

Cold, hard steel

The myth of the modern surgeon

Agnes Arnold-Forster

Manchester University Press

Published by Manchester University Press
Oxford Road, Manchester M13 9PL

www.manchesteruniversitypress.co.uk

British Library Cataloguing-in-Publication Data
A catalogue record for this book is available from the British Library

ISBN 978 1 5261 5662 4 hardback

First published 2023

Typeset by Newgen Publishing UK
Printed in Great Britain by TJ Books Ltd., Padstow

To my partner, Ben

Contents

Acknowledgements

This book was researched and part-written while I was Research and Engagement Fellow on the Wellcome Trust Investigator Award, Surgery & Emotion (108667/Z/15/B), and I am first and foremost indebted to the Trust for its funding, to the project's Principal Investigator Michael Brown, and to my colleagues Alison Moulds, James Kennaway, and Lauren Ryall-Waite. Due to the nature of academic precarity, I completed the book while working on a series of other postdoctoral projects and I am grateful to my various PIs and line managers for their generosity, intellectual support, and patience. My thanks to Thomas Dixon, Victoria Bates, Thomas Schlich, Annmarie Adams, and Martin Gorsky.

Many other academics have provided crucial intellectual, social, and emotional support throughout this process. Caitjan Gainty, Anna Maguire, Jacob Moses, Samuel Schotland, and Jacob Steere-Williams are owed particular gratitude for reading drafts of chapters or related articles, discussing with me the vexed relationship between surgery and emotion, and just generally being good, kind, and curious friends. Parts of this book appear elsewhere in journals and I am grateful to the editors of the *Bulletin of the History of Medicine* and *History Workshop Journal* for allowing me to reproduce elements of those articles and to the peer reviewers for their critical and constructive feedback.

I would also like to thank various surgeons by name, as well as those whom I interviewed who preferred to remain anonymous. Simon Fleming, Greta Lachlan, and Sam Gallivan have been particularly thoughtful and open interlocutors between me and the weird world of surgery. I am grateful to anyone who took the time to speak to me about their experiences of the profession, whether in a full-length oral history interview, or briefly over Twitter. I am particularly indebted to the Royal College of Surgeons and the Royal College of Nursing and to Hayley Kruger and Sarah Chaney for being such valuable points of contact.

I could not have written this book without the support of my friends and family. My parents Rebecca Jewell and Jake Arnold-Forster have been unrelentingly generous and encouraging, ensuring I always have delicious things to eat and people to complain to. My siblings Theo Arnold-Forster and Dora Arnold-Forster are equally loving, if slightly better at taking me, their big sister, down a peg or two. My friends Isabel Asquith, Phoebe Arnold, Bronya Arciszewska, Rita Conry, and Isabelle Fraser have no idea what I do all day, but are the best ever anyway.

Last, but certainly not least, this book is dedicated to my partner Ben. I wrote most of this book while living in Montreal, Canada, in the middle of a pandemic, with him, but thousands of miles away from everyone else I know and love. I was homesick and struggling to complete a major piece of research while libraries and archives remained closed. He was everything I needed him to be and more.

Abbreviations

BMA	British Medical Association
BMJ	*British Medical Journal*
EWTD	European Working Time Directive
GMC	General Medical Council
NHS	National Health Service
RCP	Royal College of Physicians
RCSEd	Royal College of Surgeons of Edinburgh
RCS	Royal College of Surgeons of England

Introduction: Sir Lancelot Spratt and the myth of the modern surgeon

There are many myths of the modern surgeon, and not all are particularly flattering. Mostly male, authoritarian, and paternalistic, the stereotypical surgeon is volatile, insistent, even abusive – and prone to unpredictable outburst of anger. He cuts first, asks questions later, and is never in doubt. He is good at 'hard' surgeries but bad at 'soft' skills like compassion and communication. Academically or technically brilliant, he lacks emotional intelligence. He operates with dispassion, but occasionally his capacity for emotional detachment tips into cruelty – causing psychological harm to both himself and his patients. He is often white and at the very least middle class. With his colleagues, he engages in the social pursuits of the upper echelons – hunting, shooting, and drinking Bordeaux.

Britain is populated by many of these larger-than-life surgeons, but by no one is this caricature better embodied than by Richard Gordon's irascible Sir Lancelot Spratt. Spratt first appeared in Gordon's 1952 novel, *Doctor in the House*.[1] Gordon was an English surgeon and anaesthetist who wrote a long series of comic novels on medical themes. Beginning with *Doctor in the House*, the books were set in St Swithin's, a fictional London hospital, and follow the capers and exploits of a young medical student Simon Sparrow.[2] The film adaptation under the same name was released in 1954 and starred Dirk Bogarde as Sparrow and James Robertson Justice as the fearsome teaching hospital surgeon Spratt. A dictatorial demagogue, he strode down hospital corridors with a gaggle of frightened trainees hurrying along behind him. In one iconic scene, Spratt stands at a patient's bedside firing questions at a group of medical students, one of whom has just examined the hapless and prone sufferer and found a lump. 'Is it kidney? Is it spleen? Is it liver? Is it dangerous?' barks Spratt, before drawing a long incision line on the patient's abdomen, then turning to the by-now highly alarmed patient to say, 'Now don't worry, this is nothing whatever to do with you.'[3]

Sir Lancelot Spratt was and is an archetype. He represented and constructed a lasting surgical stereotype that can be traced through film, fiction, and professional debate from the 1950s to the present. This book anatomises this myth, investigates the many strategies British surgeons have deployed to complicate or overturn it, and asks how these characters and caricatures have altered real surgeons' feelings, experiences, and the meanings they attach to their work. Ranging across the twentieth century, but focusing on the period following the foundation of Britain's National Health Service in 1948, it explores how these myths have shaped the self-image of practitioners, informed public perceptions of surgeons, transformed the doctor–patient relationship, and intervened in the interactions between different healthcare professionals. The central contention of this book is that while they might be fictional and sometimes even absurd, these stereotypes have shaped the surgical experience in twentieth-century Britain and continue to inform the nature and conditions of surgical identity and surgical work today.

This book is, therefore, about both representations and experience – and the changing relationship between the two. Revealing or demonstrating the 'relative throw – the weight or significance' of popular culture on ordinary people in the past is an unresolved challenge to the cultural historian.[4] This book takes up this challenge and seeks to explain why and how the Spratt stereotype lasted so long and proved so enduring. While some people today might not remember Sir Lancelot himself, almost all surgeons will recognise the stereotype he informed: *Doctor in the House* was the most popular box office film of 1954 in Great Britain, seen by one-third of the national population – or 15,500,000 people. The many sequels were viewed by yet more millions. Media studies scholars have long argued that film and television have the power to shape cultural norms, teach personal values, and offer 'a universal curriculum that everyone can learn'.[5] Numerous studies have noted the peculiar popularity of medical dramas, as well as the ways in which viewers use entertainment programmes as a source of knowledge about healthcare and its constituent professionals.[6] I would hazard that most people learnt more of what they do know about healthcare and operating theatres from things like *Grey's Anatomy* and *Casualty* than from school, university, or the real-life doctors and nurses they encounter in GP practices or on hospital wards. There is also an increasing and multidisciplinary recognition of the power of fictional, filmic, and televisual representations to shape professional identities and surgical self-image.[7] In other words, culture and everyday experiences inform each other.[8] Or as teacher and sociologist Lesley Scanlon puts it, 'the two become indistinguishable … having significant impacts on the way we view ourselves as professionals and the way we view other professionals both individually and collectively'.[9]

Indeed, while *Doctor in the House* and its sequels might not have set out to explicitly tackle the ethics and issues of surgical professionalism, they constructed and confirmed a mythology of surgery that continues to exist and still enjoys substantial cultural capital.[10] An article published as recently as 2014 by the Royal College of Surgeons of England described the surgical stereotype thus:

> Decisive, efficient, and a realist, but as an impersonal and autocratic person. Egocentric, he is more interested in rapid actions and immediate results than in interpersonal relationships. He works hard, expresses himself physically, is always in motion, and is incapable of relaxing.[11]

Implying a profession dominated by heterosexual men committed to their craft, a year later, the *Health Service Journal* referenced the adage 'knife, life and wife' in their description of twenty-first-century surgeons' experiences of work.[12] Clearly, Spratt is still with us.

Spratt was, of course, fictional, and there were likely many consultants working in post-war Britain who were kind rather than cruel, compassionate rather than detached, and democratic rather than dictatorial. There were also many surgeons who combined Spratt-like tendencies with other characteristics – complex humans with feelings and flaws. However, there is also evidence to suggest that the Spratt stereotype was not a total invention. As this book will explore, in post-war Britain, surgeons trained as part of a 'firm' – a hierarchical structure of senior and less-senior practitioners. The firm orbited around both the hospital ward and the hospital bar.

Surgeons often lived in, or very close to, the hospital, and the consultant wielded considerable power over his juniors and had substantial autonomy in his dealings with patients and hospital administration. This hierarchical structure allowed for Spratt-like individuals to practice unimpeded and conduct themselves as they wished and, according to doctors, health policymakers, and journalists, carbon copies of Sir Lancelot stalked the wards of the real-life hospital in the mid-century.

In their recollections of surgical training, practitioners today refer to Spratt as a living and breathing figure, someone who dominated their first years in the profession. In 2005, Graham Reed recalled his early experiences of hospital life:

> When I first entered medicine hospital doctors often did not become consultants, particularly in surgical specialties, until they were well into their 40s. In true Lancelot Spratt style consultants then had an impressive retinue: senior and junior registrars, senior house officers, and – in one instance I can remember – a 'first assistant.'[13]

A plastic surgeon born in 1946 described his first experiences of hospital work in the early 1970s. The world he recalled has much in common with the world of *Doctor in the House*: 'The surgeons were the role models. They were powerful, they were charismatic, very charismatic people, and they *did* things.' He worked as part of a firm and his consultant, 'was a very powerful and charismatic man … who every King's [College Hospital] man of my age revered. Not a man you cross.' He described the firm in terms that would not be unfamiliar to a character in a Richard Gordon novel:

> The firm system was you knew where you stood. You were working in a small group of people everybody knew you and you knew all your patients. And if you didn't know a patient then your consultant would soon expose it. So in one way you had to be thick skinned but that was how you learned.[14]

After all, Gordon likely used some of the features of hospital life he observed as an anaesthetist, and the characteristics of the surgeons he worked with, to create his demagogic anti-hero.

These real-life Spratts were not, of course, all bad. Today, surgeons often reflect fondly on this era of surgical history and they have as many, if not more, positive as negative things to say about their authoritarian consultants. However, Gordon's contribution was not the creation of a realistic character, but the construction of a mythology that could be deployed in the making, maintenance, and critique of the surgical identity. Indeed, as Spratt gradually disappeared from television and cinema screens, he became less a way to describe current colleagues and superiors, and more an archetype who embodied a troubling, if enduring, version of surgical professionalism.

Thus, late twentieth-century healthcare practitioners and policymakers frequently reference the Spratt stereotype when outlining the characters and working styles that they would rather not want to see on current and future hospital wards. In 1978, doctor Peter Banks wrote an article where he asked, 'What is a good doctor?' He posed several potential answers: 'One who spends adequate time with his patients?'; 'One who can make up his mind …?'; 'One who uses the resources of the medical team?', before concluding with, 'One with a personality strong enough to influence the patients? A Sir Lancelot Spratt in every office? Heaven forbid!'[15] In 2003, an orthopaedic surgeon under investigation for bullying other staff defended himself by referring to the 'classic *Doctor* comedy films', and insisting, 'I didn't operate like a Sir Lancelot Spratt-type surgeon.'[16] Spratt increasingly epitomised the opposite of what it meant to be a good surgeon in post-war Britain.

While I contend that Sir Lancelot Spratt offers us an insight into the interplay between cultural representations and clinical practices and identities, I am not trying to suggest that he is solely culpable for surgical culture or even surgical stereotypes in twentieth- and twenty-first-century Britain. As a result, this book will also explore what else was responsible for the construction of the surgical identity and the maintenance of certain surgical myths. What was it about surgical training, surgical culture, and surgical social life that made and remade the surgical identity and how has that training, culture, and social life interacted with broader historical changes? British healthcare was transformed in the second half of the twentieth century and the changing reception and perception of the Spratt-esque surgical stereotype took place against this backdrop.

The National Health Service was established by Clement Attlee's post-war Labour government in 1948 and it profoundly altered the relationship between surgeons and the state. The service was consolidated in the 1950s and 1960s, but just as doctors had begun to get used to the idea, everything changed again. The Conservatives won an election in June 1970 and Keith Joseph took over as Secretary of State for Health and Social Services. Joseph published a White Paper in August 1972 proposing a radical reorganisation of the NHS that was incorporated into the National Health Service Reorganisation Act of July 1973. Labour returned to government in February 1974 and implemented the planned reorganisation, which was designed to unify the health service, facilitate better cooperation between health and local authorities, and achieve better organisational management. These administrative and managerial changes fundamentally impacted the way that doctors and nurses worked and transformed the nature and conditions of surgical labour.

This book looks at how the changing policies and politics of the NHS shaped surgical stereotypes, identities, and experiences. As historian Christopher Lawrence has shown, for many surgeons the past looms large. Indeed, many of his arguments about nineteenth-century practitioners and their tendencies to deploy their collective history to cultivate their professional identities apply to surgeons of the twenty-first century.[17] They spend a lot of time reflecting on their own professional histories and drawing comparisons between how it once was and how it is now. Today, many surgeons are preoccupied with the differences between what they see as the 'traditional' styles of surgical work and the managed, bureaucratic, and individualistic experiences on wards today. While there is some debate over when the shift from 'traditional' to today occurred, the managerialism introduced by the 1974 reorganisation and its crystallisation under Margaret Thatcher in the 1980s is frequently targeted as the culprit. These comparisons between then and now are often nostalgic in tone.

As I have suggested, Spratt was not an irredeemable figure, and for every negative aspect of the stereotype, there were elements that surgeons campaigned to keep. For many, the hierarchical structure that characterised surgery in the 1950s and 1960s meant that decisions about patient care could be made efficiently. Moreover, freedom from managerial or administrative oversight gave consultant surgeons a sense of autonomy that served as an emotional buffer against the stresses and strains of long working hours. However, the reforms of the 1970s meant that surgeons spent more time doing paperwork than they had before. For some, this meant a reduction in clinical or operative labour – the labour they had devoted decades to training for and which was the source of their professional identity and sense of self. Sir George Godber, Chief Medical Officer from 1960 to 1973, made various observations about the ill effects of 1970s NHS reform. He lamented the new administrative and bureaucratic burden shouldered by hospital workers and lambasted the amount of 'office work' clinical staff now had to do.[18]

Godber also criticised managerialism. Keith Joseph 'had had some business experience and was determined that the management of the NHS should be professional'. To this end, he recruited professional management consultants, McKinsey & Co.[19] For surgeons, this was a largely negative development. Reorganisation was seen to erode the traditional hierarchies of the firm and practitioners lamented their loss of independence. One surgeon put it thus:

> In spite of the pressures in the 80s and 90s, a sense of being in control of one's own destiny mitigated against much of the stress. I have lived through 35 years of erosion of autonomy and a burgeoning weight of governance, that, in turn, contributes to a sense of jeopardy and peril.[20]

In addition, the firm system – while critiqued by many – also offered many junior and senior surgeons a sense of belonging and community. Godber was not alone, therefore, in arguing that reorganisation had had ill effects on doctors' happiness: 'The frustration which every doctor has experienced seeing the service of which he was so proud being destroyed by ministerial and administrative unwisdom has had its effect on morale.'[21]

Despite these critiques, and as the 1980s continued, hospitals only became more heavily managed and the 1990s witnessed further political and NHS policy transformation. In 1997, Tony Blair won a landslide general election for Labour, and a year later his party published the White Paper, 'The New NHS: Modern. Dependable'.[22] In many respects, 'The New NHS: Modern. Dependable' represented an evolution rather than revolution in the management of the NHS. It did, however, further alter the way hospital doctors worked. It included a new contract for consultants which aimed at increasing their accountability and restricting their freedom to work in the private sector. It ushered in a new emphasis on the provision of twenty-four-hour, consultant-led care across all subspecialties; recommended a reduction in the working hours of junior doctors; and proposed to 'break down the old hierarchical ways of working'. The White Paper also proposed a new consideration of European Union directives restricting the working hours of doctors.[23] The European Working Time Directive (EWTD) forty-eight-hour working week entered law in European Union countries in 1998 and a phased approach to implementation was agreed for doctors in training in the UK, which steadily reduced working hours to fifty-eight in 2004, fifty-six in 2007, and forty-eight in 2009.[24]

Developments also included the Calman Reforms of medical post-graduate training that introduced shorter, more intensive training programmes and required consultants to take a more active role in educating their juniors (reducing the time available for treating patients). Consultants were not, overall, keen on these new reforms, and they expressed in often fraught terms the damaging effects of new policies on their emotional health and ability to work effectively. If 1974 was a watershed moment for some, 1997 was the key turning point for others. Surgeons focus on the introduction of the EWTD and its supposedly debilitating effect on practitioner well-being. Indeed, the past often poses a paradox for modern surgeons. While Graham Reed's method of deploying Spratt to represent an outdated and harmful 'old style' of healthcare and hospital work was common in the late twentieth and early twenty-first centuries, and particularly in the debates surrounding the introduction of the new consultant contract, there were also many who lamented this old style's departure.

These New Labour policies were – both implicitly and explicitly – designed to rid hospital wards of the Sir Lancelot Spratt stereotype. As a result, senior surgeons' mistrust of the new emphasis on consultant-led care and the reduction in working hours of junior doctors was not looked upon kindly by some quarters of the press. In a 2002 *Daily Mail* article, professor of health economics Alan Maynard quoted Aneurin Bevan: 'the only message understood by a doctor is written on a cheque'.[25] Below a picture of Sir Lancelot Spratt from the film *Doctor at Large*, Maynard raged that consultants get

> the best of both words ... Featherbedded by the state, but with access to lucrative private work. The BMA with its affluent, articulate, middle- and upper-class membership ... enjoys a unique influence over the establishment and the public, which is ruthlessly exploited to ensure that its members remain well paid but unaccountable.[26]

Spratt represented an anachronistic and now untenable way of working and embodied an autocratic, hierarchical, and financially lucrative profession seemingly out of touch with the twenty-first-century world and workforce. Indeed, the *Financial Times* called the consultants' intransigence 'the last roar of a dinosaur'.[27] It warned that senior doctors who opposed the deal because it compromised professional autonomy and clinical freedom may have to accept that 'the days of the autonomous consultant à la Sir Lancelot Spratt are long gone'.[28] The paper quotes an anonymous manager saying that consultants should accept being managed 'as happens in any other walk of life'.[29]

Other histories of surgery

As has probably already become clear, this book is not a history of surgical ideas, surgical innovation, or even a history of surgical practice. It is, instead, a history of *surgeons* (both fictional and real) – a social, cultural, and emotional history that offers a new narrative of the surgical identity. It is this focus on people – and particularly their *feelings* – that marks this book out from other texts in the history of surgery. Surgeons have shown a long-standing and vivid interest in their own past and have produced numerous valuable accounts of the technical history of their work. Many of the practitioners I have met are hobbying historians with a specific and extensive interest in the lineage of their profession, subspecialty, or preferred instrument, procedure, or institution. Such interests have proven profoundly useful for the professional historian of science, technology, and medicine – partly because surgery remains a relatively understudied part of healthcare history. This is odd not only because surgery occupies a central place in medicine's history, but because – and as Thomas Schlich has observed – its practice is now routine in twenty-first-century life.[30]

In 2017, Schlich edited a handbook of the history of surgery that offered a range of new perspectives on the subject and identified a variety of new avenues for research.[31] Schlich credits the social history of medicine for this expanded field of vision. Since the 1970s, historians have turned towards a wider range of social groups involved in surgery:

> Practitioners and their patients, the patients' families, nurses, manufacturers and dealers of instruments, regulators and legislators and so on – as well as to the various institutions – hospitals, schools, colleges, universities, professional organizations – that played a role in its history.[32]

Schlich also credits the social history of medicine with establishing a new critical response to the traditional medical historiography that 'seemed to centre too much on the triumphal progress of medical science'.[33] Traditional histories of surgery – some written by surgeons themselves – tended to focus on heroic individuals and were often personal and professional biographies of practitioners. This book is different to these traditional accounts because it pays little attention to the 'great men' of surgery – the only famous surgeons you will find in these pages are fictional. It also devotes barely any space to the profound achievements of twentieth- and twenty-first-century operative practice – skating over innovations such as minimally invasive and robotic surgery. Thus, unlike other accounts of surgical technique and innovation, this book focuses on the social lives, cultural representations, and emotional complexities of 'ordinary' surgeons, both past and present.[34]

The social history of medicine's key contribution was to redress the balance and focus on the patient experience and the patient narrative. In doing so, it made crucial correctives to the power dynamics of medical history. However, it also cleaved a division between traditional histories of eminent practitioners on the one hand and textured accounts of patients and everyday healthcare experiences on the other. As a result, histories of 'rank and file' clinical professionals and their ordinary working lives are more uncommon. Additionally, most of those that do exist focus on the nineteenth century.

My focus on the history of surgeons' professional identities means that this book is in dialogue with the work of other scholars who have also attended to the question of what has made surgeons into the things they are, even if those scholars have mostly attended to the periods before the Second World War. Sally Wilde's work on surgery at the turn of the twentieth century (1890–1910), for example, reveals that the rising popularity of the profession and practice was not so much due to better surgical outcomes as it was on increased confidence in the possibility of better surgical results, and the various, compelling ways in which this confidence was communicated by doctors.[35] As my book will show, confidence became a key attribute of the myth of the modern surgeon. Along similar lines, Della Gavrus' work on American neurologists and neurosurgeons in the first half of the twentieth century shows how these practitioners used rhetoric to perform a shared and oppositional identity predicated on either a historical past or therapeutic utility.[36] And yet, historical studies of analogous subjects in the post-war period are relatively scarce.

Surgeons and their feelings

The research underpinning this book comes from three years spent as a research and engagement fellow on the project 'Surgery and Emotion'.[37] Blending histories of work, medicine, and the emotions, my research has mapped out the personal and professional landscape of modern operative practice.[38] I have questioned stereotypes of surgical dispassion and their place in historical narratives and contemporary culture. My work has revealed that emotions are central to the expectations patients have of their practitioners, key to the development of surgical identities, and fundamental to the relationships between different members of the surgical team.[39]

Readers and researchers intuitively understand that undergoing surgery can be a troubling experience for patients. However, relatively few historians have considered the emotional demands of clinical labour on healthcare professionals, and much of the existing work in this area attends to the 'high feelings' that accompany experiences such as patient death, rather than more 'mundane' or quotidian emotions.[40] One exception to this tendency to focus on patient experience is historian and Surgery and Emotion Principal Investigator Michael Brown, who, along with Lynda Payne, Peter

Stanley, and Joanna Bourke, has written about the period before the advent of anaesthetics in the middle of the nineteenth century.[41] Then, surgical interventions were undertaken with little or no pain relief and occasioned great physical suffering and emotional distress. Stanley elaborates how surgeons learned to overcome the dread of inflicting pain, without being able to preclude it entirely, and explores the richly sourced negotiated relationship between surgeon, patient, and her family or friends.[42]

However, and as Brown has argued, rather than producing detachment or dispassion in surgeons, such intense experiences gave rise to a range of feelings from pity and sympathy to anxiety, regret, and anger. He combats pervasive stereotypes of the Victorian surgeon as a barbarous butcher who cared little for the suffering of his patients, and instead presents a more nuanced account of the affective landscape of the early nineteenth-century operating theatre.[43] Taking a similar approach but attending to a very different era, this book seeks to understand how surgeons conceived of themselves and their work in terms of feeling. I will push beyond clichés of 'clinical detachment' to explore the emotional complexities of the surgical encounter, the surgical career, and the surgical identity.

When I first joined the research project in 2017, I anticipated a study of the high feelings associated with surgical care and the affective aspects of the doctor–patient relationship. While I thought I was going to be investigating the past and present of compassion, sympathy, anxiety, doubt, and grief – in oral history interviews and at professional engagement events – surgeons overwhelmingly wanted to talk about the more 'ordinary' emotions associated with surgical work. As a result, rather than exploring the intense emotions that accompany experiences such as patient death, my project became a study of stress, burnout, frustration, and fatigue – the affective landscape of professional identity, problematic colleagues, and paperwork. Inter- and intra-professional bullying, annual leave, and the impact of the EWTD on surgeons' wellbeing were far more pressing problems for the surgeons I met and worked with.

For every surgeon who could speak movingly about their first experience of death was another who could barely remember a single moment of emotional intensity with a patient. Those same surgeons could, however, recount with verve their frustrations with rotas, handovers, and bureaucracy. This observation is not a criticism of the surgeons in question, but rather a comment on the assumptions historians of medicine – myself included – make about healthcare professionals and our unwitting tendency to reify medical exceptionalism. We tend – like so many others – to mark healthcare work out as unlike labour of any other kind. Healthcare work is almost invariably presented as a calling, vocation, or labour of love, and it is easy to assume that the associated feelings will be radically different to the feelings that attend other paid employment. Different jobs do, of course, elicit different feelings – but lots of roles also share 'emotional regimes' and sources of frustration.[44]

Over the past five years or so, these sources of frustration in the surgical workplace have attracted new attention from surgeons, professional organisations, and health policymakers. There is a consensus that surgery is in the midst of a crisis of emotional ill health and depleted wellbeing. Recent studies have revealed a high level of burnout among doctors and medical students in the United Kingdom, and new and persistent pressures have led to a supposed epidemic in serious psychological and emotional conditions. This epidemic has prompted a range of responses from those responsible for professional standards and training in Britain. From working with surgeons and researching these responses, a rough taxonomy of the 'crisis' in surgical wellbeing is possible. The key emotional problems in contemporary surgery are stress, burnout, bullying, and the perceived erosion of individual autonomy and 'resilience' because of structural changes to the NHS over the past two decades.

One of my key motivations to write this book was to find out where this crisis came from and to explore what, if anything, a cultural history of the profession might be able to contribute to current practitioners. My approach, inspired by other historians of medicine and emotion, has been to consider workplace distress and wellbeing as historically contingent. For example, and as Mark Jackson argues, the version of stress that was conceptualised by scientists and clinicians in the late nineteenth century onwards was shaped by specific social mores, economic trends, and by changing political contexts. Rather than an unchanging emotional state, stress as we know it today is a dynamic product of modern life.[45] Histories of burnout and resilience make similar contributions.[46]

Moreover, while understanding the myths that dominate modern and contemporary surgery might allow us to further delineate how professional identity was developed and maintained, it also gives us insight into the emotional consequences of certain professional behaviours and responses. For example, a key component of the surgical stereotype is the emotional range expected or required. Spratt was capable of anger, derision, and indifference – but not care, compassion, or collegiality. He also had little time for introspection, reflection, or emotional 'self-care'. As a result, this book will investigate the connections between certain emotional expectations and the realities of surgical work. Attending to feelings helps us access the meanings and values surgeons applied and apply to their work and gives us insight into the relationship between policy change and experience.

This book looks at how the myths of modern surgery interact with the surgical experience. Do they attract or deter medical students and foundation-year doctors to or from the specialty? How do they shape surgeons' identities and experience of their practice? Is there any truth to these stereotypes? Are there any surgeons who aspire to match them? What have individuals and the professional community done to address, nuance, or overturn them? And how do these stereotypes alter public perception of surgeons, affect the doctor–patient relationship, and intervene in intra-professional communication? These aims are also particularly relevant now. In the aftermath of a catastrophic pandemic, when government, organisations, and administrators are intensely concerned with the nature and conditions of clinical work, the emotional costs of surgical care, and the changing politics of workplace wellbeing, this book attempts to intervene in pressing conversations about contemporary healthcare policy, practice, and professionalism.

If the myths of modern surgery are as harmful as I suggest, then why have they survived? The key to this conundrum, I argue, is something already mentioned. For every negative aspect of the surgical stereotype, there were elements that surgeons campaigned to keep. For every unflattering myth, there was a countervailing alternative that cast the profession in a glowing light. Medical paternalism and authoritarianism have increasingly fallen out of favour, but they are entwined with the more positive attributes of efficiency, expertise, and quick decision making. Excessive working hours and fatigue are entangled with the ideals of a devoted, committed profession suffused with vocational zeal. While an all-encompassing professional life might render surgery a community that excludes parents, for example, it also offers others a sense of profound belonging. The 'old boys' club' might be male dominated, upper class, and overwhelmingly white, but it can also provide crucial emotional support to its members.

If the mythology of modern surgery was singular and straightforward, it might already have been radically transformed. But the surgical stereotype is messy. As off-putting as it is appealing, practitioners can, sometimes at least, take what they wish, and leave the things that do not serve their needs. One of the many problems with this is that not everyone in the profession can agree on what the positive and negative attributes of the surgical stereotype are, and not all of the attributes can be easily disentangled from their more compromising alternative. Another issue is that some of the aspects work better for some surgeons than others. The ideals of devotion, vocation, and commitment are easier to uphold if you do not have caring responsibilities, and the collegiality of the 'old boys' club' is more accessible to some ethnicities and social classes than others. The myths of modern surgery have made modern surgery. To undo them means undoing much of what is familiar, even meaningful and appealing, to current practitioners.

Methods and sources

In researching and writing this book, and to move beyond a history of technique and innovation, I drew on a diverse array of approaches to understanding the modern and contemporary surgical world. These include quantitative studies of recruitment, retention, and pay; qualitative surveys of the surgical experience conducted by co-professionals seeking empirical evidence for their subjective suffering; and laboratory-based investigations into the biomarkers of surgical stress and fatigue.[47] As this is partly a history of work and professional identity, I have drawn on sociologies of labour and organisational change.[48] I have also used literary analyses of medical fiction and surgical memoirs alongside cultural studies of film and television.[49] This reliance on multiple different kinds of academic literature – and not just history – is required partly because the story I am telling is so contemporary. While there are studies of surgery, medicine, and healthcare in the middle and later decades of the twentieth century, the scholarly literature on the past thirty years has tended to emerge from disciplines such as sociology, health policy, cultural studies, and literature.[50] Engaging with these investigations and analyses also, I hope, makes this book accessible to people without professional historical training and allows me to intervene in diverse discussions and debates.

The ability to write this book has depended on close collaboration with medical students, trainees, and currently practicing surgeons. This book takes seriously Felicity Callard and Des Fitzgerald's claim that we can 'make more interesting interventions by … collaborating *with* people in [the] sciences, rather than simply scrutinizing them',[51] particularly in a moment in which the sciences seem 'ever more richly and capaciously *social* in both their orientation and their practice' (emphasis in the original).[52] Collaborating with surgeons has required me to become comfortable with an array of different approaches and source materials – I have had to learn how to 'speak their language' by familiarising myself with their journals and academic conventions. I have also used them and their lives as sources for my historical work. I have conducted approximately thirty oral history interviews with currently practicing and recently retired British surgeons. Oral history is often used to address subjects that are missing from existing archives, and its practitioners have sought to record the experiences of the dispossessed, disempowered, and marginalised.[53] This valuable tendency has meant, however, that oral history interviews with doctors – with their substantial social and financial capital – are relatively rare.[54] My corpus constitutes one of the only existing collections of semi-structured interviews with British surgeons.

Social media has become a key site for surgical sociability in the twenty-first century.[55] As a result, I did much of my recruitment of participants via Twitter – issuing calls for participants and engaging with surgeons on the platform. This proved productive partly because it allowed me to connect with practitioners from across the United Kingdom, particularly during the pandemic when travel was restricted and interviews had to take place over the phone or online. In addition, I could circumvent traditional specialty or hospital hierarchies and speak to surgeons from a range of different career stages and states of employment. However, there were some drawbacks as, in my experience, practitioners convinced by the value of social media tend to be younger and more socially progressive, thus potentially skewing the perspectives I gathered. To redress this, I also recruited via publications in more traditional venues like the *British Medical Journal* and the *Bulletin of the Royal College of Surgeons*. Together, these two approaches – alongside word-of-mouth and attending professional events – resulted in a diverse mix of interviewees.

The oldest participant was born in the 1930s, and so the interviews cover surgical experiences from the 1950s to the present day. Most of my participants were male, but around a third were women (reflecting the demographics of the profession), and around a quarter were people of colour (again, roughly corresponding with the ethnic make-up of British surgery). I interviewed consultants, specialty trainees, and doctors straight out of medical school in the first few years of their professional lives. I also interviewed people from a range of different specialties – from trauma and orthopaedics to neurosurgery. As discussed in Chapter 4, different surgical specialities have their own unique stereotypes and cultural associations.

A semi-structured interview is open, relatively free form and allows new ideas to be brought up during the interview process. I began by asking participants about medical experiences in childhood, before moving chronologically through their lives according to a predetermined (although flexible and responsive) framework of themes. We discussed their decisions to embark on a medical career path, their early exposure to anatomical dissection, their first time on the hospital ward, their own experiences of ill health, why they were drawn to surgery as a specialty, and their relationships with their colleagues, patients, and families. The interviews each lasted for about an hour and were recorded and then transcribed. My theoretical approach to the analysis of the interviews is primarily historical and draws on the ample literature on reflexivity and memory. I pay as much attention to the questions they cannot answer as to those they can, and stay attuned to *how* they say something, not just *what* they say.

Due to my use of oral history interviews and my efforts to engage with the professional community, I have spent plenty of time with surgeons while researching and writing this book. They are valuable repositories of information and engaging primary sources. They are also often interesting and reflective people, offering insights and analysis alongside personal, professional, and historical detail. This book is a product of their insight, my analysis, and the relationship between researcher and subject. These relationships have been fundamental for my understanding of the past and present of British surgery and I am indebted to those men and women who gave up their time to talk to me.

Structure

This book is made up of seven chapters and a conclusion. The first three chapters are devoted to delineating the post-war surgical stereotype and its reverberations through both popular and surgical culture. Drawing on written sources such as records from professional societies and social clubs alongside some oral history recollections, I flesh out the real-life corollaries to the Spratt caricatures. I also offer some alternatives to the detached demagogue, and using surgical textbooks and conduct guides reveal the nuanced and sensitive debates taking place in professional circles about the nature of the surgical identity and the behaviour expected from newly trained practitioners. In chapters 4, 5, 6, and 7 I rely on medical journal articles and oral history interviews to trace how ideas of emotional detachment and dispassion have permeated later twentieth-century surgical cultures and how they have shaped surgical practice, affected the diversity of the profession, and influenced the emotional wellbeing of surgeons themselves. I interrogate the changing nature of surgical professionalism and the surgical career against the backdrop of major transformations in the structure of the National Health Service and explore how experiences of surgical work altered with developments in organisational ideologies and social and cultural shifts.

In the first two chapters, 'Self-made myths' and 'Surgeons in film, fiction, and on TV screens', I look at sources written by practitioners for practitioners alongside cultural representations to delineate the construction of the 'ideal' and infamous surgeon, interrogate the sources of surgical stereotypes, and examine instances where suggestions for good surgical behaviour contrast with caricatures. Textbooks were written by senior surgeons and designed to be read by practitioners at the outset of their careers. They devoted chapters to outlining anatomy, diagnosis, suturing, wound dressings, and aftercare. However, they also all dedicated an opening chapter or preface to the elaboration of the surgical identity and to setting out their vision of surgical behaviour. These introductions are replete also with emotions. Thus, I argue that such texts shaped assumptions and expectations about the emotional expression and affective behaviour of surgeons and were as attentive to non-technical skills as they were to the development of expertise and the acquisition of knowledge. In Chapter 2 I anatomise the stereotype embodied by Sir Lancelot Spratt and search for evidence of his existence in other fictional genres and cultural outputs.

As discussed, in post-war Britain, surgeons trained as part of a 'firm' – a hierarchical structure of senior and less-senior practitioners. Community, professional bonds, and social interaction were key features of past surgical life, and while they likely sustained the emotional health of some healthcare practitioners, they also drew boundaries around the surgical profession and cultivated cultures and communities with deeply problematic characteristics. In Chapter 3, 'Surgical conduct and surgical communities', and using the archives of surgical associations, clubs, and professional societies, I reveal the crucial role of socialising in the development and maintenance of professional identities and the definition of what it meant to be a surgeon. This definition depended not just on surgical skill, but on the ability to wine, dine, and fire a gun.

In chapters 4 and 5, 'Gender in surgery' and 'Race and ethnicity in surgery', I argue that the construction and maintenance of the surgical stereotype as male and white has had a lasting impact on who is allowed access to the profession, what kind of healthcare professionals patients will anticipate or tolerate, and the expectations of appropriate conduct both in and out of the operating theatre. These chapters build on work done by historians and sociologists such as Claire Brock, Mary Ann Elston, Julian M. Simpson, Stephanie J. Snow, and Aneez Esmail, who have investigated the social, cultural, and legislative reasons underpinning the racial dynamics and male-dominated nature of modern British surgery.[56] Using written sources as well as oral history interviews, and building on the evidence put forward in Chapter 3, I argue that surgeons in post-war Britain participated in activities open primarily to white, English-speaking men from affluent social backgrounds.

In Chapter 6, 'Surgical time', I use oral history interviews to interrogate the changing nature of surgical professionalism and the surgical career against the backdrop of major transformations in the structure of the National Health Service. Key to image, identity, and stereotype of the surgeon is the notion that surgical work is in some way distinct from other kinds of labour or employment. Surgery and related professions are understood as 'vocations' or 'callings', not careers like any other. This exceptionalism is used to justify and rationalise excessive temporal commitments on behalf of practitioners, and ideas about different 'surgical time' are crucial to surgeons' professional identity. This chapter will explore this aspect of the surgical stereotype. Not only were surgeons expected to devote substantial *quantities* of time to their professional lives, but they were required to maintain blurred boundaries between their working and leisure hours. How has the surgical stereotype responded to the reshaping of working time and its meanings in the managed healthcare bureaucracies of late twentieth-century Britain?

In Chapter 7, 'Military myths and metaphors', I use oral history interviews alongside articles in the medical press to interrogate the changing cultural script of the surgical identity and investigate how experiences of surgical work altered with developments in organisational ideologies and broader social and cultural shifts. Starting with a longer history of military metaphors in post-war surgical discourse, this chapter focuses on the twenty-first-century emergence of resilience rhetoric in British surgery and interrogates the increasingly prevalent assumption that resilience is something surgeons should possess or learn.[57] Building on the claims of the previous chapter about the reshaping of working time and its meanings in the managed healthcare bureaucracies of contemporary Britain, I argue that resilience developed as a popular and pervasive concept in surgery just as the emotional landscape of the British hospital was undergoing a profound transformation in the first few years of the twenty-first century.

In the conclusion I critically appraise the surgical memoir and its contribution to the development and maintenance of the surgical stereotype. There is an expanding collection of surgical memoirs where writers present a range of thoughts and feelings pertaining to the stress, strain, and sorrow associated with a clinical career. These candid and compassionate books belong to a relatively new genre. Twenty years ago you would be hard pressed to find a single published autobiographical account by a surgeon. Those that you might uncover tended to be narrative retellings of biographical detail, professional achievements, and innovative successes. Instead, thick with emotional commentary, these recent surgical memoirs integrate accounts of professional and personal life and attest to the affective intensity of modern operative practice. They describe moments of doubt, failure, and regret, and ruminate on the urgency and uncertainty of surgery.

These first-hand accounts, however, must compete with the pervasive and persistent stereotype in which surgeons are men (and sometimes women) who cultivate detachment and who are unable or unwilling to engage with their patients. Indeed, the blurb to the genre's most famous member, Henry Marsh's *Do No Harm*, compels the reader to challenge their assumptions of neurosurgery as a 'precise and exquisite craft, practised by calm and detached surgeons'.[58] This final, concluding chapter of the book will explore the tension between these two images: the dispassionate caricature contained in popular culture and patient imagination on the one hand, and the empathetic intellectual portrayed in the surgical memoir on the other. Indeed, as with so many other elements of surgical culture, memoirs seek both to disrupt the mythology of modern surgery and simultaneously, albeit inadvertently, confirm it.

Notes

1 Richard Gordon, *Doctor in the House* (London: Michael Joseph, 1952).

2 *Doctor in the House* was preempted by the physician Edward Berdoe, who in 1887 adopted the pseudonym Aesculapius Scalpel to scandalise the medical profession with his novel *St Bernard's: The Romance of a Medical Student*. Sarah Chaney, 'Dying Scientifically: Sex and Scandal in Victorian Medicine', *The Lancet*, 379:9831 (2012), 2042.

3 John Spencer, 'Some Activity but Still Not Much Action on Patient and Public Engagement', *Medical Education*, 50 (2016), 3–23, 3.
4 Lesley Scanlon, 'White Coats, Handmaidens and Warrior Chiefs: The Role of Filmic Representations in Becoming a Professional', in Lesley Scanlon (ed.), *"Becoming" a Professional: An Interdisciplinary Analysis of Professional Learning* (Dordrecht: Springer, 2011), 109–127.
5 George Gerbner and Larry Gross, 'Living with Television: The Violence Profile', *Journal of Communication*, 26:2 (1976), 172–199; and see George Gerbner et al., 'The Mainstreaming of America: The Violence Profile', *Journal of Communication*, 30:11 (1980), 10–29.
6 J. D. Brown and K. Walsh-Childers, 'Effects of Media on Personal and Public Health', in J. Bryant and D. Zillman (eds), *Media Effects: Advances in Theory and Research* (Hillsdale, NJ: Erlbaum, 1994), 389–415.
7 See Jessica Miller, 'Passionate Virtue: Conceptions of Medical Professionalism in Popular Romance Fiction', *Literature and Medicine*, 33:1 (2015), 70–90; and Scanlon, 'White Coats, Handmaidens and Warrior Chiefs', 109.
8 Phenomenological film theory advocates the 'notion of film as experience', that is, the viewer is cast as 'an active agent' and makes sense of a film 'by relating it to the stock experiences of their life-worlds'. Scanlon, 'White Coats, Handmaidens and Warrior Chiefs', 109.
9 Scanlon, 'White Coats, Handmaidens and Warrior Chiefs', 110.
10 Miller, 'Passionate Virtue', 70.
11 N. Stobbs and E. Ward, 'Do Modern-Day Surgeons Break the Stereotype and Show Emotional Intelligence in their Leadership?', *Bulletin of the Royal College of Surgeons of England*, 96 (2013), 5–8, 6.
12 Jyoti Shah, 'Knife, Life, and Wife: Old Stereotypes Persist in Surgery', *Health Service Journal* (1 December 2015), www.hsj.co.uk/women-leaders-network/knife-life-and-wife-old-stereotypes-persist-in-surgery/7000785.article (accessed 13 May 2020).
13 Graham Reed, 'Hospital Doctors Need a New Career Structure', *British Medical Journal*, 330:7504 (2005), 1397.
14 Interview with male surgeon; interviewed by author, 23 March 2018.
15 Peter Banks, 'Part IV: Decompartmentalizing Art and Science', *CMA Journal*, 119 (1978), 1239.
16 Geoffrey Lakeman, 'Spoons OK for Ops, Say Bosses', *Daily Mirror* (21 February 2003), 28.
17 Christopher Lawrence, 'Democratic, Divine and Heroic: The History and Historiography of Surgery', in Christopher Lawrence (ed.), *Medical Theory, Surgical Practice: Essays in the History of Surgery* (London: Routledge, 1992).

18 Wellcome Library, History and Origins of the NHS, GC/201/A/1/63.
19 Ibid.
20 Correspondence with author, 4 February 2019.
21 Wellcome Library, History and Origins of the NHS.
22 Secretary of State for Health, 'The New NHS: Modern. Dependable' (Department of Health and Social Care (December 1997), https://assets.publishing.service.gov.uk/government/uploads/system/uploads/attachment_data/file/266003/newnhs.pdf.
23 Ibid.
24 Richard Canter, 'Impact of Reduced Working Time on Surgical Training in the United Kingdom and Ireland', *The Surgeon*, 9 (2011), 6–7.
25 Rebecca Coombes, 'Press: The Consultant Contract', *British Medical Journal*, 325:7372 (2002), 1120.
26 Ibid.
27 Ibid.
28 Ibid.
29 Ibid.
30 Thomas Schlich, 'Introduction: What is Special about the History of Surgery', in Thomas Schlich (ed.), *The Palgrave Handbook of the History of Surgery* (London: Palgrave Macmillan, 2017), 1–24, 8.
31 Thomas Schlich (ed.), *The Palgrave Handbook of the History of Surgery* (London: Palgrave Macmillan, 2017).
32 Schlich, 'Introduction: What is Special about the History of Surgery', 9.
33 Ibid.
34 For the latter, see Thomas Schlich and Christopher Crennner (eds), *Technological Change in Modern Surgery: Historical Perspectives on Innovation* (Rochester, NY: University of Rochester Press, 2017); and Christopher Lawrence (ed.), *Medical Theory, Surgical Practice: Studies in the History of Surgery* (London: Routledge, 1992).
35 Sally Wilde, 'Truth, Trust, and Confidence in Surgery, 1890–1910: Patient Autonomy, Communication, and Consent', *Bulletin of the History of Medicine*, 83:2 (2009), 302–330.
36 Delia Gavrus, 'Men of Dreams and Men of Action: Neurologists, Neurosurgeons, and the Performance of Professional Identity, 1920–1950', *Bulletin of the History of Medicine*, 85:1 (2011): 57–92.
37 Surgery and Emotion, www.surgeryandemotion.com (accessed 20 May 2021).
38 Agnes Arnold-Forster, '"A Small Cemetery": Death and Dying in the Contemporary British Operating Theatre', *Medical Humanities*, 46 (2020), 278–287, 283.

39 Ibid.; Agnes Arnold-Forster, 'Resilience in Surgery', *British Journal of Surgery*, 107:4 (2020), 332–333; Agnes Arnold-Forster, 'Sexism in Surgery: Little has Changed', *BMJ Opinion* (24 January 2018), https://blogs.bmj.com/bmj/2019/01/24/agnes-arnold-forster-sexism-in-surgery-little-has-changed/ (accessed 20 May 2020); Agnes Arnold-Forster, 'Doctors' Wellbeing: Learning from the Past Can Help Improve the Future', *British Medical Journal*, 363 (2018), https://doi.org/10.1136/bmj.k4101 (accessed 15 February 2023).

40 My thinking on the relationship between emotions and work is indebted to Professor Claire Langhamer. Claire Langhamer, 'Feelings, Women and Work in the Long 1950s', *Women's History Review*, 26:1 (2016), 77–92; Claire Langhamer, 'Who the Hell are Ordinary People? Ordinariness as a Category of Historical Analysis', *Transactions of the Royal Historical Society*, 28 (2018), 175–195.

41 Joanna Bourke, *The Story of Pain: From Prayer to Painkillers* (Oxford: Oxford University Press, 2014); Michael Brown, *Emotions and Surgery in Britain, 1793–1912* (Cambridge: Cambridge University Press, 2022); Michael Brown, 'Surgery and Emotion: The Era Before Anaesthesia', in Thomas Schlich (ed.), *The Palgrave Handbook of the History of Surgery* (London: Palgrave Macmillan, 2017), 327–348; Michael Brown, 'Redeeming Mr Sawbone: Compassion and Care in the Cultures of Nineteenth-Century Surgery', *Journal of Compassionate Health Care*, 4:13 (2017), 1–7; Lynda Payne, *With Words and Knives: Learning Medical Dispassion in Early Modern England* (Burlington, VT: Ashgate, 2007); Peter Stanley, *For Fear of Pain: British Surgery, 1790–1850* (Amsterdam: Rodopi, 2003).

42 Stanley, *For Fear of Pain*.

43 This stereotype is present in Lindsey Fitzharris's popular biography of nineteenth-century surgeon Joseph Lister. Lindsey Fitzharris, *The Butchering Art: Joseph Lister's Quest to Transform the Grisly World of Victorian Medicine* (London: Penguin, 2017). See also Agnes Arnold-Forster, 'Review of *The Butchering Art: Joseph Lister's Quest to Transform the Grisly World of Victorian Medicine*', *Reviews in History* (2018), https://doi.org/10.14296/RiH/2014/2256 (accessed 25 March 2020).

44 William Reddy, *The Navigation of Feeling: A Framework for the History of Emotions* (Cambridge: Cambridge University Press, 2001).

45 Mark Jackson, *The Age of Stress: Science and the Search for Stability* (Oxford: Oxford University Press, 2013).

46 Matthew J. Hoffarth, 'The Making of Burnout: From Social Change to Self-Awareness in the Postwar United States, 1970–82', *History of the Human Sciences*, 30:5 (2017), 30–45.

47 For a selection, see Shelly Luu et al., 'Waking up the Next Morning: Surgeons' Emotional Reactions to Adverse Events', *Medical Education*, 46 (2012), 1179–118; Ruth McDonald, Justin Waring, and Stephen Harrison, 'At the Cutting Edge? Modernization and Nostalgia in a Hospital Operating Theatre Department', *Sociology*, 40:6 (2006), 1097–1115; Abi Rimmer, 'Working Time Restrictions May Have Increased Tensions Between Trainees and Consultants, Studies Find', *British Medical Journal*, 348 (2014).

48 See Paul S. Adler, Linda C. Forbes, and Hugh Willmott, 'Critical Management Studies', *The Academy of Management Annals*, 1:1 (2007), 119–179; Yiannis Gabriel, 'Organisational Nostalgia: Reflections on the Golden Age', in S. Fineman (ed.), *Emotions in Organisations* (London: SAGE, 1993); Tim Strangleman, 'The Nostalgia of Organisations and the Organisation of Nostalgia: Past and Present in the Contemporary Railway Industry', *Sociology*, 33:4 (1999), 725–746; Tim Strangleman and Ian Roberts, 'Looking Through the Window of Opportunity: The Cultural Cleansing of Workplace Identity', *Sociology*, 33:1 (1999), 47–67.

49 See Catherine Baker, 'Beyond the Island Story?: The Opening Ceremony of the London 2012 Olympic Games as Public History', *Rethinking History: The Journal of Theory and Practice*, 19:3 (2015), 409–428; Julia Hallam, 'Grey's Anatomy: Scalpels, Sex, and Stereotypes', *Medical Humanities*, 35 (2009), 60–61; Hannah Hamad, 'Contemporary Medical Television and Crisis in the NHS', *Critical Studies in Television: The International Journal of Television Studies*, 11:2 (2016), 136–150; Susan E. Lederer 'Surgery and Popular Culture: Situating the Surgeon and the Surgical Experience in Popular Media', in Thomas Schlich (ed.), *The Palgrave Handbook of the History of Surgery* (London: Palgrave Macmillan, 2017), 349–367; Elena C. Strauman and Bethany C. Goodier, 'The Doctor(s) in House: An Analysis of the Evolution of the Television Doctor-Hero', *Journal of Medical Humanities*, 32:1 (2011), 31–46; Scanlon, 'White Coats, Handmaidens and Warrior Chiefs'; Estella Tincknell, 'The Nation's Matron: Hattie Jacques and British Post-war Popular Culture', *Journal of British Cinema and Television*, 12:1 (2015), 6–24.

50 Rachel Prentice, *Bodies in Formation: An Ethnography of Anatomy and Surgical Education* (Durham, NC: Duke University Press, 2012).

51 Felicity Callard and Des Fitzgerald, *Rethinking Interdisciplinarity across the Social Sciences and Neurosciences* (London: Palgrave Macmillan, 2015), 2.

52 Ibid.

53 Valerie J. Janesick, 'Oral History Interviewing: Issues and Possibilities', in Patricia Leavy (ed.), *The Oxford Handbook of Qualitative Research* (Oxford: Oxford University Press, 2014).

54 One exception is the British Library's 'Oral Histories of Medicine and Health Professionals', www.bl.uk/collection-guides/oral-histories-of-medicine-and-health-professionals (accessed 14 August 2018).

55 Janet W. C. King and Stephen J. Wigmore, 'How Surgeons Should Behave on Social Media', *Surgery*, 38:10 (2020), 623–626.

56 Claire Brock, *British Women Surgeons and their Patients, 1860–1918* (Cambridge: Cambridge University Press, 2017); Mary Ann Elston, 'Medicine: Half our Future Doctors?', in Rosalie Silverstone and Audrey Ward (eds), *Careers of Professional Women* (London: Routledge, 1980), 99–139; Mary Ann Elston, *Women and Medicine: The Future* (London: Royal College of Physicians, 2009); Julian M. Simpson, Stephanie J. Snow, and Aneez Esmail, 'Providing "Special" Types of Labour and Exerting Agency: How Migrant Doctors Have Shaped the UK's National Health Service', in Laurence Monnais and David Wright (eds), *Doctors Beyond Borders: The Transnational Migration of Physicians in the Twentieth Century* (Toronto: University of Toronto Press, 2016), 208–229.

57 Arnold-Forster, 'Resilience in Surgery'.

58 Henry Marsh, *Do No Harm: Stories of Life, Death and Brain Surgery* (London: Hachette, 2014).

1

Self-made myths

Surgeons are invested in their professional past. They tend to venerate their predecessors and see contemporary achievements as part of a long lineage of past successes and heroic figures. Prominent surgeons, long dead, populate a kind of surgical aristocracy. They gave their names to procedures and instruments and are crucial to the individual and collective identity of the profession. Post-war surgery was (and in some ways continues to be) a profoundly hierarchical community, one where seniority is respected, where individuals and interventions carry the weight of their ancestors, and where professional positions were as much inherited or bestowed as they were earned. History, therefore, matters to surgeons, and the myths of the twentieth-century practitioner were shaped by the events and identities of the nineteenth.

In Britain today, where the NHS is everything, the reputation of nineteenth-century healthcare suffers badly by comparison. The Victorian era was an 'age of agony' – a 'grisly world' – according to popular historian Lindsey Fitzharris.[1] Past surgical care has had particularly bad press, and the stereotype of surgeons working under Queen Victoria has been made from gory and sensationalist stories. Take the myth of the surgeon Dr Robert Liston as one example. He was 'abrupt, abrasive, argumentative', 'an incorrigible bustler, even for a surgeon'. He had a reputation for 'speedy wizardry' and his technique was a sight to behold. He would spring across 'the blood-stained boards upon his swooning, sweating, strapped-down patient like a duellist, calling, "Time me, gentlemen, time me!"'[2] In one such episode, he killed three people during a single surgery. While amputating a patient's leg, his flaying knife accidentally removed his assistant's finger. The patient died from an infection, as did the sorry assistant, while someone watching the operation died from shock after Liston's knife slashed through the poor man's coat tails. It remains the only operation in surgical history with a 300 per cent mortality rate.[3]

While influential and remarkably persistent – it appears in medical journals, history books, and in almost every biography of Liston ever written – this story is probably not true. The only evidence it ever happened comes from a book called *Great Medical Disasters* written in 1983 by the author Richard Gordon (the same man responsible for the fictional Sir Lancelot Spratt). As Michael Brown has pointed out, there are no primary sources from the 1840s to confirm Liston's apocryphal operation even ever actually took place.[4] But when you are dealing with myths and legends, shaky evidentiary foundations matter not. Indeed, this story nevertheless embodies and embeds the still pervasive idea that nineteenth-century surgeons were not just emotionally detached, but barbaric and indifferent to the suffering of their patients.

The flaws in this assumption do not mean that nineteenth-century hospitals were not dangerous places or associated in the public psyche with poverty and risk. Anyone who could afford private healthcare stayed as far away from these institutions as possible, but for the poor who required medical intervention, including surgery, the hospitals were often their only option. Some of the most famous hospitals in Britain were medieval in origin, but most were set up in the eighteenth century by philanthropic gentlemen in collaboration with eminent surgeons and physicians. The three endowed hospitals – St Bartholomew's, St Thomas's, and Guy's – could subsist on the income from their large investments and land holdings without appealing to the community. The rest relied on public charity and the generosity of the local gentry. Who worked at the voluntary hospitals depended on the size, wealth, and prestige of the institution concerned. At the three endowed hospitals, there were three principal physicians and three principal surgeons (generally fellows of the royal colleges of physicians and surgeons) who attended to their cases several times a week. The senior surgeons and physicians mostly worked without a regular salary – and any payment, if made at all, was small and mainly symbolic.

Working at a voluntary hospital was attractive partly because practitioners could earn extra money training more junior surgeons (young men would pay senior surgeons for the opportunity to act as their apprentices or 'dressers'), but mainly for the prestige and opportunities for clinical learning that working at these institutions could afford. Surgeons who attended voluntary hospitals earned their income elsewhere – in private practice. *The Times* said that connection with a great hospital was the main ambition of London physicians and surgeons: 'It gives professional status; it brings fees for tuition … it often leads to a large and lucrative practice; and, indeed, without it there is scarcely a possibility of a very high position being attained.'[5] However, the popular and reforming medical press frequently lambasted the surgeons attached to these prestigious institutions for their incompetence and cupidity,[6] in part because these appointments often required nepotistic connections to attain them, and some seemed to be more inherited than earned.

In the eighteenth century, there was a clear distinction between physicians – doctors who dealt with the internal workings of the human body – and surgeons – practitioners who removed lumps, bumps, and legs. Surgeons were trained by apprenticeship and had only recently divested themselves from their barber brothers. In contrast, physicians traditionally trained at either Oxford or Cambridge and received broad, humanistic educations replete with classical literature, ethics, and physiology. However, this conventional hierarchy was increasingly under threat and as the nineteenth century got underway, surgeons were newly articulating themselves as equal – if not superior – to physicians. To do so, and to differentiate themselves from the barber or butcher, they frequently emphasised restraint, insisted on the unity of medicine and surgery, and claimed the ability to cure increasingly complex diseases, like cancer.[7]

In other words, they were battling against their own version of the surgical stereotype that Richard Gordon was trading on. The idea that surgeons were crass, ill-educated, and brutal was widespread in early nineteenth-century Britain, and to combat this notion, surgeons engaged in a busy programme of self-promotion and image reform. Throughout the century, they debated with intense ferocity what it meant to belong to the profession, demarcating who could and could not be allowed entry with new regulations and legislations, as well as changing cultural norms and rhetorical styles. Historians such as Michael Brown have focused on this 'cultural history' of professionalisation and looked towards surgeons' and physicians' use of language in constructing an external image and coherent identity. He argues that 'the medical profession of the early nineteenth century was less a structural category than an imaginative concept, a point of individual and collective self-identification'.[8] The professionalisation of surgery was, therefore, accomplished by using a rhetorical arsenal that not only elevated their craft to the 'scientific' level and gentility of internal medicine, but also crafted a new persona associated with feelings.

Contrary to popular belief, the early decades of the nineteenth century (before the introduction of anaesthesia in the 1840s) was an intensely emotionally expressive era.[9] This had much to do with the limited curative power of surgery at the time. For both surgeons and patients, operations were seen as a last resort and both approached the table, 'painful and risky as it was', as something of a 'shared tragedy'.[10] Perhaps because they were more accustomed to failure than surgeons are today, nineteenth-century practitioners were more likely to express pity, sadness, and regret. In addition, the culture of the early nineteenth century, the 'Romantic era', maintained and fortified such forms of emotional reflection and self-fashioning. For example, Scottish surgeon Charles Bell (1774–1842) wrote to his wife that he got 'wearied – exhausted by the sufferings of others'. Such exhaustion derived from his emotional entanglements with his patients, and it was central to his personal and professional identity. As he once told his brother, 'I have had a most miserable time since I wrote to you, from the failure of an operation, and the death of a most worthy man. I shall regret it as long as I live. It is very hard, more trying than anything that any other profession can bring a man to.'[11]

The real early nineteenth-century surgeon had, therefore, very little in common with Richard Gordon's fictionalised Liston. As the century continued, however, the emotional cultures of medicine, surgery, and society changed. These changes made possible the persistence of earlier ideas about the profession, but also allowed new myths to emerge and take hold. Though doctors and surgeons continued to experience intense emotions, the improved efficacy of medicine and the introduction of surgical technologies such as anaesthesia and antisepsis reduced the scale of suffering and death. Moreover, as the Romantic era's 'sentimental cultures' made way for more 'stoic forms of manliness and professional identity', it became less acceptable for men to express their emotions, and medical practitioners were no longer encouraged to discuss the affective consequences of healing.[12]

The late nineteenth-century surgeon continued, therefore, to be marked by contradictions. On the one hand, his image was coloured by a commitment to humanitarianism, the increasing contribution of his profession to the social good and the national project, and the life-saving technical arsenal he was rapidly acquiring. Aided by more complimentary representation and galvanised by the introduction of anaesthesia and antisepsis, the early twentieth-century surgeon was an increasingly vaunted public figure. On the other hand, that same surgeon struggled to strip himself of his profession's association with barbarity and accusations of avarice and self-interest. Despite many generations of self-promotion and image management, even present-day popular historians publish books that adhere to early nineteenth-century critiques of surgeons and their unfeeling ways.[13]

There are two main reasons for this. First, surgeons are themselves partly responsible because, and as discussed, they habitually place themselves in a lengthy professional chronology. But rather than just celebrating their ancestors, they also use their predecessors' supposed 'barbarity' to elevate their current position. The past is a flexible resource. In the stories they tell about themselves, surgeons often narrate a 'rags-to-riches' tale from miserable butchery to scientific surgery – contrasting their own humanitarianism and technical skill with their forerunners' brutalism. In essence, it served twentieth-century surgeons' needs to denigrate the emotional qualities of their nineteenth-century predecessors because it made them look good by comparison. And second, just as surgeons became increasingly life-saving, they were also implicated in a healthcare system coming under greater critical scrutiny.

The Citadel

As in the nineteenth century, the early twentieth-century surgeon's reputation relied on the character and condition of the health service he operated within. Between 1900 and 1948, British healthcare moved towards a mixed economy of mutual payment schemes, local authority services, and not-for-profit providers, with limited space for commercial medicine.[14] Despite the complexity of the system, there was much to commend. By 1942, eleven million people were members of hospital contributory schemes (which entitled them to hospital care provided they paid in a proportion of their salary) and it was generally believed that the level of hospital care was improving.[15] In 1911, the new National Insurance Act provided access to general practitioners (GPs) for manual labourers and those workers earning below a certain threshold.[16] Changes to that threshold meant that by 1936 half of the adult population had their primary care covered and by 1938, 19,060 doctors were included in the National Insurance 'panel'.[17] This system was not, of course, without its flaws. Fees for GPs were increasing, especially for those who earned just above the income threshold. The families of National Insurance members were excluded, including wives and children, as was hospital treatment (including surgery), meaning many had to pay additional fees or rely on free clinics for mothers and children, and pharmacists for treatment advice.

These flaws were best, and perhaps most famously, captured by A. J. Cronin's 1937 novel, *The Citadel*.[18] For his fifth book, Cronin drew on his experiences practising medicine in the coal-mining communities of the South Wales Valleys. His publisher presented the book as a social exposé, an attack on an unreformed British institution.[19] Thus, while surgeons might have become relatively vaunted professionals by the end of the nineteenth century, their reputation was sullied by their necessary association with a healthcare system that was seen as less and less fit for purpose. Throughout his book, Cronin lambasts the acquisitive, avaricious, and self-interested nature of the healthcare professions and critiques the close links between medicine and social class, or the 'status system'.[20] The hero of the tale, Andrew Manson, begins his career as a GP in the small, fictitious Welsh mining town of Drineffy. He is then seduced by the promise of easy money from wealthy, healthy clients in London – the 'citadel of greed and ignorance'[21] – before returning to his principles and campaigning against the villainous, inept surgeons he encounters on Harley Street.[22] *The Citadel* is, according to historian Ross McKibbin, a 'sustained attack on the whole of British medicine'.[23]

Cronin particularly targeted those at the top of the medical hierarchy – the 'grandees' whose driving concern was money and who encouraged 'illnesses' in their 'wealthy, idle, hypochondriac, mostly female patients'.[24]

While much changed in terms of the efficacy of hospital medicine and the social status of surgeons as the nineteenth century gave way to the twentieth, the 'incompetence and chicanery' of metropolitan medicine is one of the most memorable themes in *The Citadel*.[25] At one point, Manson complains,

> The way I look at it is this ... the whole layout is obsolete ... Nobody but the good old B[ritish] P[ublic] would put up with this – like our roads, for instance, a hopeless out-of-date chaos ... half the hospitals are shrieking that they are falling down! And what are we doing about it? Collecting pennies.[26]

From the moment of its publication in July 1937, *The Citadel* was an extraordinary success. By November it had sold over 150,000 copies in Britain, unprecedented sales in interwar publishing. Until the end of the year, it was printed in weekly editions of '10,000 or so'.[27] This is partly because, and as McKibbin has argued, Cronin reflected a reality.[28] He presented 'a picture of British medicine immediately recognisable or acceptable to his readership'.[29] In interwar Britain, the country's health system was coming under increasingly sustained critique. The newly funded British branch of the Gallup organisation asked as one of its first 'political' questions whether people favoured the hospitals becoming a 'public' service (i.e. nationalised), with the majority (71 per cent) voting in favour.[30] In the same year that *The Citadel* was published (1937), Political and Economic Planning, a carefully non-partisan organisation founded in 1931, brought out a famous report on Britain's health system which was, despite its even-handedness, very damming.[31] However, surgeons benefited from this early twentieth-century health system. They had plenty of opportunities for clinical practice, a variety of sources of income, and ample autonomy to conduct themselves as they wished (within reason, of course). As a result, many of them were sceptical about the coming of a new, state-funded and state-managed healthcare system.

The origins of the NHS

The NHS had its origins in the nineteenth century, when the provision of health was seen by many as fundamental to the workings of a civilised society. The example of the army medical services during the First World War emphasised the importance of centralised organisation in healthcare delivery, and at the government's request, in 1920 Lord Dawson produced a report on how a health service might be organised.[32] In 1939, an emergency medical service was created – further demonstrating the potential of the state to administer care and successful interventions. The 1942 Beveridge Report set out plans for Britain.[33] It identified the country's ills and laid the foundations of the post-war Welfare State. In 1945, Labour came to power with a huge majority and set in motion an extensive programme of welfare reforms – including a National Health Service. The NHS was planned as a three-tier, or tripartite, system. At the top was the Minister of Health and below were the three tiers designed to work symbiotically in service of patients' needs.

The voluntary and municipal hospitals were nationalised and organised into fourteen regional groups run by Regional Hospital Boards.[34] These boards supervised local hospital management committees, doctors in hospitals received salaries, and all treatment was free. Teaching hospitals were directly controlled by the Minister of Health, as these hospitals should serve the whole country rather than just their local area. General practitioners, dentists, opticians, and pharmacists were self-employed professionals with a contract with the NHS to provide services so that patients did not have to pay directly. The GP continued to be the first port of call for most patients – providing treatment or referring them on to other parts of the health service for specialised care. The third tier, the local authority health services controlled by a Medical Officer for Health, ran community clinics that provided services such as immunisation, maternity care, and school medical services.

For patients, the benefits of the new NHS were obvious, even if they were not always realised. For surgeons, the advantages were less apparent. Some bitterly opposed the NHS, imagining the service as an economically dangerous bureaucratic machine that 'crushed medical independence and risked pushing the country towards dictatorship'.[35] In 1946, the British Medical Association objected to surgeons and physicians being relegated to the status of 'salaried' workers. They asserted, 'The medical profession is, in the public interest, opposed to any form of service which leads directly or indirectly to the profession as a whole becoming full-time salaried servants of the State or local authorities.'[36] One professional wrote to the *BMJ* to say,

> If I am to be one of the victims of … the Government's major surgery I should prefer some preliminary investigation, accurate diagnosis and possibly premedication to help me to survive the operation. Safe surgery takes into account the patients' (in this case the doctors') constitutions and idiosyncrasies.[37]

Oppositions to the NHS on behalf of doctors and surgeons were varied, but many circulated around the pervasive idea – inherited from the nineteenth century – that medical men had, and were entitled to, a degree of independence. By the middle of the twentieth century, surgeons were at the top of the hospital pecking order and senior practitioners had a remarkable amount of autonomy of thought and action. The new NHS was seen to compromise that intellectual and professional independence by subsuming the authority of the surgeon beneath that of the state.

Despite the anxieties and protestations of surgeons and other doctors, the Health Service Bill was passed in 1947 and the NHS was established in 1948. Nearly ten years later, however, practitioners were still grumbling about the perceived effect the service had had on their work, professional identity, and relationships. Eric Linklater published an article in the *BMJ* in 1955 arguing that the 'social revolution has also done something to change the relationship between doctor and patient'.[38] He complained, 'Under the benign provision of the National Health Service the doctor's skill has become a sort of public reservoir from which all may drink at any time so long as they pay their water rate; and from which many are allowed to drink free.'[39] This, he suggested, had changed the 'public character' of the doctor by implicating his responsibility with that of the welfare state. Linklater was pleased, however, to note that this change had not been so dramatic nor so malignant as his predecessors had predicted in 1946: '[Doctors] have – or the great majority have – resisted the temptation to which they were exposed: the temptation to become Civil Servants … They realised the basic incompatibility between the ideal of the Civil Servant and the ideal of the physician.'[40]

The century between the introduction of anaesthesia (1848) and the foundation of the NHS (1948) had altered the practice of surgery in profound and long-lasting ways. However, the period was also one of remarkable continuity in perceptions of surgery and the self-image of surgeons – even if the details had changed. The twentieth-century surgeon inherited a great deal from his (he remained overwhelmingly male) nineteenth-century ancestors. Both valued their authority over other members of hospital staff and their patients. Both cherished their intellectual and professional autonomy, valorised the skill required to perform their craft, and prized the supposed objectivity of science. Surgery had become much safer, and while this had probably made the operating theatre less terrifying for prospective patients, it had – perhaps paradoxically – reduced the opportunities for surgeons to express their emotions and engage with people about their feelings. As a result, the surgeon in 1948 had more in common with late nineteenth-century practitioners, shaped by the marshal masculinity of the imperial age and informed by the value society placed on stoicism and professional cool.

But the world had changed. Healthcare had been nationalised, new operative techniques had been introduced, new psychological and emotional ideas were circulating, and more and more women were qualifying as surgeons. New social and political pressures were also coming down the road. The scale of the surgical job was due to expand, there was a newly literate and engaged public keen to exert their own influence on the surgical identity as readers, viewers, and consumers, and the healthcare professions were set to become increasingly ethnically diverse. The stereotypes of the nineteenth century are relatively well known, but just as historians have started to complicate those caricatures, they must do the same for the twentieth. Indeed, there has been crucial, careful work that dissects the rhetoric and normative values of nineteenth-century practitioners, and some that delineates the self-presentation of their early twentieth-century descendants.[41] But what about surgeons in the new NHS? How were they seen by the non-medical public, how did they see themselves, and how did they want themselves to be seen?

Surgery's golden age

The decades immediately after the Second World War, from the late 1940s to the 1960s, was an exciting time to be a real-life surgeon. Following Joseph Lister's 'revolutionising' innovations in the late nineteenth century and his popularisation of antisepsis, surgery became safer. While many patients continued to die from infection and blood loss, the development of blood transfusion and antibiotics such as penicillin in the early 1940s further reduced operative risks. The application of X-rays allowed practitioners to plan their surgery more effectively by allowing them to see beneath the skin. Safer gases and intravenous anaesthetics replaced unpredictable chloroform. Surgery became more specialised – and its practice became both more complex and more routine.

This was a 'golden age' of surgery. Or at least it was according to surgeons themselves. They told tales of great men with their great inventions. Similarly, contemporary accounts written by current surgeons emphasise the achievements of their colleagues and recent predecessors. In his slim 1948 volume, *Recent Advances in Surgery*, Harold C. Edwards wrote, 'The progress of surgery in all its many and varied branches has been well-nigh immeasurable during the past decade, and the surgeon of to-day is reaping to an unprecedented extent the fruits of the labours of his fathers.'[42]

While it might have been a 'golden age', the mid-twentieth century was also an era of intense flux for British surgery. Many practitioners had participated in the Second World War – both at home and on the battlefield – and there was an acute awareness that the conflict had reshaped the surgical landscape: 'Lessons of war, learned at fighting speed, have added much to the general advance and, in many instances, expedited.'[43] Accounts written by practitioners and professional historians alike tend to focus on these various professional developments and technical acquisitions.[44] But we know much less about the social, political, and cultural dynamics of the profession and its practice in post-war Britain. These dynamics were also under pressure in the years immediately following the Second World War and particularly in the context of the new NHS.

In the 1950s and 1960s, surgeons spent plenty of time writing for each other. They used textbooks to expand upon the real or ideal nature of the profession, wrote strident letters to medical journals and the mainstream press, and penned articles accounting for the current conditions of surgical work. These various texts might not give us much insight into the inner emotional lives of surgeons in the decades immediately following the foundation of the NHS. They do, however, allow historians to investigate how surgeons thought members of their profession should feel and behave. Textbooks were generally written by senior surgeons and designed to be read by practitioners at the outset of their careers. These were places where surgeons went to speak to members of their own community. They were intended for a like-minded audience and did not, necessarily, need to justify the fundamental value or utility of surgery (which anyway by the 1940s was an uncontroversial assertion) or the core benevolence of its practitioners. Authors of these textbooks devoted sections to outlining anatomy, diagnosis, suturing, wound dressings, and aftercare. However, they also all dedicated an opening chapter or preface to the elaboration of the surgical identity and to setting out their vision of ideal surgical behaviour.

In these prefaces or introductions, they also acknowledge the limited ability of a textbook to teach the practice of surgery or guarantee an appropriate emotional attitude among students or trainees. In his 1953 book, *An Approach to Clinical Surgery*, Gerald H. C. Ovens, wrote, 'It is not the intention of this book to teach you how to behave towards patients or to expound the patient-doctor relationship … Such things cannot be learnt from books.'[45] He went on to say, 'No book can teach you the art of dealing with a patient, the "bedside manner."'[46] The pedagogical limitations of the textbook were widely acknowledged in part because of the belief that surgery was both a science and an 'art'. In an article published in the *BMJ* in 1955, Eric Linklater wrote,

> Here, I suppose, is the chief reward and prime difficulty of your profession: its practice is scientific (at least, one hopes so), but the practitioner should transcend the scientist. For the scientist relies on measurement and analysis, on observation and deduction; but the physician, who is dealing also with imponderables and qualities that can neither be analysed nor filtered, should also be something of an artist, who is inductive and capable by instinct of assessing the imponderable.[47]

Surgeons, more so even than other doctors, recognised that surgical practice was just that, a 'practice', one that could be learnt and developed only through observation and apprenticeship. It was a craft – 'primarily a practical art'.[48] In his 1958 edited text, *An Introduction to Surgery*, David H. Patey wrote, 'the student during this part of his career acquires simple techniques which every doctor should possess, e.g. the stitching and dressing of a wound, the giving of an intravenous infusion, or the passing of a catheter'.[49] In his chapter on operating theatre cleanliness, he emphasised the development of haptic and habitual knowledge: 'While learning these techniques and assisting in the operating theatre, the student develops the habit of asepsis.'[50] This acknowledgement of the limitations of written instruction at the beginning of every textbook also explains why these are not ideal sources for the researcher seeking historical experience.

Surgical textbooks and medical journal articles were not straightforward reflections of 'real life'. Instead, they are texts that represent a normative ideal of the post-war British surgeon. They were themselves constructions – idealised narratives of surgical conduct and identities. As such, they are revealing about the myths of surgery that were circulating in the early years of the NHS and, in many ways, these texts conform to the conventional surgical stereotype presented in this book's introduction. They promoted a vision of surgical identity that orbited around authority, paternalism, and emotional detachment.

Authority and paternalism

Hierarchy is key to the myth of the modern surgeon. The surgeon must also have a natural tendency towards leadership – he should have a flair for authority and be able to direct not only more junior surgeons, but other members of the hospital workforce like nurses and technicians.

In fiction, this flair for authority was recast as authoritarianism and the stereotype of the surgical demagogue is pervasive. Today, surgeons are socialised to respect and reproduce hierarchy from the very start of their medical school training, where they learn not to challenge authority. One participant in a study conducted in 2016 said, 'There's very much the patriarchal thing of the consultant, you never question them and you're there to do exactly what they say.'[51] The relationship between surgeon and patient often remains similarly hierarchical, although more has been done to challenge that dynamic in recent decades. As the *BMJ* observed in 2015, 'the accepted model that has guided us for centuries is "doctor knows best"' and in 2001, the American Medical Association proposed, 'Only your physician has the necessary experience and expertise to diagnose and treat medical conditions.'[52]

Rigid hierarchies between different healthcare professionals, and between doctor and patient, have been around for decades, if not centuries. While they began their careers close to the bottom of the hospital's pecking order, right from the outset surgeons in post-war Britain were trained with the assumption that they would eventually reach the top of the institutional hierarchy. In 1968, Leonard I. Stein published an influential article in the *American Journal of Nursing*, called 'The Doctor–Nurse Game', in which he described the hospital as a 'rigid organizational structure with the physician in clear authority'. The surgeon, in this account, was maintained as an 'omnipotent leader'.[53] The importance of surgical authority appeared in British publications too, with textbooks insisting that the surgeon must, therefore, be self-assured: 'he can help both his patient and himself by discussion, explanation, and by imparting an atmosphere of confidence'.[54]

A degree of paternalism was, according to mid-century surgeons, essential to manage the emotions and health of patients. And nowhere was paternalism more prominent than in the care of cancer patients. Despite the development of chemotherapies in the early decades of the twentieth century, even after the Second World War surgeons were the first (and sometimes last) port of call in cases of malignancy. Cancer had retained its fearsome reputation and carried plenty of emotional baggage. As a result, it was a disease that required careful management – and some of that management had as much to do with patient feeling as with operative technique. Some of the tools surgeons suggested to ameliorate patient concern seem – to twenty-first-century readers – overly paternalistic or patronising. Gerald H. C. Ovens suggested that a surgeon might want to 'refer to various conditions without giving away to the patient what he is talking about', and identified cancer as a diagnosis for which trainee surgeons might like to find synonyms so as not to 'frighten the patient'.[55] However, he cautioned against using 'malignant' as one of those synonyms: 'this word must never be used in front of patients as it always frightens them'.[56] He reflected on his own experience: 'Four times in my life I have, under pressure, deliberately told patients they have cancer and every time I have subsequently regretted it. I will never do so again.'[57] Even in cases where patients insisted on being told their diagnosis – however dire – Ovens thought that the surgeon knew better: 'In spite of most people's protestations that "I would like to know the truth," that is not really so; they only ask because they are afraid of the truth.'[58]

The question of whether or not surgeons and other healthcare professionals should inform patients, particularly those with terminal illnesses, of their diagnoses, was a live topic in the 1950s and 1960s, and Ovens was not alone in thinking that perhaps it might be best to keep the dying in the dark. In 1960, romance novelist and ex-nurse Elizabeth Gilzean proposed a book to the publishing house, Mills & Boon, in which the heroine dies from cancer but is never told her diagnosis. She got the idea from Arthur Hailey's 1959 novel, *The Final Diagnosis*, and she thought that the ethical dilemma of whether healthcare professionals should inform patients of terminal prognoses well suited to the romance genre.[59] However, Gilzean's potential publishers were not so certain that this question would make for thrilling escapism. Their concerns did, however, acknowledge the powerful influence romance fiction could exert on the attitudes and behaviours of readers. The editor of the magazine *Woman's Day* 'felt that the idea might give anxieties to many patients in hospital'.[60]

Emotional detachment

For much of the twentieth century, commentators on the role and identity of the surgeon placed high value on detachment because so many believed – or at least insisted – that emotions could interfere with a surgeon's ability to effectively and efficiently carry out their work. Historians of emotion call this an 'emotional regime' (the dominant mode of emotional expression and thought in different times and cultural contexts), the unspoken code of emotional conduct.[61] Various recent medical ethicists and professionals have argued that doctors, and particularly surgeons, must maintain 'distance' from their patients to 'generate objectivity in diagnosis and treatment'.[62] This notion is also widespread in the public sphere. A 2017 article in *Prospect* magazine included this passage:

> Emotional detachment from the fraught contexts in which they have to make life-and-death decisions can result in better choices being made. Being immune to stress might actually benefit patients by facilitating empathy. Too much emotion can lead physicians and other care-givers to turn away from their patients, in fear or disgust. A calm, analytical logic enables surgeons to reach out their hands to help.[63]

Evidently, emotional detachment is a key feature of the mythology of the modern surgeon – one that permeates lay and professional discussions, both past and present. The question of whether surgeons should maintain a degree of distance from their patients is, therefore, a recurring theme in the history of surgical representation and behaviour. Indeed, the profession has long struggled to achieve an appropriate balance between emotional distance and proximity.

In 1889, William Osler gave a valedictory address at the University of Pennsylvania. He advised medical graduates to display 'imperturbability', which he defined as 'coolness and presence of mind under all circumstances'. Patients so valued 'calmness amid storm', he warned, that the physician who failed to embody 'immobility, impassiveness, or … phlegm', would quickly lose their trust. Osler suggested this was a 'bodily endowment', adding regretfully that some young doctors were inherently incapable of this affective disposition, which would hinder their career development.[64] Osler's admonition continues to be quoted regularly by medical writers searching for ways to promote the value of emotional calmness, even as they apply it to storms quite different from those encountered or imagined by Osler.[65] For Osler, maintaining emotional coolness was a way of upholding authority and professional power.[66]

Since Osler, this idea has gathered pace and influence and researchers have increasingly emphasised how institutions and professions establish and maintain particular affective temperaments. Pioneering work by sociologist Renée Fox noted the historical importance of 'detached concern' in mid-twentieth-century medical training and practice. Fox first derived her concept from fieldwork in research clinics. Clinical researchers on the wards of the Peter Bent Brigham Hospital had to balance their concern for the patients' humanity with the 'equanimity' of the experimenter. Fox argued that such a posture both served scientific functions and afforded psychological protections as physicians administered interventions that they were unsure would work.[67] In other words, detached concern was an emotional posture that was co-constitutive with the identity of a physician-scientist. Subsequent work by Fox, with psychiatrist and psychoanalyst Howard Lief, noted how this almost paradoxical stance towards patients, combining the 'counterattitudes' of objectivity and empathy, was cultivated in medical education. Lief and Fox proposed a sequence of socialisation phases that tracked from the anatomy lab to the hospital wards. Yet these steps did not simply represent increased detachment. Rather, standardised rituals of twentieth-century medical education emphasised both attachment with the patient and detachment with the sick body in ways that initially appeared contradictory to students. Too much detachment could lead to cynicism, dejection, or other forms of emotional paralysis. The ability to balance countervailing commitments across medical school experiences thus became the mark of the successful professional.[68]

Over the ensuing decades, it became evident that detached concern was a historically specific pedagogical and professional stance that would shift in response to social, cultural, and political changes. The growth of biomedical experimentalism in the 1950s necessitated both epistemic and emotional forms of distancing. By the 1970s, however, Fox observed that some medical students placed much greater emphasis on 'feeling with the patient' and accepted the necessity for detachment with greater ambivalence.[69] Indeed, in the twenty-first century, 'clinical empathy' is held up by many as a pedagogical goal and moral virtue.[70] But this emphasis on emotional labour, medical sociologists have argued, connotes historical shifts in the corporate and consumer-minded organisation of healthcare.[71] Fox and Lief's model of emotional detachment was, therefore, complex, nuanced, and changeable, far more so than the caricature of dispassion presented in popular culture or by many surgeons themselves.

This more simplistic notion of 'detached concern' or 'imperturbability' continues to predominate in discussions about surgical behaviour and ethics today.[72] While many twenty-first-century surgeons might not seek to become or present themselves as unfeeling, they often see emotional detachment – or detached concern – as a desirable professional characteristic. As Jodi Halpern suggests, doctors often argue that detachment is needed not only for practitioners to avoid 'burning out', but more importantly, to provide objective medical care.[73] Surgeons also frequently express the idea that they need to detach to protect themselves from compassion fatigue, as they care for one suffering person after another under great time constraints, and they assume that detachment is necessary to concentrate and perform painful procedures. For Hedley Atkins in the 1950s, the surgeon did not need to be an academic genius, but he must at least possess 'a rather more than normal degree of common sense'. This common sense was required to 'inhibit his emotional responses to the sometimes tragic situations which confront him and to get on with the job which needs to be done'.[74]

Complicating the surgical stereotype

However, texts written by surgeons for surgeons in the years immediately following the foundation of the NHS tell a more complicated story of hierarchy, paternalism, and emotional detachment than you might expect. They reveal that most mid-century surgeons did not want to see themselves as Sir Lancelot Spratt figures, and they did not think that was the right way for their colleagues and students to behave. In contrast to the homogenising caricatures in the introduction, these texts written by surgeons for surgeons reveal a more nuanced image of the idealised doctor–patient relationship in this period, and contradict some of the most pervasive assumptions of professional dispassion.

Take Cecil Augustus Joll as an example. Joll was born in Bristol in 1885, the second son of a dental surgeon and 'his wife'. He achieved a 'brilliant career' in science at Bristol and London universities, before studying medicine and dentistry. He served a series of resident posts, including senior house surgeon and senior resident officer at Leicester Royal Infirmary, and in March 1912 was appointed senior resident medical officer at the Royal Free Hospital in London. Less than two years later, he was elected assistant surgeon and became senior surgeon in 1931. During his lengthy career, he was also senior surgeon to the Royal Cancer Hospital and the Mille Hospital in Greenwich. He was a general surgeon, with special expertise in thyroid surgery. He published widely, was twice a Hunterian professor, and an active member of both the Royal College of Surgeons of England and the British Medical Association. During the heavy air raids on London in 1940 and 1941, he slept every second night at the Royal Free, which was severely bombed, and spent alternate weekends there. He made ritual of carving the Christmas turkey for his surgical ward every year, and insisted on doing so at his last Christmas, in 1944, when his health was already failing.[75]

He died in 1945, aged just 59, and the *BMJ* published a series of obituaries and tributes from colleagues, patients, and students.[76] These texts attest as much to Joll's emotional talents as they do to his dexterity and operative skill. Catherine Evans wrote a 'few words of appreciation' after being treated by Joll for her thyroid problems. She said, 'Those who have not suffered from thyrotoxicosis may not realise the mental as well as physical stresses and strains which have to be borne by the patient.'[77] As a result, her testament to Joll focused on his abilities to soothe: 'Cecil Joll had that great gift of inspiring complete confidence, trust, and optimism in his patients, and this gift combined with his superb surgical skill, made him the ideal surgeon.' This account of an 'ideal' 1940s surgeon, common in the pages of the medical press, contrasts with stereotypes of indifference and dispassion.

Written about the same time as Richard Gordon was magicking up a very different myth of the modern surgeon – that of Sir Lancelot Spratt – these sources offer, therefore, an alternative and more humane image of the surgeon and prompt an alternative set of questions. How did words written *by* surgeons *for* surgeons frame the 'ideal' practitioner? What characteristics must he have, how should he relate to his colleagues and patients, and what sort of emotional standards should he adhere to? Thus, in the many and various representations of surgeons in post-war Britain, emotions played a key role. These feelings were, however, complex. For every authoritarian, autocratic, and paternalistic demagogue, there was another, emotionally intelligent practitioner seemingly invested in the hopes, fears, and personhood of his patient. These texts caveated the image of the surgeon as an authoritarian leader with limited affective capacity and put across a version of surgical professionalism that made space for feelings and the therapeutic value of emotions.

Surgeons from this period frequently reflected on their own power, influence, and authority. Despite instructions to keep crucial healthcare information away from patients, surgical textbooks also attempted to limit the surgeons' authority over patients and mostly insisted on a more collaborative approach to care and treatment. Surgeons tried to caveat the authoritarian tendencies of their co-professionals in their own books, and while they could not quite let go of the idea that the surgeon should probably be in a position of power and retain a degree of influence over their patients, the crass stereotype of the consultant surgeon storming down hospital corridors barking at patients referred to only by their inflicted body part or condition is very unlike the nuanced and emotionally alert practitioner presented in the pages of textbooks and the medical press. As it is something of an unflattering caricature that is perhaps not all that surprising, however, even more moderate versions of that stereotype were rejected by surgeons who were keen to emphasise the participatory relationship between doctor and patient and the value of professional humility.

While he might wield 'authority as a technical expert' and can give 'orders', he was in 'no position to enforce them or to penalize a patient for not carrying them out'. His authority was, therefore, 'confined exclusively to matters concerning the patient's health'. He may counsel them on occupation, diet, and physical activity, but he 'trespasses on his legitimate rights and does more harm than good by telling a patient that all she needs is a husband, a child, or sexual intercourse'.[78] He should demonstrate humility, and the surgeon must also not allow his authority to tip over into self-aggrandisement and he should be careful to only ever act within his means: 'The surgeon's training must teach him to resist the temptation to "show off"; that is to engage in a piece of technique which is not at that stage of the operation the very best for the patient under the circumstances but is one which he is especially adept at performing.'[79]

Another way that the surgical textbooks and prescriptive literature contravened the pervasive and persistent stereotypes was in their emphasis on the patient and their rights and responsibilities. They modelled a version of 'patient-centred' care, even if they would not have described their behaviour in such terms. 'Patient-centred' or 'person-centred' care is a type of healthcare that became increasingly popular and prevalent – at least in theory – in the late twentieth century. It is a way of practicing medicine, nursing, and social care in which the patient actively participates in their own treatment in close cooperation with their health professionals. It contrasts to 'traditional treatment models', where patients are viewed as passive receivers of medical intervention.[80] We might expect that surgeons working in post-war Britain might conform to this 'traditional treatment model' and, while in some ways they did, in others they subverted expectations and prefigured (or rather, laid the groundwork for) later developments in healthcare theory and practice.

While today's version of 'patient-centred' care would advocate for complete honesty with patients about their diagnosis and prognosis, and mid-century surgeons were undeniably paternalistic in cases of cancer and other terminal illnesses, those same surgeons also imagined their interactions with patients as a partnership. For example, in his 1946 textbook, Frederick Christopher advocated for a mutual and sustained relationship between doctor and patient: 'It is essential for the surgeon really to know his patient and to give the patient an opportunity in turn to know the surgeon.'[81] Similarly, Hamilton Baily and R. J. McNeill Love emphasised the patient's 'point of view' and drew readers' attention to the differences between how a surgeon and a lay person might perceive an operation: 'An operation should be regarded from the patient's point of view and not just treated as "another case"; the mental preparation is just as important as the physical.'[82] Patey also emphasised the value of the patients' thoughts and feelings: 'the student will rapidly learn that the understanding of the individual patient may often be far more important than his classification as a diagnosed case'.[83]

In *An Approach to Clinical Surgery*, Ovens insisted that when practising surgery 'you are dealing with living human beings who think and feel and have minds of their own'.[84] He insisted that in clinical work – and unlike Richard Gordon's Spratt – surgeons were not dealing with 'a case or a specimen' and that they must never allow their 'scientific interest' to 'obscure the personal relationship between [the surgeon] and [the] patient'.[85] Like other authors, Ovens drew a distinction between what could be learnt from a book and what had to be developed during practice:

> It is not the intention of this book to teach you how to behave towards patients or to expound the patient-doctor relationship, although here and there some tips are given. Such things cannot be learnt from books, but only from the example and precepts of seniors and from those who are experienced in the art.[86]

He went on to narrow the distinction between doctor and patient: 'The briefest and best guide is to treat the patient as you would wish to be treated yourself if you were ill, with kindliness, patience and understanding.'[87]

The self-representation of surgeons was emotionally diverse, and textbooks avoided simplistic models of emotional detachment. Instead, a surgeon must have a 'natural liking for his fellow men' and should be able to respond emotionally to their suffering.[88] Atkins wrote, 'The last acquired quality of the surgeon which must be considered, indeed, it is often the last to be acquired, is a capacity for sympathetic understanding of his fellow men. The surgeon not infrequently has to be the constant visitor of a dying man.'[89] He had to express authentic feelings, not just perform a compassionate attitude: 'His bearing and his behaviour in these circumstances are important professional attributes. These attitudes, although polished by experience and training, must not be false and must, to be effective, spring from a genuine sympathy with mankind.'[90] Post-war surgical textbooks and conduct guides provide a complex and multifaceted version of surgical professionalism, one that highlighted rather than denigrated the therapeutic power of the emotions. These books reveal that feelings played a key role in surgical practice and identity – even at a moment when the profession was supposedly preoccupied with technical skill, innovation, and progress, and even at a time when the popular stereotype of emotional dispassion was at its most robust and widespread.

As a result, and while these textbooks might have offered up an emotionally distant vision of ideal surgical behaviour, they also acknowledged the importance of empathy and framed the ability to understand and ameliorate patients' feelings of distress and disempowerment as a key part of the surgeons' therapeutic arsenal. If the treatment of cancer provided the surgeon with an opening for paternalism, it also offered practitioners the opportunity to give emotional support: 'The treatment of patients with incurable cancer is an important and often difficult aspect of medical practice. The physician can bring relief in many ways to the patient and his family, and it may be said with respect to the true physician that this will be his "finest hour." '[91] In his *Fundamentals of General Surgery*, John Armes Gius wrote that the surgeon must pay 'special attention' to 'the alleviation of pain, fear, worry, anxiety, insomnia, depression, suicidal tendencies and psychoses'.[92] He argued that surgeons must understand patient feelings because 'the management of the psychologic and emotional disturbances encountered in patients with cancer' was as much a part of the 'over-all treatment as is ... the maintenance of nutrition'.[93] In similar but more general terms, in an article for the *BMJ*, Eric D. Wittkower and Kerr L. White wrote, 'The practice of medicine not only consists in the application of biological knowledge but also demands considerable degrees of social and psychological understanding, described as bedside manners and psychotherapy.'[94]

Surgeons spent a great deal of time figuring out the various ways that feelings could help or hinder their professional goals. They were not, however, doing so in a vacuum and nor were they the only members of the medical profession participating in new discussions about the psychological side of clinical practice or care. As Victoria Bates has observed, calls to '(re)humanize hospitals' increased over the post-war period in Britain, Europe, and the United States of America. These efforts advocated a kind of hospital design that addressed patients' 'emotional and holistic needs', rather than seeing people as solely biomedical entities.[95] Movements like this were not just confined to hospitals, but also permeated primary care. In the late 1950s, Michael Balint and his wife Enid began holding psychological training seminars for GPs in London.[96] These took the form of case presentations and small-group discussions, led by a psychoanalyst. These seminars were supposed to be 'safe places' where doctors could talk about interpersonal and emotional aspects of their work.

Psychotherapy and psychoanalysis were powerful post-war forces and offered surgeons a language and conceptual framework to articulate and interpret their professional responsibilities.

Following correspondence with the physician and writer Georg Groddeck, Freud had developed a special interest in psychosomatic concepts, and by the 1950s his influence had permeated even the traditionally positivist surgical profession. As Michael Brown has shown, in the nineteenth century surgeons believed that emotional management of patients was one of their key responsibilities because they thought that patient feelings during and after operations had the capacity to affect survival.[97] The lessons from psychosomatic medicine were not, therefore, new – but they did offer an updated language with which to express this very old aspect of the surgical identity.

In 1952, P. T. O'Farrell gave the British Medical Association's 120th Annual Meeting's presidential address. He reported on the research in psychosomatic medicine that had demonstrated the close and influential relationship between 'emotional factors' and the 'aetiology of so-called "organic" diseases'.[98] While he cautioned that 'enthusiasm for psychosomatic medicine may become exaggerated' – 'one author has gone so far as to state that all medicine will be psychosomatic in the future' – he also admitted that 'there should be no dichotomy between the psyche and the soma in the causation and investigation of disease'.[99] He outlined the 'ample evidence' that some symptoms were 'unrelated to any structural organic changes', deducing that 'emotional factors can cause disturbance of bodily functions'.[100] He argued that while psychosomatic medicine was not a specialty, it was a 'common-sense approach to the investigation and treatment of disease'.[101] In the 1950s, this 'common-sense approach' infiltrated British surgery and shaped surgeons' professional identity.[102]

There is also some evidence to suggest that 1950s surgeons were interested in their own emotions. Ovens offered empathetic advice to those surgeons just starting out on their professional journeys and reminded readers that they could find support in their colleagues and co-professionals: 'At first you will find it difficult to adjust yourself to this relationship and you are likely to be confused and embarrassed, but you can comfort yourself with the knowledge that your difficulties are appreciated and everyone is out to help you.'[103] He acknowledged the power imbalance between surgeon and patient: 'You start with the enormous advantage of great prestige; to him [the patient], the most immature medical student is just as much a doctor as the most senior member of the staff, though perhaps not such a good one; he does not know that you have only just started in the hospital.'[104] Both the nursing and medical staff remembered 'their own difficulties when they began' and as members of a teaching hospital were 'accustomed and prepared to help' junior surgeons in their 'difficulties'.[105]

Indeed, Ovens devoted considerable space in his textbook to the emotional experiences of the surgeon, not just the patient:

> The 'bedside manner' ... largely consists in the ability of putting the patient (and his relations) at their ease, and the prerequisite for this is to be at ease yourself. At first you will find this difficult; you will naturally be nervous, hesitant and uncertain of what to do. But do not worry; appear confident even if you do not feel it. Be patient and gentle. You, like every other doctor, will acquire the manner in time.[106]

However, he also offered practical tips to help put the patient at ease and ameliorate their worries: 'Learn your patient's name as early as possible and thereafter always refer to him by name. It is probably already written on the patient's case-paper ... Treat them as a person and not as a case.'[107] He suggested that surgeons sit down beside their patients, make themselves comfortable, and 'see that he is comfortable too. By literally and metaphorically getting down to his level, you are much more likely to win his confidence.'[108] In response to a crying child – 'from fear or temper' – the surgeon reader must 'ignore the howls and continue your procedure' (unless the crying is from pain), and 'continue talking to him in a gentle, low voice and you will very soon stop the noise in order to hear what you are saying!'[109] If that fails, small babies can 'usually be quietened by being given something to suck, the tip of a finger if necessary'.[110]

Conclusion

Surgical textbooks and medical journal articles offer a glimpse into the social and cultural dynamics of the surgical profession in post-war Britain. These were prescriptive texts – idealised narratives of surgical conduct and identities – efforts to nudge trainee surgeons towards certain ways of behaving. Written by surgeons, they offered a positive representation of the profession. However, while they might have been constructions, even fictionalised descriptions, they show how surgeons *thought* they ought to behave. Thus, while this period of medical history – the 'golden age' of surgery – is often dominated either by accounts of invention, progress, and technical innovation, or by accounts of emotionally detached, paternalistic, and heroic practitioners, the self-image of surgeons was more complex.

This chapter has used these sources to examine two prominent and enduring aspects of the surgical stereotype. First, the surgeon as authoritarian or paternalistic, and second, the idea that surgeons were, or at least should be, emotionally detached. In contrast to these caricatures, these books and articles reveal a more nuanced and humane image of the idealised doctor–patient relationship in this period, and contradict some of the most pervasive assumptions of professional dispassion. As much space was devoted to the importance of the patients' feelings, care was taken over what the physical consequences of emotional ill health might be, and there was a frank acknowledgement of the troubling nature of surgical work for the surgeons themselves.

Evidently, the surgeon of the mid-twentieth century refrained from aligning himself too closely with the Sir Lancelot Spratt model, and did not necessarily think that was the right way for his colleagues and students to behave. This chapter has, therefore, demonstrated that the fiction of emotional detachment has always been precisely that – a fiction. Finding a real-life surgeon who embodied all that Spratt was is, of course, impossible. And, trying to identify a historical moment when the surgeon was everything the continuing stereotype makes him out to be is an equally futile task. However, much like the efforts of nineteenth-century surgeons to reform their image and shed their associations with the unfeeling practitioners of previous generations, these post-war attempts to position the surgeon as emotionally literate and affectively complex had limited impact on popular representations and the pervasive stereotypes of surgical dispassion.

In the next chapter, I will look at these popular representations and examine the extent to which these more nuanced profiles of the surgeon made their way into the mainstream. As discussed, crass and simplistic stereotypes of emotional detachment and paternalism predominated in the public sphere, and continue to inform patients', practitioners', and medical students' perceptions of surgery and its constituent professionals. While a reputation for calmness, kindness, and an intuitive sense of patients' needs might make your profession seem enlightened, nuanced, and capable, these ideals competed with other, equally beneficial, aspects of the surgical myth, namely heroism, clinical competence, scientific objectivity, manual dexterity, autonomy, and expertise. The latter ultimately dominated the former.

Notes

1 Lindsey Fitzharris, *The Butchering Art: Joseph Lister's Quest to Transform the Grisly World of Victorian Medicine* (London: Penguin, 2017), 15.
2 Richard Gordon, *Great Medical Disasters* (London: Hutchinson & Co., 1983), 13.
3 Ibid., 15.
4 Michael Brown, 'Robert Liston, the "Fastest Knife in the West End"? Part 1: Historical Myth-Making', *Surgery & Emotion*, http://www.surgeryandemotion.com/blog/view/robert-liston-the-fastest-knife-in-the-west-end-part-1-historical-myth-making (accessed 6 April 2023).
5 'London Hospitals and Dispensaries', *The Times* (30 January 1869).
6 'Gratuitous Medical Practice', *The Lancet*, 2 (1854), 217; 'Canvassing for Hospital Appointments', *British Medical Journal*, 2:1194 (1883), 981.
7 Agnes Arnold-Forster, *The Cancer Problem: Malignancy in Nineteenth-Century Britain* (Oxford: Oxford University Press, 2021).
8 Michael Brown, *Performing Medicine: Medical Culture and Identity in Provincial England, c. 1760–1850* (Manchester: Manchester University Press, 2011), 6; See also, Michael Brown, 'Medicine, Reform and the "End" of Charity in Early Nineteenth-Century England', *English Historical Review*, 124 (2009), 1353–1388.
9 Agnes Arnold-Forster, 'Gender and Pain in Nineteenth-Century Cancer Care', *Gender and History*, 32:1 (2020), 13–29; Michael Brown, 'Surgery and Emotion: The Era Before Anaesthesia', in Thomas Schlich (ed.), *The Palgrave Handbook of the History of Surgery* (London: Palgrave Macmillan, 2017), 327–348.
10 Agnes Arnold-Forster and Michael Brown, 'Healthcare Workers and their Emotions in the Time of Covid-19', *Surgery and Emotion*, www.surgeryandemotion.com/blog/view/emotions-healthcare-workers-and-covid-19 (accessed 31 May 2021).

11 Quoted in Carin Berkowitz, *Charles Bell and the Anatomy of Reform* (Chicago: Chicago University Press, 2015), 103.
12 Arnold-Forster and Brown, 'Healthcare Workers and their Emotions'.
13 Fitzharris, *The Butchering Art*.
14 See George Campbell Gosling, *Payment and Philanthropy in British Healthcare, 1918–48* (Manchester: Manchester University Press, 2017); Martin Gorsky, John Mohan, and Tim Willis, *Mutualism and Health Care: British Hospital Contributory Schemes in the Twentieth Century* (Manchester: Manchester University Press, 2006).
15 Ross McKibbin, 'Politics and the Medical Hero: A. J. Cronin's "The Citadel"', *English Historical Review*, 123:502 (2008), 651–678, 664.
16 Anne Digby and Nick Bosanquet, 'Doctors and Patients in an Era of National Health Insurance and Private Practice, 1913–1938', *Economic History Review*, 41 (1988), 74–94, 74.
17 Barry Doyle and Rosemary Wall, 'What was Healthcare Like before the NHS?', *The Conversation* (3 July 2018), https://theconversation.com/what-was-healthcare-like-before-the-nhs-99055 (accessed 28 April 2020).
18 A. J. Cronin, *The Citadel* (London: Picador, 2019).
19 McKibbin, 'Politics and the Medical Hero', 656.
20 Ibid., 662.
21 Ibid., 660.
22 Ibid., 659.
23 Ibid., 660.
24 Ibid.
25 Ibid.
26 Cronin, *The Citadel*, 325.
27 McKibbin, 'Politics and the Medical Hero', 661.
28 Ibid., 663.
29 Ibid., 665.
30 Ibid.
31 Ibid.
32 Ministry of Health: Consultative Council on Medical and Allied Services, *Interim Report on the Future Provision of Medical and Allied Services* (London, 1920), www.nhshistory.net/Dawson%20report.html (accessed 28 April 2021).
33 William Beveridge, *Social Insurance and Allied Services* (London: His Majesty's Stationery Office, 1942).
34 Charles Webster, *The National Health Service: A Political History* (Oxford: Oxford University Press, 2002), 18.
35 Andrew Seaton, 'Against the "Sacred Cow": NHS Opposition and the Fellowship for Freedom in Medicine, 1948–72', *Twentieth Century British History*, 26 (2015), 424–449, 425.

36 Ibid.
37 E. Gerard Housden, 'The Health Service Bill', *British Medical Journal*, 1 (1946), 846–847, 847.
38 Eric Linklater, 'Prometheus and To-Morrow', *British Medical Journal*, 2:4955 (1955), 1517–1520, 1519.
39 Ibid.
40 Ibid.
41 See Rob Boddice, *Humane Professions: The Defence of Experimental Medicine, 1876–1914* (Cambridge: Cambridge University Press, 2021); Joanna Bourke, 'Pain, Sympathy and the Medical Encounter between the Mid-Eighteenth and the Mid-Twentieth Centuries', *Historical Research*, 85:229 (2012), 430–452; Brown, *Performing Medicine*; Delia Gavrus, 'Men of Dreams and Men of Action: Neurologists, Neurosurgeons and the Performance of Professional Identity, 1920–1950', *Bulletin of the History of Medicine*, 85:1 (2011), 57–92.
42 Harold C. Edwards, *Recent Advances in Surgery*, 3rd edition (London: J. & A. Churchill, 1948), v.
43 Ibid.; see also Leo Bergen, 'Surgery and War: The Discussions About the Usefulness of War for Medical Progress', in Thomas Schlich (ed.), *The Palgrave Handbook of the History of Surgery* (London: Palgrave Macmillan, 2017), 389–407.
44 Peter J. Kernahan, 'Surgery Becomes a Specialty: Professional Boundaries and Surgery', in Thomas Schlich (ed.), *The Palgrave Handbook of the History of Surgery* (London: Palgrave Macmillan, 2017), 95–113.
45 Gerald H. C. Ovens, *An Approach to Clinical Surgery* (London: J. & A. Churchill, 1953), 2.
46 Ibid., 108.
47 Linklater, 'Prometheus and To-Morrow', 1519.
48 David H. Patey (ed.), *An Introduction to Surgery* (London: Lloyd-Luke, 1958), 5.
49 Ibid.
50 Ibid.
51 Sophie Crowe, Nicholas Clarke, and Ruairi Brugha, '"You Do Not Cross Them": Hierarchy and Emotion in Doctors' Narratives of Power Relations in Specialist Training', *Social Science and Medicine*, 186 (2017), 70–77, 72.
52 Dave de Bronkart, 'From Patient Centred to People Powered: Autonomy on the Rise', *British Medical Journal*, 350 (2015), 1–3, 1.
53 Leonard I. Stein, 'The Doctor–Nurse Game', *American Journal of Nursing*, 68:1 (1968), 101–105, 105.
54 Patey, *An Introduction to Surgery*, 8.

55 Ovens, *An Approach to Clinical Surgery*, 295.
56 Ibid.
57 Ibid.
58 Ibid.
59 Arthur Hailey, *The Final Diagnosis* (New York: Doubleday, 1959).
60 Letter from Alan W. Boon to Elizabeth Gilzean, 1 November 1960, MB/AB/1/035d.
61 William Reddy, *The Navigation of Feeling: A Framework for the History of Emotions* (Cambridge: Cambridge University Press, 2001).
62 Natalie J. Lewis et al., 'Emotional Intelligence Medical Education: Measuring the Unmeasurable?', *Advances in Health Sciences Education*, 10:4 (2005), 339–355.
63 Joanna Bourke, 'Some Surgeons may be Psychopaths – But that's no Bad Thing', *Prospect* (21 June 2017), https://prospectmagazine.co.uk/magazine/two-new-books-explore-how-surgeons-must-be-resolute-and-merciless (accessed 18 May 2021).
64 William Osler, *Aequanimitas: With Other Addresses to Medical Students, Nurses and Practitioners of Medicine* (Philadelphia: P. Blakiston, 1922), 4.
65 Matthew L. Edwards, 'On William Osler, Psychiatry, and the Law: Reflections on "Aequanimitas" at 130 Years', *American Journal of Psychiatry Residents' Journal*, 15:1 (2019), 3; Daniel K. Sokol, 'How to Be a Cool Headed Clinician', *British Medical Journal*, 344 (2012), e3980; David L. Anders, 'Aequanimitas Centennial', *Southern Medical Journal*, 82:11 (1989), 1403–1404. Edwards and Sokol both reference *Aequanimitas* in the context of medical malpractice proceedings. On the cultural history of 'coolness' in the US, see Peter N. Stearns, *American Cool: Constructing a Twentieth-Century Emotional Style* (New York: New York University Press, 1994).
66 Reddy argues that 'emotional regimes' are maintained by empowered classes and prevailing norms. Reddy, *The Navigation of Feeling*.
67 Renée C. Fox, *Experiment Perilous: Physicians and Patients Facing the Unknown* (Glencoe, IL: Free Press, 1959).
68 Harold I. Lief and Renée C. Fox, 'Training for "Detached Concern" in Medical Students', in Harold I. Lief, Victor F. Lief, and Nina R. Lief (eds), *The Psychological Basis of Medical Practice* (New York: Harper & Row, 1963), 12–35. On 'affective neutrality' in medical education, see Allen C. Smith and Sherryl Kleinman, 'Managing Emotions in Medical School: Students' Contacts with the Living and the Dead', *Social Psychology Quarterly*, 52:1 (1989), 56–69; Mary-Jo DelVecchio Good and Byron J. Good, 'Disabling Practitioners: Hazards of Learning to Be a Doctor in American

Medical Education', *American Journal of Orthopsychiatry*, 59:2 (1989), 303–309. Charles S. Bryan has argued that Osler's call for coolness was not at the expense of empathy: '"Aequanimitas" Redux: William Osler on Detached Concern versus Humanistic Empathy', *Perspectives in Biology and Medicine*, 49:3 (2006), 384–392.

69 Renée C. Fox, 'Is There a "New" Medical Student?: A Comparative View of Medical Socialization in the 1950s and the 1970s', in *Essays in Medical Sociology: Journeys into the Field* (New York: John Wiley & Sons, 1979), 100.

70 Jodi Halpern, *From Detached Concern to Empathy: Humanizing Medical Practice* (New York: Oxford University Press, 2001).

71 Alexandra H. Vinson and Kelly Underman, 'Clinical Empathy as Emotional Labor in Medical Work', *Social Science & Medicine*, 251 (2020), 112904; Carter Hardy, 'Clinical Sympathy: The Important Role of Affectivity in Clinical Practice', *Medicine, Health Care and Philosophy*, 22:4 (2019), 499–513; Kelly Underman and Laura E. Hirshfield, 'Detached Concern?: Emotional Socialization in Twenty-First Century Medical Education', *Social Science & Medicine*, 160 (2016), 94–101.

72 Philip F. Stahel, *Blood, Sweat and Tears: Becoming a Better Surgeon* (Shrewsbury: TFM, 2016), 18–19.

73 Halpern, *From Detached Concern to Empathy*, xxi.

74 Ibid.

75 Royal College of Surgeons of England, 'Joll, Cecil Augustus (1885–1945)', *Plarr's Lives of the Fellows* (23 July 2013).

76 'Cecil Joll, M.D., M.S., M.Ch., F.R.C.S.' *British Medical Journal*, 1:4387 (1945), 168; H. W. Loftus Dale, 'Cecil Joll. M.Ch., F.R.C.S.', *British Medical Journal*, 1:4388 (1945), 202–203; G. Gordon-Taylor, 'Cecil A. Joll, F.R.C.S.', *British Medical Journal*, 1:4389 (1945), 238–239.

77 P. Catherine Evans, 'Mr. Cecil A. Joll', *British Medical Journal*, 1:4391 (1945), 314.

78 Eric D. Wittkower and Kerr L. White, 'Bedside Manners', *British Medical Journal*, 1:4876 (1954), 1432–1434, 1433.

79 Hedley Atkins, *The Surgeon's Craft* (Manchester: Manchester University Press, 1965), 35.

80 The Health Foundation, 'Person-Centred Care Made Simple: What Everyone Should Know About Person-Centred Care' (London: The Health Foundation, 2016).

81 Frederick Christopher (ed.), *A Textbook of Surgery by American Authors*, 4th edition (Philadelphia and London: W. B. Saunders, 1945), 1456.

82 Hamilton Baily and R. J. McNeill Love (eds), *Surgery for Nurses* (London: H. K. Lewis, 1946), 423.
83 'The actual complaint may be minor compared with the mass of fears and misunderstandings in the patient's mind' (Patey, *An Introduction to Surgery*, 7).
84 Ovens, *An Approach to Clinical Surgery*, 1.
85 Ibid.
86 Ibid., 2.
87 Ibid.
88 Atkins, *The Surgeon's Craft*, 30–31.
89 Ibid., 36.
90 Ibid.
91 John Armes Gius, *Fundamentals of General Surgery* (Chicago: Year Book Medical Publishers, 1962), 241.
92 Ibid.
93 Ibid.
94 Wittkower and White, 'Bedside Manners', 1434.
95 Victoria Bates, '"Humanizing" Healthcare Environments: Architecture, Art and Design in Modern Hospitals', *Design for Health*, 2 (2018), 5–19, 11.
96 Rhodri Hayward, *The Transformation of the Psyche in British Primary Care, 1870–1970* (London: Bloosmbury, 2015).
97 Brown, 'Surgery and Emotion: The Era Before Anaesthesia'.
98 P. T. O'Farrell, 'British Medical Association One Hundred and Twentieth Annual Meeting, Dublin, 1952 President's Address: Topics, Thoughts, and Tendencies', *British Medical Journal*, 2 (1952), 53–57, 55.
99 Ibid.
100 Ibid.
101 Ibid.
102 Ibid.
103 Ovens, *An Approach to Clinical Surgery*, 1.
104 Ibid.
105 Ibid., 1–2.
106 Ibid., 108.
107 Ibid.
108 Ibid., 109.
109 Ibid.
110 Ibid.

2

Surgeons in film, fiction, and on TV screens

Elizabeth Gilzean was born in Lachine, just outside Montreal, Canada to French-Canadian and English-Scottish-Dutch parents. She trained as a nurse before working in Bermuda during the Second World War, treating the sick and injured. In 1945, she moved to Birmingham with her English husband and continued nursing under the NHS. She started writing romantic novels for the famous publishing house, Mills & Boon, before quitting nursing to write full time in April 1957.[1] Gilzean mostly wrote 'Doctor–Nurse' romances, which traditionally involved a love affair between a male doctor or surgeon and a female nurse, although she frequently subverted the genre. She was an avid letter writer, especially to her editor Alan W. Boon, and her personality and irreverent sense of humour leap from the pages and pages of their correspondence. Her letters to and from Boon are warm and affectionate. He often invited her for lunch or dinner in London and they exchanged witty and friendly banter. She wrote to him in March 1957:

> I am hurt, deeply hurt. On Wednesday evening, Olive leaned across the coffee bar and said to me: 'How long have you been calling him Alan?' In true Mills & Boon fashion I sighed deeply and said sadly: 'Never. He hasn't asked me to.' There was a gleam of pride in Olive's eyes when she replied: 'He asked me to call him Alan the last time I was in London.' 'T'aint fair. What's she got that I haven't got? I shall certainly have to put you in my next book and I doubt very much if you will be allowed to get the girl![2]

Despite the frivolity of much of her correspondence, Gilzean brought a wealth of knowledge about hospitals, nursing, and surgery to her books and prided herself on the authenticity and accuracy of her novels.

In June 1958, she wrote to Boon, wanting to discuss one of her books' characters. This character was everything the myths made surgeons out to be – emotionally detached, taciturn, even gruff. She justified her characterisation with her own real-life experience of hospital staff and their emotional dynamics: 'Most surgeons have the knack of shutting out their personal lives as if while on duty they are playing a part that has no link with real life.'[3]

'Doctor–Nurse' romances were, therefore, one of the many places that fictional surgeons appeared in post-war Britain. These characters were made up, but, as the example of Elizabeth Gilzean and her writing demonstrates, they were also often based on reality or drawn from the creator's own experiences of hospitals, operating theatres, and healthcare more generally. In this chapter, I will examine the emergence and presence of the surgical stereotype in film, fiction, and television programmes and explore its relationship to the version of surgical professionalism contained in texts written by surgeons themselves. Were more popular representations similarly complex? Or did they align with, and then reinforce, the stereotype of the paternalistic, avaricious, and emotionally detached surgeon the textbooks were trying to frustrate? And, perhaps most importantly, why does it matter?

While it is difficult to extrapolate public perception from popular representation (and this book tries to avoid doing this as much as possible), 'Doctor–Nurse' romances, medical soap operas, and satirical and serious books and films were read and watched by millions. Indeed, I argue that these representations had an impact on lay expectations of professionals and I am not alone in doing so. Elena C. Strauman and Bethany C. Goodier suggest that cultural representations provide non-medical people with a map for understanding the unfamiliar world of healthcare and that these representations offer audiences a glimpse behind the (operating) theatre curtain.[4] Michael Pfau, Lawrence J. Mullen, and Kirsten Garrow argue that television has become an important vehicle for the construction of professional roles irrespective of the viewer's own 'real-life' experiences.[5] Joseph Turow warns doctors and other healthcare workers to be aware that their patients often come to their offices with years of dramatic, romantic, and comedic stories about the medical system 'swimming in their heads'.[6] He argues that healthcare professionals should consider how these fictional portrayals affect the 'mental scripts' patients bring to appointments. Film portrayals of surgeons may create public expectations of similar behaviours, attitudes, values, and practices that inform their real-life interactions with doctors.[7]

These claims depend on the idea that societies have a 'repertoire of identities' from which individuals draw to construct their personal and professional selves. This repertoire relies on multiple sources, or a 'cumulative cultural text' which embraces an ever-changing parade of songs, stories, poems, films, television programmes, memoirs, paintings, photos, and novels. These images and scripts play back to healthcare workers what it is to be a professional and at the same time shape public perception of professional identity. It is not possible, therefore, in the media-saturated world we all inhabit, for a surgeon to make sense of their own professional identity without reference to these public and professional representations. Surgeons on screen have also become a powerful teaching tool in a more specific sense. Clinical educators have recognised the potency of filmic representations in 'professional becoming', and many incorporate these images in formal education programmes. Spratt himself regularly appears in lectures on surgical communication skills to demonstrate a paternalistic, doctor-centred approach to medicine.[8] I have sat through multiple talks by eminent surgeons and physicians in which they show clips from *Doctor in the House* to emphasise how far we have, and have not, come since the 1950s.

There are so many possible examples of mid-century medical writing, film, and television that this is, of course, a selection and by no means the only places where surgeons – both fictional and real – appeared. They do, however, offer a nice cross-section of post-war British society, and I take seriously culture that might otherwise be dismissed as 'light-weight' or 'women's fiction'.[9] I also think it is important to examine these popular representations alongside and in conversation with surgeons' own reflections on their profession and reputation. To do so, I not only interweave discussions from surgical and non-surgical sources, but also look for moments where the two intersect, for example moments when surgeons commented explicitly on popular representations in medical journals, or when writers drew on their professional clinical experience to inform and flesh out their fictional characters and caricatures.

Popular representations under the NHS

In Chapter 1 I discussed the novel *The Citadel*, which painted a harsh and critical picture of British healthcare and its constituent professionals. After the foundation of the NHS, however, popular representations changed. In post-war Britain, various cultural products – ranging from romantic fiction to TV dramas – presented doctors, surgeons, and nurses to an increasingly adoring public. As Mathew Thompson has argued, these portrayals 'helped promote sympathy for the service'.[10] Their use of humour and romance 'provided a valve for the release of tensions of class and gender that was important in building affection for the system, despite its shortcomings and its inheritance of a hierarchical culture'.[11]

These new and altered cultural representations of healthcare tell us much about the medical past and I am not the first historian to gravitate towards popular culture as potentially illuminating primary source material. Films, fiction, and television programmes help us 'democratise the past' and give us tantalising insight into what ordinary people thought about healthcare and its practitioners.[12] Usually, historians of medicine focus on conventional historical materials, such as those written by healthcare professionals and published in esoteric journals and textbooks. In contrast, and while this is not the primary aim of this book, more popular outputs help bring the patient into the picture and emphasise her interactions with doctors and healthcare systems – interactions that are 'seldom addressed in more conventional approaches'.[13]

Film, fiction, and television are all useful sources for me, but at the time these popular representations also served several, crucial, purposes. For one, they sought to demystify the hospital and reveal how patients experienced surgery and other clinical processes and procedures. And, in the case of some of these popular representations, they tried to do so in a comic and relatable way.[14] Many, also, endeavoured to promote the healthcare professions and embarked on a deliberate programme of positive representation. Some of this was already going on in the 1930s. As McKibbon has observed, reviewers of *The Citadel* were concerned that its criticisms of healthcare and the medical professions went too far. One journalist in the *Times Literary Supplement* wrote,

> All over the country today are county and municipal officers who care less for fees than for healing; in general practice are insignificant men and women living devoted, anxious lives with only fourteen days a year away from the clamorous telephone by day and night. In Harley Street are men who might stand by Lister without shame. Above all, in the research departments of many a hospital are heroes and martyrs. They should have been made an offset to Dr. Cronin's 'selected types'.[15]

The film censors, when they saw the initial script of the film, were even more critical. The chief censor, J. C. Hanna, was anxious that 'the confidence of the nation in the medical profession' should not be shaken. His assistant, Mrs N. Crouzet, agreed: 'There is so much that is disparaging to doctors in this book, that I consider it unsuitable for production as a film.'[16]

While doctors, nurses, and surgeons appeared in popular culture throughout the nineteenth century and into the twentieth, the new NHS prompted a proliferation of cultural representations of hospitals, general practice surgeries, and their staff. Indeed, as surgery increasingly relocated from the home to the hospital and into highly specialised spaces within the hospitals, 'it paradoxically loomed larger in popular culture'.[17] Writing about the American context – but about things with plenty of resonance on this side of the Atlantic as well – Susan E. Lederer argues that the middle decades of the twentieth century, long regarded as a 'golden age' for medicine, were also a 'golden age' for popular representations of medicine.[18] If clinical characters had appeared in Victorian crime novels and early twentieth-century satirical fiction, it was after the foundation of the NHS that surgeons became popular celebrities.[19]

'Doctor–Nurse' romances

In the first few decades of the NHS, the public myths and popular representation of surgeons varied widely. Those who appeared in televised soap operas were idealised, self-abnegating heroes. In contrast, those in comedy films, middle-brow fiction, and romantic novels were often detached and dispassionate, ranging from the merely unsympathetic to the cruelly sadistic. Mills & Boon were the most prolific publishers of romantic fiction in twentieth-century Britain. Today, they have 3.2 million devoted readers in the United Kingdom and 50 million worldwide. They sell 200 million novels every year, and a Mills & Boon paperback is sold in a UK bookshop on average every 6.6 seconds.[20] Founded in 1908 as a publisher of general fiction, as well as etiquette guides and manuals for modern living, it quickly became clear that romances were their bestsellers. Mills & Boon love stories were indeed widely read. They were sold in ubiquitous high street shops like Woolworths and WH Smith and distributed through public and private lending libraries. In 1972, they sold 26,800,000 English-language novels globally, and in 1973 sales exceeded 30 million.

Despite the global reach of their books, Mills & Boon saw themselves as a British institution. And they offered a very narrow definition of Britishness. Mills & Boon heroines from the mid-twentieth century were invariably white. While this might not be all that surprising considering the nature of popular culture in post-war Britain, the clinical setting of these novels means that the absence of Black and Brown protagonists requires further explanation. As I will discuss in chapters 4 and 5, the foundation of the NHS saw an expansion of female participation in the labour market and a much more ethnically diverse healthcare workforce. Indeed, the advent of the NHS in 1948 coincided almost exactly with the post-war mass movement to Britain of once-colonial populations. Against this backdrop, the absence of Black and Brown Mills & Boon heroines is more notable. As Hsu-Ming Teo has observed, 'white women – primarily of British heritage – were naturalised as the heroines of romance', because historically, 'white women function as emblematic objects of heterosexual desire'.[21]

Around 1950, the publisher introduced a new sub-genre – the 'Doctor–Nurse' romances. These books soon flourished, and by 1957 they constituted a quarter of the publisher's sales.[22] While Mills & Boon did not mandate that its authors have relevant expertise, just like in the case of Elizabeth Gilzean, the 'Doctor–Nurse' romances were almost always written by women with healthcare backgrounds who drew on their real-life experiences of hospital life in their efforts to portray romantic, but authentic, characters. And yet, despite this gloss of reality, the hospitals in these many thousands of novels were populated by stereotypical figures who embodied romantic ideals and gendered extremes. Surgeons, and to a lesser extent doctors, were famed for their authoritarian and autocratic attitudes and their detachment from patient suffering. While many of these qualities might be considered unappealing, some of them were used by Mills & Boon authors to emphasise doctors and surgeons as ideal male romantic leads.

Even in romantic fiction otherwise devoted to positive portrayals of healthcare professionals, surgeons were repeatedly described as being emotionally detached or restrained – characteristics that applied to both their jobs and to their romantic affairs. Both authors and fictional characters were ambivalent about the pros and cons of emotional detachment. In *Love Unspoken*, a romantic novel serialised in the magazine *Woman's Own*, the surgeon hero was described: 'At thirty Philip Redwood was nearing the peak of his profession. There were some who said he was ruthless in his determination to get to the top, but he was oblivious of the criticism levelled against him, oblivious too, of the idolatry of the younger nurses in the hospital.'[23] Redwood's professional peak aligned with his emotional invulnerability. Completely focused on his work and professional advancement, he represented the ideal man to the hospital's female staff members (and by implication, the readers of *Woman's Own*).

Emotional detachment from patients was mirrored by an indifference in love and female affection. In Hilda Pressley's *Staff Nurses in Love*, the heroine ruminates anxiously about the unobtainable hero: 'She thought of Dr Kendal, that rather forbidding, taciturn physician. She could not imagine any woman, nurse or not, finding her way to his heart.'[24] Elizabeth Gilzean described the hero of her new novel in a letter to Boon as 'detachedly cold-blooded' and said that he exploits the nurse-heroine's affections 'quite shamelessly'.[25] Stereotypes of virile masculinity and clinical professionalism frequently overlapped.

While most of the heroines in medical romances were nurses, some were physicians or even surgeons. Many of the female clinicians exhibited high degrees of emotional intelligence and acuity, much more than the traditional, macho stereotype usually allowed. Madeline Keys from Hilda Nickson's 1962 *Surgeons in Love* was both the main love interest and a remarkably compassionate surgeon:

> The scalpel poised, Madeline paused for a brief second … to allow the fact that the patient really was anesthetized to seep into her brain. The incision was the part of operating she liked least, and only by pausing and telling herself that the patient would feel no pain … could she begin with confidence.[26]

However, Madeline was also a talented and devoted surgeon: 'A love of surgery was in her bones and in her blood as well as in her fingers.'[27] Her fellow surgeon, Francis Meyland, remarks on one of her operations, 'That was well done indeed.'

Mills & Boon were invested in creating relatable, but aspirational, female characters. As a result, they not only created female surgeons – male surgeons otherwise dominated the profession in both fiction and in real life (more on this in chapters 3 and 4) – but they also consistently portrayed those women as highly accomplished and technically excellent clinicians. In Elizabeth Gilzean's *No Time for Love*, the heroine Noel Aston is

> tall and slender whose quiet grey eyes … give little hint of the brilliance that has brought her through her medical exams with honours, seen her through her eighteen months of walking the hospital wards, got her past the obstacle of the Primary Examination for her F.R.C.S., and has obtained for her the coveted post in the Surgical Research Unit at St Almonds Hospital.[28]

As well as skilled and intelligent, fictional female surgeons were also capable of appropriate levels of emotional detachment. Madeline admonished a nurse for unnecessary displays of sentiment: 'Sister, we only let ourselves down when we give way to our feelings and let our emotions run away with us.'[29] She is repeatedly complimented by her male colleagues for her ability to keep her head under pressure. Her anaesthetist 'told her it was the neatest incision he had ever seen and that her coolness and aplomb filled him with admiration'.

The representation of male surgeons in these novels was also more complex than they might seem at first glance, and the emotional landscape of fictional surgery in post-war Britain was neither consistent nor stable. Instead, cultural representations offered an array of emotional models. While some romance novels portrayed gruff, emotionally restricted surgical heroes, many of the authors also subverted the stereotypical clinical identities and engaged in a process of creative refashioning. Just as the novels constructed caricatures of masculinity, they also portrayed male healthcare professionals – including surgeons – who were capable of care and compassion. This complicates claims by some scholars who suggest that in these novels, medicine was exclusively a heroic and interventional enterprise practiced by granite-jawed young surgeons. Care and compassion were presented as not only essential to the hero's appeal as a potential lover or husband, but also as a crucial facet of their professional identity.

Elizabeth Gilzean was well aware of the need to balance her surgical hero's tendencies towards detachment, dispassion, even cruelty, against his capacity to love and care for any future wife. She wrote to her editor Alan W. Boon in 1957 articulating this dilemma: 'I have to find that tender scene to counteract the hero's apparent brutality.'[30] Tenderness was, however, also a valued professional characteristic. In the emotional landscape of romantic fiction, the best surgeons had to be emotionally literate as well as technically brilliant. In *Surgeons in Love*, Madeline Keys described her love interest as 'a good surgeon, kind and considerate', implying that to be a 'good surgeon' you must also be 'kind and considerate'.[31] This portrayal subtly contradicted pervasive and contemporaneous professional stereotypes that represented the surgeon in particular as male, overconfident, and unfeeling. 'Doctor–Nurse' romances did, therefore, attempt to shape people's expectations of doctors, and offered an alternative portrayal of the emotionally detached surgeon to the one presented by the likes of Sir Lancelot Spratt.

Carbolic soap operas

These alternative portrayals also carried over into the relatively new genre of television, and particularly to the emerging medical soap opera. The substantial increases in healthcare spending and major advances in biomedicine that took place in 1950s Britain were accompanied by a new kind of film and television: the healthcare drama – sometimes referred to as a 'carbolic soap opera', in reference to the cleaning product's astringent smell and its associations with healthcare settings. Like medical romance fiction, these television programmes praised the doctor and surgeon, presenting him in a positive light, and emphasising his emotional complexities alongside clinical abilities. *Emergency Ward 10* was one of British television's first major soap opera series, shown on ITV from 1957 to 1967. The series was set in the fictional Oxbridge General and was the first hospital-based television drama to establish a successful format combining medical matters with storylines centring on the personal and romantic lives of doctors and nurses. It offered viewers innovative plot lines and was the first to introduce the British public to a pacemaker, made in the USA but not yet in use in the UK. In 1964, it attracted attention for its portrayal of an interracial relationship between surgeon Louise Mahler and Doctor Giles Farmer, showing the second ever kiss on television between a Black and a white actor.[32]

Emergency Ward 10 was one of the many medical soap operas screened on both sides of the Atlantic that was deeply respectful 'of the growing power and authority of the medical institutions'.[33] The programme was particularly invested in the production of the surgical hero. While this character type conformed to many of the stereotypes outlined in this book's introduction – paternalistic, distant, in a position of leadership – in order to appeal to his audience's emotions, he was also compassionate and caring. In *Life in Emergency Ward 10*, the film version of *Emergency Ward 10*, a new registrar joins a small county hospital, accompanied by a revolutionary heart lung machine that he had brought over from America. He must win over his colleagues, including the senior house surgeon, and the British doctor who had anticipated getting the foreign registrar's appointment for himself. In a series of scenes, an older patient dies on the table and a young boy undergoes an urgent operation to correct a hole in his heart. The movie was a real tear-jerker. An advertisement included a quotation from the magazine, *Woman's Mirror*: 'The film that will make a million women cry.'

As Rebecca Feasey has argued, *Emergency Ward 10* (and its film spin-off) prompted audiences to trust competent healthcare staff and believe in the advances in medical technology by emphasising the 'central and capable figure' of the male doctor-hero, who was 'at the centre of authority in the hospital'. The depiction of the doctor-hero was 'so reassuring during this period' that he came to be perceived as 'the most trusted and respected figure on television'. After all, he was 'god-like', a 'matinee idol … with a great bedside manner', 'a handsome paragon of masculine virtue', 'an emblematic figure for the brave new post-war world', and the personification of a 'benevolent, kind and caring healthcare system'.[34] Sociologist John Turow summarises these early programmes and encapsulates this tension between life-saving and self-interested: 'the driving assumption behind TV's premier doctor series was that the physician was the unquestioned king of healthcare in a society where medicine was an infinitely expandable commodity'.[35]

These complimentary portrayals were, therefore, no coincidence. Much like the producers who translated *The Citadel* to the screen, both those responsible for 'Doctor–Nurse' romances and television dramas like *Emergency Ward 10* were committed to positive representations of the healing professions. In 1958, J. D. Davidson, managing editor of a women's magazine, agreed: 'I have a theory that fiction must never disturb the faith and trust a woman feels for doctors and/or nurses.'[36] He was particularly concerned that the newly popular and prevalent medical romances had the capacity to undo readers' devotion to the health service and that authors must endeavour to do the opposite – to inculcate them into the value of medicine and the positive moral character of healthcare professionals, surgeons included. In romantic fiction and on television, surgeons were overwhelmingly portrayed as committed, technically skilled, and capable professionals.

Both Mills & Boon and the makers of *Emergency Ward 10* were also deeply invested in medical authenticity and accuracy. In ITV's 1959/60 Annual Report, the programme was described as an 'established documentary drama series', implying that it at least attempted to accurately reflect real life. Antony Kearey, *Emergency Ward 10*'s producer, was proud of the research that went into his hospital series: 'A panel of special advisers is permanently on call.'[37] They were dramas, but they were also supposed to be realistic. The series creator, Tessa Diamond, had some grounding in healthcare when writing the series, as her father had been the Deputy Medical Officer of Health in Kingston-Upon-Hull and her uncle was a doctor.[38] As a result, *Emergency Ward 10* was indebted to the advice of healthcare professionals. Doctors were keen to formalise this relationship. As early as 1951, the British Medical Association resolved that a 'close liaison should be established between the BMA and the BBC to control the selection of subjects and the scripts of material presented to the public'. Ten years later, they proposed the appointment of a full-time Medical Editor at the BBC, a doctor with 'experience in the problems of communicating medicine to the lay public'.[39] It is no surprise, therefore, that the programme buttressed the power and social capital of doctors, shaped positive images of healthcare professionalism, and crafted heroic surgical characters. The British viewing public were so taken by the series that they used to address letters to the fictional hospital seeking medical advice.

The Millstone

Unlike romance novels and carbolic soap operas, the independent authors of middle-brow fiction had a bit more latitude to craft complex and even off-putting surgical characters. Margaret Drabble's 1965 novel, *The Millstone*, tells the story of Rosamund Stacey, a young female academic who was brought up by middle-class, well-intentioned socialists.[40] Set in the 1960s, against the backdrop of the emerging Women's Liberation Movement, Rosamund has some freedoms (as much a product of her class and race as of her newly politicised gender) but not others. She meets a man, has sex, and becomes pregnant. She experiments with self-induced, back-alley, and authorised abortions, but ultimately decides to carry the baby to term, give birth, and become a parent. The book manages to be, therefore, 'both radical and a paean to motherhood'.[41] It is a fascinating novel with much to say about womanhood, motherhood, and life in 1960s London. As many of its scenes take place in doctors' consulting rooms and on hospital wards, it is also a novel which represents the social and emotional world of mid-century medicine.

Operations to correct congenital heart defects symbolised technological advance in mid-century surgery and were frequently reported on in the popular press. This coverage told stories of heroism and success against the odds, and framed surgeons as life-saving risk-takers. An article published in *Woman's Own* in 1954 described the case of Pamela, an American child who underwent open heart surgery while being kept alive by cardiopulmonary bypass: 'In her desperate bid for the right to live, baby Pamela needed the help of a miracle. And it came – in time – when doctors discovered this wonderful new method of heart surgery.'[42] Articles like this one that romanticised the role of surgery were a regular feature of *Woman's Own*, a British magazine with a circulation of millions. Octavia, Rosamund's daughter in *The Millstone*, undergoes a similar operation. However, Rosamund's encounters with the surgeons who eventually operated on Octavia were shrouded in mystery and marked by a similar kind of disregard for plain communication and compassion embodied by Sir Lancelot Spratt.

As is hopefully clear by now, cultural representations of surgeons in the post-war period were varied. And yet, they all – in one way or another – played with and expanded upon the idea that surgeons were authoritarian figures on the hospital ward that exerted unusual power and influence over their patients. The surgeon Rosamund met recommended an operation, but only 'murmured' something about the diagnosis.[43] Octavia's disease or deformity is never actually identified in the novel, partly because the surgeon makes little effort to explain to Rosamund what is wrong with her daughter or delineate what they are going to do to help her. From references to 'pulmonary artery', however, it seems that she undergoes surgery to correct a congenital heart defect. As the surgeon goes on to say, operations of this type on babies so young were progressing quickly but still in their very early stages: 'As little as five years ago, in an infant of this age, I should have said that the chance of survival was about five to one. Now we would put it at four to one, I think.'[44]

Along with paternalism, heroism, and power, emotional detachment was another pervasive theme in cultural representations of surgery in post-war Britain. In *The Millstone*, surgery saves Octavia's life. However, surgery and its practitioners occupy ambivalent positions in Drabble's narrative. The surgeon who offers to operate on Octavia is presented as detached and indifferent – an emotional style that damages his relationship with Rosamund and only intensifies her suffering. She says that while he was describing the operation, 'I could see that he was not really attempting to explain.'[45] She goes on to reflect, 'It has never ceased to amaze me that they showed, at this stage, so little professional sympathy; I see now, and suspected then, that his only emotion was professional curiosity. She was an odd case, my baby, a freak.'[46]

Throughout, *The Millstone* reflected and reinforced the pervasive stereotype of the masculine, stoic, and dispassionate surgeon. The surgeon Rosamund encounters also practised precisely the kind of paternalistic and emotionally detached healthcare that the surgical textbooks advocated. However, unlike Osler and the medical sociologists discussed in the previous chapter, Drabble *critiques* the detachment displayed by her novel's surgeon anti-hero and considers the harm it could cause patients and their loved ones. The surgeon in this book is simultaneously taciturn, paternalistic, and unfeeling, and the man who saves Rosamund's daughter's life. While it acknowledges the social utility of modern medicine, it is also critical of the healthcare system and its inability to accommodate emotional expression or communicate effectively with patients and loved ones.

Doctor in the House

Last, but certainly not least, the stereotype of the surgeon as taciturn, paternalistic, and unfeeling was crystallised in *Doctor in the House*, Richard Gordon's first medical-themed book, published in 1952. Gordon was an English surgeon and anaesthetist and his comic novels centred around the experiences of a medical student turned trainee who shared a name with the author in the books, but was rechristened Simon Sparrow in the films. The fictional Gordon spends his student days at a fictional London teaching hospital, St Swithin's, trailing behind the irascible Sir Lancelot Spratt. He initially aspires to become a surgeon himself, but in the series' third novel, *Doctor at Large* (1954), leaves his first job as a St Swithin's junior casualty house surgeon to assist a GP in the Midlands. All the books trade in surgical stereotypes and Gordon relies on familiar caricatures for much of his humour. In this case – as with all the others – the book's genre dictates the kind of surgeon that it creates. Subtlety and emotional complexity are difficult to play for laughs – just as an unfeeling automaton makes for an unappealing romantic lead.

However, even in the satirical *Doctor in the House* novels, surgical characters demonstrate a keenness for their profession and practice. When the fictional Gordon is appointed junior casualty house surgeon at St Swithin's, he is one of two men in the position. They shared a commitment to their profession and to the improvement of their craft – even if that commitment was described in irreverent ways: 'Both of us had the same enthusiasm for the knife as the Committee of Public Safety for the guillotine.'[47] And both were anxious to attain the lofty heights of the surgical career, even if 'the casualty-room at St Swithin's was not likely to fire in any young man the inspiration to be a second Louis Pasteur or Astley Cooper.'[48]

In one iconic scene of *Doctor in the House*, described in this book's introduction, Sir Lancelot Spratt stands at a patients' bedside firing questions at a gaggle of medical students, one of whom has just examined the hapless and prone sufferer and found a lump. He interrogates the student over what, exactly, the lump might be – raising several potentially deadly possibilities. Spratt concludes that the only solution is major abdominal surgery, a suggestion unlikely to reassure the by-now highly alarmed patient. He turns to the supine sufferer with the off-the-cuff dismissal: 'Now don't worry, this is nothing whatever to do with you.'[49] Surgical practitioners in Gordon's books – at least the ones that seem to succeed – display varying degrees of indifference to the patients they treat. The fictional Gordon's colleague, Bingham, had 'the true surgeon's mentality' for 'it never occurred to him that interesting signs and symptoms were attached to human beings'.[50] He gleefully refers to maladies rather than people – ' "I've got a couple of septic fingers, a lipoma, and four circs. lined up for minor ops. already." He rubbed his hands, as if contemplating a good dinner',[51] and seems to feel actual joy at other people's suffering: 'There's a kid with a smashing ductus, too. Murmur as loud as a bus. Could hardly take my bally stethoscope away.'[52]

This is a general rather than specific lack of interest in the humanity of patients – one shared, at least in Gordon's world, by the whole surgical profession. When he first graduated from medical school, fictional Gordon's landlady says, 'They used to let the learners do the poor people who couldn't afford to pay, but the Government's gone and stopped all that with the National Health Service.'[53] This suggests not only that surgeons saw at least some of their patients as expendable sources of clinical experience, but that the introduction of the NHS was supposed to have improved the lot of poor people undergoing surgery.

Gordon's novels were, of course, comedies and played serious subjects for laughs. It is unlikely that he – a health professional himself – believed that real surgeons were as uninterested in their patients as some of his characters might make you think, but the success of these novels and the ease with which he reaches for such stereotypes suggests that these ideas circulated widely in post-war British thought. Moreover, Gordon and other authors drew on their own clinical experiences in their construction of characters. In January 1958, Gilzean went on a tour of psychiatric hospitals to research the latest treatments for mental illness as background for a future book.[54] She ended up spending nearly ten days 'observing life in mental hospitals, treatments, staff, and so on'.[55] She hoped that this research would ensure that her proposed book would be 'steeped in the proper background' and have 'the authenticity' that would appeal to editors and readers alike.[56]

The surgeons respond

Doctors, nurses, and other healthcare professionals were involved in the research, writing, and production of medical novels, films, and TV programmes. But influence did not travel in just one direction and the relationship between professional and popular culture in this period is better described as a dialogue, or feedback loop. Surgeons were interested in medical-themed popular culture, and some were complimentary about their educational efforts. In 1961, the *BMJ*'s parliamentary correspondent quoted Lord Taylor from a debate in the House of Commons about medical advertising. While the MP had some concerns about broadcasting false claims about patent medicines, he had different feelings about medical TV: 'I do not object to "Emergency Ward 10" or "Matters of Medicine," and I believe that both in documentaries and fiction they do a good job of health education.'[57] While some, like Lord Taylor, wanted to bring entertainment and education together – using the former to promote the latter – others sought alternative approaches. In the United States, and as historian Martin Pernick has observed, one response to the 'troublesome allure' of medicine's motion pictures was instead to 'sharpen the distinction between entertainment and education'.[58] It is also worth pointing out that attitudes to television and film differed, and in the 1950s there were emerging anxieties about TV specifically, and its potentially malign effects on audiences.

In 1961, the Committee of the Council of the British Medical Association submitted a memo about medicine on radio and television to the government's Committee on Broadcasting. They approved, in principle, of radio and television broadcasts 'on medical subjects' and believed that it was in the 'public interest' that the 'work of doctors and their contribution to the community should be made known to the public at large'.[59] They were particularly fond, somewhat unsurprisingly, of programmes which presented the doctor as 'a person of integrity, both just and compassionate, and medicine itself as a humane and scientific discipline'. They were pleased with the media portrayals of medicine thus far: 'Indeed, the public "image" of the doctor, as seen in these programmes, is one with which doctors can generally be satisfied.'[60] They cautioned, however, that the constraints of drama and good storytelling might 'pervert' this positive public image: 'morally perfect heroes make less interesting reading than those who are morally imperfect'. Nonetheless, programmes like *Emergency Ward 10* received a very positive write-up: 'This programme has helped to relieve many members of the public of anxiety and fear about hospital treatment.' Seduced by the soap opera's flattery, the BMA was pleased that it presented doctors as 'likeable human beings'.[61]

However, not everyone was so impressed. Considering the efforts to which some medical dramas and publishers went to construct and uphold the glowing reputation of healthcare professionals, it is somewhat surprising that some doctors held the books and programmes in such low regard. A scathing article in the *BMJ* reported on the 1959 Hunterian Oration, a biennial lecture given at the Royal College of Surgeons of England: 'Not long after … [the lecture], gossip-column writers described with glee a party in Lincoln's Inn Fields where stars of the *Emergency Ward 10* film drank cocktails with the College's famous skeletons.'[62] The article's author did not approve of the college for extending this invitation: 'As the President … is the most unassuming and modest of men, it was obvious there must be something desperately wrong with the present state of the College for him to assent to this kind of publicity.'[63] He thought that perhaps the college could raise the money it needed 'without losing its dignity', and clearly thought very little of the public association with medical drama:

> This Journal has a great respect for the present President of the Royal College of Surgeons of England. No one who knows him can doubt that his first concern is for his college and the last is for himself. He is not in private practice, and therefore does not stand to gain any professional advantage from the present series of publicity stunts of which he is the unwitting centrepiece. Doubtless they are as distasteful to him as they may be pleasing to the ingenious minds which have thought them up.[64]

Any funds this ill-conceived alliance might procure was not, in the author's opinion, worth the loss of reputation it would doubtless result in: 'It would be a pity if the College, in achieving its target of £3m., found that in the process it had lost something more precious than money.'[65]

Complaints about *Emergency Ward 10* were a common feature of the *BMJ*'s letters page. C. M. Ottley wrote in 1960, 'Sir, May I raise yet another protest against the television programme, "Emergency Ward 10"?' He saw no 'possible advantages' and lamented 'the disservice it does to patients, potential and actual, and to us who have to advise and treat them'.[66] He was preoccupied with the programme's potential to elevate patient anxiety: 'A small relative asked to see an operating theatre, and I allowed her to look into an unoccupied one. She took a long look and then said in a relieved tone, "But it's not frightening at all. In the telly it was dreadful." '[67] He thought television's necessary sensationalism could frighten people with the conditions and illnesses they might see on screen: 'Recently, the management of an expectant mother with chronic rheumatic carditis was cloaked with mystery, doubtless necessary for dramatic effect, but terrifying for a real-life character so placed.'[68] J. M. Armitt had similar concerns about the programme's efforts to dramatise healthcare and the impact those efforts might have on patients. He argued that most people's interaction with the NHS was for mild or mundane complaints, not the high drama of innovative surgeries: 'Their general practitioner is their contact with the Health Service.'[69]

Doctors were not, however, opposed to all fictionalised clinical settings and S. H. F. Howard thought that 'Richard Gordon's boisterous, if somewhat Rabelaisian, humour makes more appeal to the healthy-minded than the insipid pseudo-cultural young men of "Emergency Ward 10." '[70] Their critique of *Emergency Ward 10* was perhaps, therefore, less about the programme's setting, and more about its class and gender connotations. Medical soap operas were supposedly lightweight, watched by women and other susceptible viewers. Clearly, the 'boisterous ... Rabelaisian humour' of *Doctor in the House* was far more macho, more upper class, and therefore far more tolerable to professionals themselves.[71]

Later cultural representations

As Mathew Thomson has argued, by the end of the 1960s the landscape of cultural representations of the NHS had shifted. Not only were broader social tensions being exacerbated, but the health service was under increasing strain. A new generation of television programmes in particular were now bolder and more critical. The popular culture that dealt with healthcare and its professionals – including surgeons – became grittier and more devoted to realism. 1986 saw the start of *Casualty*, a medical drama that is still on TVs today. Set in the fictional hospital Holby City's emergency department, the programme was and remains high-stakes drama, with plenty of critical accidents and love affairs. The surgeons that have appeared in *Casualty* over its multiple-decade run are diverse, but many conform to the surgical stereotype: brusque, impatient, arrogant, but somehow still charming.

Unlike programmes like *Emergency Ward 10*, *Casualty* turned NHS shortcomings into storylines, focusing on problems in service delivery, low staffing, waiting times, and limited resources. Against this backdrop, however, the surgeons, physicians, and nurses were mostly portrayed as devoted healthcare professionals, struggling with a broken system beyond their control. Thus, while the programme and its spin-off *Holby City* (1999–2022) were more critical than earlier cultural representations of the NHS, they nonetheless continued to present NHS *staff* as broadly beyond reproach. Gruff, stand-offish, and emotionally detached maybe, but never in danger of harming their patients, and never motivated by anything other than devotion to clinical excellence.

This transformation of the health service from backdrop to an anti-hero with agency became an increasingly common feature of early twenty-first-century medical popular culture. In 2017, junior doctor-turned-comedian Adam Kay published his memoir *This is Going to Hurt* about his experiences of his chaotic NHS job. In 2022, the book was turned into a BBC television series of the same name. While the book was more funny than miserable, the television version, though in many ways a faithful adaptation, was the reverse. The suffering on screen was unyielding. Kay, played by Ben Whishaw, was not an entirely unsympathetic character – he was racked with guilt over his medical errors and misjudgements and he at least tries to rectify the damage he does to his colleagues, boyfriend, family, and friends – but he is very hard to like. While some of his colleagues are likeable, others embody some of the worst elements of the Spratt stereotype. Nigel Lockhart, the chief Obstetrics and Gynaecology consultant, is aloof, domineering, self-interested, and authoritarian. But it is Kay himself who behaves the worst. He treats a junior trainee, Shruti, with cruelty. Patients suffer because of his vengeful treatment and callous lack of interest. He speaks to and about the women he is supposed to be looking after with disregard, mocking their pain, humiliation, and occasional ignorance. Amid all this cruelty, however, it becomes clear that the real villain is the NHS itself. So much so, that in the series' crescendo scene, when Kay is hauled in front of the GMC and is threatened with being struck off the medical register, he makes an impassioned speech about the health service, describing it as a brutalising regime that strips its staff and patients of their humanity. Kay is allowed to remain a doctor, and viewers are left believing that the problems are systemic and structural, rather than individual.

Conclusion

The modern surgeon made in the fictional world of the post-war British hospital was a complex character. He was simultaneously gruff, granite-jawed, paternalistic, emotionally detached, and also calm, compassionate, and committed to the social good. He was, in the words of the BMA, a man of integrity. While there were some surgeons uneasy about the way they were represented, in venues that operated beyond their control, many were complimented by the myths made by romantic, serious, and satirical fiction, as well as by television and film. And it is this that explains the prevalence and persistence of some of these modern myths. The constraints and opportunities of romance and drama as genres required the authors and screenwriters to inject some complexity and humanity into the stereotypical surgeon in order to make him likeable, even lovable. Paternalism could fade into decisiveness and machismo and emotional detachment could be read as professionalism. The myths made by popular culture therefore had buy-in from the surgeons themselves. Indeed, as evidenced by their own coverage of medical television, and their involvement in the creation of medical popular culture, healthcare practitioners were active participants in the public articulation of their professional identities.

But even in the more straightforward send-up of the satirical *Doctor in the House* franchise, there was something in the mythology that appealed to real-life surgeons. There were elements of even the crassest surgical stereotype that suited the self-image of practitioners. As suggested by the positive write-up *Doctor in the House* received in the medical press, surgeons were willing to overlook implied critiques of their inhumanity for the sake of 'boisterous … Rabelaisian humour'. In Chapter 3, I will show how these aspects of the surgical identity were associated with white men from socially elite backgrounds – and demonstrate that surgery continued to be predominantly populated by people from this demographic, well into the second half of the twentieth century.

Notes

1 'Biography', MB/AB/1/035a.
2 Letter from Elizabeth Gilzean to Alan W. Boon, 9 March 1957, MB/AB/1/035a.
3 Letter from Elizabeth Gilzean to Alan W. Boon, 3 June 1958, MB/AB/1/035b.
4 Elena C. Strauman and Bethany C. Goodier, 'The Doctor(s) in House: An Analysis of the Evolution of the Television Doctor-Hero', *Journal of Medical Humanities*, 32:1 (2011), 31–46.
5 Michael Pfau, Lawrence J. Mullen, and Kirsten Garrow, 'The Influence of Television Viewing on Public Perceptions of Physicians', *Journal of Broadcasting & Electronic Media*, 39:4 (1995), 441–458.

6 Joseph Turow, *Playing Doctor: Television, Storytelling, and Medical Power* (Ann Arbor: University of Michigan Press, 2010).
7 Lesley Scanlon, 'White Coats, Handmaidens and Warrior Chiefs: The Role of Filmic Representations in Becoming a Professional', in Lesley Scanlon (ed.), *"Becoming" a Professional: An Interdisciplinary Analysis of Professional Learning* (New York: Springer, 2011), 113.
8 Daniel Darbyshire and Paul Baker, 'A Systematic Review and Thematic Analysis of Cinema in Medical Education', *Medical Humanities*, 38 (2012), 28–33, 28.
9 Critics of romance fiction argue that they offer only 'retrograde' and 'limited' views of women's lives. Lisa Appignanesi, 'Happily Ever After', *New Statesman* (13 July 1984), 24.
10 Mathew Thomson, 'Representation of the National Health Service in the Arts and Popular Culture', in Jennifer Crane and Jane Hand (eds), *Posters, Protests, and Prescriptions: Cultural Histories of the National Health Service in Britain* (Manchester: Manchester University Press, 2022), 237.
11 Ibid., 238.
12 Susan E. Lederer, 'Surgery and Popular Culture: Situating the Surgeon and the Surgical Experience in Popular Media', in Thomas Schlich (ed.), *The Palgrave Handbook of the History of Surgery* (London: Palgrave Macmillan, 2017), 349–367, 350.
13 Ibid.
14 Ibid., 357.
15 Ross McKibbin, 'Politics and the Medical Hero: A. J. Cronin's "The Citadel"', *English Historical Review*, 123:502 (2008), 651–678, 662, fn 48.
16 Ibid.
17 Lederer, 'Surgery and Popular Culture', 350.
18 See Alison Moulds, *Medical Identities and Print Culture, 1830s–1910s* (London: Palgrave Macmillan, 2021).
19 Lederer, 'Surgery and Popular Culture', 350.
20 Francesca Segal, 'Who Said Romance was Dead?', *The Observer* (27 January 2008), www.theguardian.com/books/2008/jan/27/fiction.features1 (accessed 18 May 2021).
21 Hsu-Ming Teo, 'The Romance of White Nations: Imperialism, Popular Culture, and National Histories', in Antoinette Burton (ed.), *After the Imperial Turn: Thinking With and Through the Nation* (Chapel Hill, NC: Duke University Press, 2003), 284.
22 James McAleer, 'Love, Romance, and the National Health Service', in Clare V. J. Griffiths, James J. Nott, and William Whyte (eds), *Classes, Cultures, and Politics: Essays on British History for Ross McKibbin* (Oxford: Oxford University Press, 2011), 174.

23 Rachel Lindsay, 'Love Unspoken', *Woman's Own* (18 March 1954), 14.
24 Hilda Pressley, *Staff Nurses in Love* (London: Mills & Boon, 1962), 13.
25 Letter from Elizabeth Gilzean to Alan W. Boon, 8 June 1957, MB AB/1/035a.
26 Hilda Nickson, *Surgeons in Love* (London: Mills & Boon, 1962), 42.
27 Ibid., 8.
28 Synopsis for *No Time for Love*, MB/AB/1/035b.
29 Nickson, *Surgeons in Love*, 68.
30 Letter from Elizabeth Gilzean to Alan W. Boon, 1 October 1957, MB AB/1/035a.
31 Nickson, *Surgeons in Love*, 46.
32 Rebecca Feasey, *Masculinity and Popular Television* (Edinburgh: Edinburgh University Press, 2008), 68–79.
33 Jason Jacobs, *Body Trauma TV: The New Hospital Dramas* (London: BFI, 2003), 4. See also Jason Jacobs, 'Hospital Drama', in Glen Creeber (ed.) *The Television Genre Book* (London: BFI, 2002), 23–26.
34 Feasey, *Masculinity and Popular Television*, 68–69.
35 Turow, *Playing Doctor*, 109.
36 Letter from Elizabeth Gilzean to Alan W. Boon, 5 December 1957, MB AB/1/035a.
37 Derek Paget, *No Other Way to Tell It: Docudrama on Film and Television* (Manchester: Manchester University Press, 2011), 188.
38 Television Heaven, https://televisionheaven.co.uk/reviews/emergency-ward-10 (accessed 18 May 2021).
39 British Medical Association, *Medicine on Radio and Television* (London: British Medical Association, 1961), 7–8.
40 Margaret Drabble, *The Millstone* (London: Weidenfeld & Nicolson, 1965).
41 Tessa Hadley, 'The Millstone: The Crucial 1960s Feminist Novel', *The Guardian* (15 May 2015), www.theguardian.com/books/2015/may/15/the-millstone-the-crucial-1960s-feminist-novel (accessed 28 April 2020).
42 William Peters, 'A New Heart for Pamela', *Woman's Own* (16 December 1954), 18.
43 Margaret Drabble, *The Millstone* (London: Penguin, 2016), 117.
44 Ibid., 117–118.
45 Ibid., 117.
46 Ibid.
47 Richard Gordon, *Doctor at Large* (London: Harmondsworth, 1975), 15.

48 Ibid., 13.
49 John Spencer, 'Some Activity But Still Not Much Action on Patient and Public Engagement', *Medical Education*, 50 (2016), 3–23, 3.
50 Gordon, *Doctor at Large*, 15.
51 Ibid., 12.
52 Ibid., 13.
53 Ibid., 10.
54 Letter from Elizabeth Gilzean to Alan W. Boon, 5 December 1957, MB AB/1/035a.
55 Letter from Elizabeth Gilzean to Alan W. Boon, 21 December 1957, MB AB/1/035a.
56 Ibid.
57 'Medical Notes in Parliament: Objectionable Examples', *British Medical Journal*, 1:5227 (1961), 755–757, 756.
58 Leslie J. Reagan, Nancy Tomes, and Paula A. Treichler, 'Introduction: Medicine, Health, and Bodies in American Film and Television', in Leslie J. Reagan, Nancy Tomes, and Paula A. Treichler (eds), *Medicine's Moving Pictures: Medicine, Health, and Bodies in American Film and Television* (Rochester, NY: University of Rochester Press, 2007), 7; Martin S. Pernick, 'More than Illustrations: Early Twentieth-Century Health Films as Contributors to the Histories of Medicine and of Motion Pictures', in Leslie J. Reagan, Nancy Tomes, and Paula A. Treichler (eds), *Medicine's Moving Pictures: Medicine, Health, and Bodies in American Film and Television* (Rochester, NY: University of Rochester Press, 2007), 19–35.
59 British Medical Association, *Medicine on Radio and Television*, 5.
60 Ibid., 6.
61 Ibid., 12.
62 'Top Surgeons', *British Medical Journal*, 1:5129 (1959), 1100.
63 Ibid.
64 Ibid.
65 Ibid.
66 C. M. Ottley, 'Emergency Ward 10', *British Medical Journal*, 1:5174 (1960), 728.
67 Ibid.
68 Ibid.
69 N. G. C. Hendry, J. H. E. Bergin, J. M. Armitt, and A. T. Seaton, 'Differences and Differentials', *British Medical Journal*, 1:5388 (1964), 984–985, 984.
70 S. H. F. Howard, 'Medicine Broadcast', *British Medical Journal*, 1:5225 (1961), 595.
71 Ibid.

3

Surgical conduct and surgical communities

In the decades immediately following the Second World War, the modern surgeon was a varied, complicated character and multiple myths co-existed. So far, I have discussed emotional detachment, masculinity (albeit only briefly), paternalism, authoritarianism, and a little bit of sexiness. But there were other elements of the surgical myth that needed making, like affluence and affability. The latter was particularly important in the context of the 'firm', which, as described in the introduction, was and in some places remains the key organising principle of a surgeon's working life. The firm was important both in the operating theatre – while surgeons were at work – and at times and in spaces of leisure and rest. As a result, the ideal surgeon was a social animal. Or at least he was if post-war obituaries are to be relied upon.

Just after Christmas in 1975, the Scottish surgeon Sir John Bruce died. He had been Regius Professor of Clinical Surgery at the University of Edinburgh and one-time president of the Royal College of Surgeons of Edinburgh (RCSEd). He was, in other words, a big deal in the British surgical world. His death was covered in the medical press and his obituaries offer a glimpse into the cultures and communities of this select group of elite professionals.[1] For example, this account of his character, written shortly after his death, attests to the importance of personality and friendship in the making of the mid-twentieth-century surgeon:

> His multitudinous friends and colleagues over the globe testify to the bonds he was able to create and countless young men of all nationalities owe much to him for furthering their careers. Indeed, this was one of his greatest qualities – a sympathy for and a receptive ear to the young of all ages; though he walked with the kings of

> his profession, and was one himself, he was the ready counsellor of successive generations of aspiring surgeons. His gregariousness and readiness of wit overshadowed to some extent his solid achievements in clinical surgery.[2]

Bruce was evidently a social and professional engineer – lubricating the careers of his junior colleagues. His 'greatest quality' was his 'receptive ear' – a 'king' of the profession not because of his surgical skill (although no doubt he possessed some), but because of his ability as a 'ready counsellor'. Indeed, the obituary made this distinction explicit. His 'gregariousness' and good humour 'overshadowed' his 'solid achievements in clinical surgery'. Far from the brash indifference of Sir Lancelot Spratt, Bruce embodied an alternative version of the ideal surgeon. He possessed attributes that made him likeable, relatable, and supportive – attributes that gained him entry to the surgical community. No doubt Bruce was everything this obituary made him out to be. However, if you read the epitaphs of other British surgeons who died shortly after the Second World War, a pattern emerges.

In 1955, Sir James Walton died aged 73. He was a 'great gentleman' and a 'most kindly chief and colleague'.[3] As many of the words in his *BMJ* obituary were devoted to his personality and 'recreations' ('fishing, tennis, and badminton'), as to his skill as a surgical diagnostician or technician.[4] The frequency with which these attributes and activities appear in written descriptions of post-war surgeons suggests that the praise given by colleagues was about more than just individual personalities and proclivities, and instead made a general statement about the surgical profession and the ideal characteristics of its members. Similar statements were made about Sir Arthur Porritt who, unlike Bruce and Walton, survived well into the 1990s. He was 'warm and friendly', and a fellow surgeon described his 'alert mind, his intuitive "feel" for others, and his sincerity', that together added 'up to a personal magnetism not given to many men'.[5] In some ways, this surgical myth contradicts other widely held assumptions about the surgical character. In his review of Lindsey Fitzharris's most recent book, a biography of the pioneering plastic surgeon Harold Gillies, retired neurosurgeon Henry Marsh observed that what distinguished Gillies from his colleagues was his 'skill as a leader in building a team'. This was a quality that is 'rare in surgeons, who are often egotistic'.[6]

But these descriptions of distinctly personable surgeons not only tell us that there are many, sometimes contradictory, layers to the surgical stereotype, but that the myth of the modern surgeon was not just a product of film and television, and that the process of becoming a surgeon happened as much off the hospital ward – on golf courses, grouse moors, and over glasses of Bordeaux – as it did in the operating theatre itself. It also suggests that the development of the surgical identity did not just happen while the man (and sometimes woman) was in medical school or training; instead, it was a lengthy process that required constant maintenance and reconfiguration. While there is some scholarship on the history of workplace socialising – and particularly its gendered manifestations and implications – most of it focuses on industrial settings or working-class communities.[7] But what about at the other end of the social spectrum? Socialising also shaped surgery – a professional community traditionally dominated by debates over changing technology and techniques.

There are obviously positive elements of these accounts of the surgical personality – these characters (and they were 'characters') were kind, generous, and friendly colleagues. However, the hobbies and habits surgeons pursued and participated in were hardly democratic. Predominantly practised by white, affluent men, the social lives of surgeons were dictated by the profession's demographics and, in turn, served as a barrier against those who did not quite fit the mould. The archives of surgical associations, clubs, and professional societies alongside oral history interviews and medical journal articles reveal quite how important these 'extracurricular' activities were in the development and maintenance of professional identities, stereotypes, and the definition of what it meant to be a surgeon in post-war Britain. From these sources, it is clear that this definition depended not just on surgical skill, but on the ability to entertain colleagues, wine, dine, and fire a gun.

That surgical success depended on a degree of social ability or ease is not that surprising. Despite what Marsh claims, surgical work is a collaborative endeavour and cooperation is built into the very fabric of professional life.[8] When the firm functioned well, says the Royal College of Physicians (RCP), it provided 'a structured development process, role modelling of professional behaviour, mentoring, and a good balance of challenge and support'. Harold Ellis, a retired professor of surgery who qualified in 1948, described his firm as being like a family. 'The firms were wonderful', he insisted.[9] However, these 'wonderful' bonds were not just made at the bedside or in the operating theatre. Instead, the firm orbited around both the hospital ward and the hospital bar. Surgeons often lived in, or very close to, their place of work and they spent social time together at dances, dinners, and professional societies. Community, shared pursuits, and friendship were, therefore, key features of past (and, indeed, present) surgical life. For those who gained entry to the profession, these were positive features that helped sustain their emotional health, gave them a sense of belonging, and supported their commitment to their craft. However, these features also drew boundaries around the surgical profession and cultivated cultures and communities with deeply problematic characteristics – cultures and characteristics that still exist within surgery and are still partially responsible for some of the profession's entrenched inequalities.

There are, therefore, further layers to the surgical stereotype that I have described thus far. As well as being emotionally detached and paternalistic, the surgeon was also white, male, socially elite, bawdy, loved fine dining and fine drinking, and participated in hobbies and extracurricular activities designed for a narrow stratum of British society. As discussed in the previous two chapters, while profoundly problematic and sometimes exclusionary, this stereotype also served surgeons, and for those who could participate in these activities and attributes, being a surgeon was often professionally meaningful, personally validating, and a great deal of fun. In this chapter, I will begin by walking through the different communities and social spaces that were occupied by surgeons, starting with the firm. After the firm, I will take us through the hospital residence – where most junior surgeons lived after graduating medical school and before marriage.[10] Hospitals were places of leisure and places to live, as well as places of work. Then, we will spend some time in the hospital bar and other social spaces – including the doctors' mess, staff common room, and the consultants' dining room.

In the second section, we leave the hospital, seeking surgeons socialising away from work. We follow them grouse hunting, onto the golf course, to society dinners, and on their international travels. In the third section, I analyse these various forms of sociability, arguing that they were key to the making and maintenance of stereotypes and the surgical identity. Not only were these professional communities supportive – protecting surgeons from some of the stresses and strains of hospital life and labour – but they were also troubling. They limited the surgical profession – narrowing the range of different kinds of people who could participate. Finally, and as I will also discuss in the next two chapters, while these barriers have weakened in recent decades, the identities and stereotypes that were developed and hardened in this post-war period have had a lasting impact on the demographic make-up of the profession and continue to influence the entrance to, and experience of, the surgical community today.

The firm

The firm crops up in almost any discussion of hospital-based healthcare that has taken place in Britain in the last century or so. It was, and continues to be, the key mechanism and organisational unit for the type of apprenticeship-style learning common in modern British clinical settings. It has become a cipher for a type of hospital culture and community that many people think has been gradually eroded by recent health service restructuring and policy interventions. Despite this ubiquity, however, the firm has attracted little sociological or historical scrutiny. Healthcare professionals – especially senior ones – tend to take it for granted. They assume that everyone will know what they mean when they say 'the firm', and they assume that their own experiences of training will map on to the experiences of others. The term and its casual usage, however, mask substantial historical, institutional, specialty, and geographical variation and obscure the ways in which the concept and its real-life manifestations have changed over time.[11]

Broadly speaking, however, the firm refers to a unit of doctors working together. It is usually made up of a single profession, and while some clinicians consider other workers to be part of the 'clinical team', nurses are not usually included in references to the firm. The unit has one, or occasionally two, permanent members – a consultant – after whom it is named. It also includes other grades of doctors who join temporarily and for varying lengths of time. There is a clear hierarchy and distribution of roles and for many it connotes a military-style structure (see Chapter 7). In a firm, Ellis described, there would be one or two consultants known as 'the chiefs', a senior trainee known as 'the registrar', a junior trainee known as the 'house physician' or 'house surgeon' who lived in the hospital, and medical students.[12] The medical students were not technically part of the firm, but the usual members took collective responsibility for the students' welfare and education, or at least they ought to have done. The firm denotes a kind of collegial and intergenerational model of learning – one which brought together 'novices who were being inducted and taught on the ward not only by consultants, but also by nurses and junior doctors who took on much of the day-to-day training of students'.[13] The firm's salience is stronger in some specialties – like surgery and acute medicine – than in others.

The firm predates the institutionalisation of medical training and the foundation of medical schools in the early nineteenth century.[14] The firm of post-war Britain is, therefore, an eighteenth-century inheritance. Back then, students paid surgeons for their apprenticeships on hospital wards. These trainees were delegated responsibility for their consultant's patients. This apprenticeship model did not solely, or even primarily, depend on explicit instruction. Rather, knowledge was transmitted through informal learning – watching and then doing – learning that, in an ideal world, relied on time spent together and the formation of trusting, professional relationships.[15] While nineteenth-century medical students had a poor reputation, and required plenty of discipline and reform, in theory the development of these relationships allowed for mutual dependability and support which in turn facilitated the transmission of how things were done.[16]

Following the foundation of the NHS in 1948, a named consultant (and their firm) oversaw all inpatients and outpatient sessions. The new health service, while transformative in many ways, perpetuated the working cultures that surgeons and other hospital doctors had long been accustomed to. As a result, the firm survived the Second World War and brought many older ideas about surgery into the second half of the twentieth century and beyond. For example, the informality and apprenticeship learning developed in the Victorian era is still a big part of surgical life and the phrase 'see one, do one, teach one' is still used to describe a form of valid and widely practised training.[17]

And yet, the post-war firm was not just a tool for training and education. It was as much a social organisation as a unit of work. To be a surgeon in the middle decades of the twentieth century meant participating in this social organisation, and professional success required adherence to a certain culture and community. This culture was dominated and determined by excessive temporal commitment, a blurring of boundaries between the personal and professional, complete institutional commitment, and classed, raced, and gendered forms of sociability such as elite and macho sporting pursuits, and eating and drinking together. As the obituaries quoted at the beginning of this chapter make clear, surgeons' personalities, not just technical skill, mattered a great deal and helped to determine their success.

Living on site

Personality mattered in part because post-war British surgeons spent a huge amount of time together, particularly when training. When, in 1963, Ronald Macbeth described hospital clinical work as 'quite literally full-time' he was not exaggerating.[18] Not only were surgeons at the outset of their careers expected to work excessive hours (see Chapter 6 for more details), but in the middle decades of the twentieth century, many healthcare professionals lived where they worked. Trainee doctors, surgeons, and nurses were often accommodated in hospital-supplied housing and it was supposed to be 'in the interests of hospitals and their patients that doctors [were] made resident'.[19] Pay was minimal beyond room, board, and laundry services, and it was assumed that most young healthcare practitioners had few other obligations outside of medical or nursing training. This dual nature of the hospital blurred boundaries between professional and domestic space and undermined the distinctions between work and home. Writers to the *BMJ*'s letters page alerted readers to the 'somewhat unique condition which doctors have accepted without demur'.[20] After all, there were few professions where it was 'a condition of the appointment that members of the staff [were] required to be resident'.[21]

Traditionally, and since well before the foundation of the NHS, board and lodging were given free to make allowances for trainees' enforced residence in hospitals.[22] From the early 1950s, however, the Ministry of Health began to mandate that charges be deducted from junior doctors' salaries to pay for their food and accommodation.[23] In response, the British Medical Association began to defend the interests of their junior members, and demanded that hospitals maintain adequate accommodation. Their investigations into the living quarters provided by hospitals revealed the less than salubrious conditions of mid-century resident doctors. In 1963, R. M. Forrester heralded a new dawn in hospital residency: 'The time has come when hospitals must make their jobs, and their accommodation, attractive. The grubby monastic cell, with its worn lino, cracked lampshade, and iron bedstead, is slowly on the way out.'[24] Rooms must not just be adequately furnished, and they should be big enough to live in comfortably. The BMA called on the Ministry of Health to specify a minimum size for a room and at one meeting the chairman invited the submission of 'horror pictures', which showed 'accommodation which fell short of the standard'.[25] One member at that meeting said he had had 'a room which contained all the things the Ministry said it should contain, only it was so small that he could hardly get in'.[26] In 1964, the BMA's Hospital Junior Staffs Group Council passed a resolution affirming that where standards of hospital residential accommodation fell short of Ministry of Health recommendations, a reduction of charges should be made.[27]

Beginning in the 1970s, British hospital residences began to be sold off or repurposed. The debates about charges in the 1950s and 1960s, and then about their potential closure in the 1970s, tell us much about how trainee surgeons felt about their living conditions and working cultures. Advocates commented on the protective sense of belonging fostered by employees living and working together, and detractors deplored their exclusionary nature (residences were difficult or impossible to occupy if you were married or had children). In his speculative account of clinical life, written in 1968, hospital chaplain George Day described how he would gain a full understanding of an institution and its employees:

> I would make a point of lunching and dining quite frequently in the resident house doctors' mess, and keeping my ears open. I would even drop in for a late-night beer or coffee – or even lose half a crown to

> them at their poker school. In this way, I would come to learn more about the hospital than the matron, the medical superintendent, and the hospital secretary all rolled into one: more about the things that matter – that is, the personalities, the clash of personalities, and the fluctuating morale. For these young chaps are in the front line of the battle, holding the fort during the hours of darkness and at weekends, when their chiefs are away.[28]

In this description, he alluded to the emotional value of the firm and hospital community. This is a portrait not just of working life, but of friendship. He identified these informal interactions, the intangible exchanges, the subtle texture of social life as 'the things that matter'.[29]

Support for the importance of these informal interactions was clamorous in the debates over hospital quarters for married junior doctors that emerged in the 1960s. Earlier in the twentieth century, surgeons tended to marry late – after they had finished their itinerant training and once they had settled on a long-term post. By the 1960s, however, more and more practitioners were marrying young, some even before they had finished medical school. D. W. Dingwall conducted a survey for the *BMJ* about the provision of married quarters for house officers in 1963. He found that 'to-day many doctors are married at the very beginning of their graduate career and … a considerable number of final-year medical students throughout the country are already married'.[30] This proved problematic for the 'life of collegiate monasticism' that had been traditionally expected of trainees.[31] References to religious orders in correspondence about hospital residence were rife and pregnant with meaning. Not only did they imply a kind of religious devotion to the job on behalf of the trainee surgeons, but they made assumptions about the gender and sexuality of these doctors.

In all the letters sent to the editor of the *BMJ* and other healthcare journals, the trainee surgeon was assumed to be male and married to a woman who waited at home. Hospitals cultivated the kind of single-sex, masculine culture and community more usually seen in monasteries, the military, or even boys' public schools. As one correspondent put it in 1963, 'The outlook of many hospital management committees that it is immoral for any houseman to have sexual relations in the hospital, be he married or no, persists.'[32]

Once students had graduated, they then embarked on a programme of training that required them to live on hospital site, attend to patients overnight, and move from institution to institution every six months or so. Few, if any, hospitals provided residential quarters for couples – 'very few hospitals in the country provide married-quarters for house officers' – and local, short-term rental accommodation was hard to find.[33] House officers must either live apart from their spouse for several months at a time or live together outside the hospital walls.

Neither of these solutions were popular. As early as 1954, W. Arklay Steel complained about the financial consequences of married couples living apart: 'Many young married doctors have to contribute to the upkeep of two establishments when they become resident, and the financial hardship and privations they must experience to make ends meet can be imagined.'[34] Nine years later, the problem remained unresolved, and surgeon Michael Hession deplored the 'considerable hardship during the pre-registration year' suffered by married junior doctors 'due to the paucity of married quarters'.[35] This hardship was both financial and a product of the 'imposition of relative chastity'.[36] He wrote, 'He is unlikely in London to be paying less than £250 per annum for his flat where his wife waits patiently for the precious half-day and the two week-ends in five which should bring her husband home.'[37] Advocates for married quarters argued that surgical trainees should be able to combine married life with hospital life: 'A married man wishing to continue in the hospital service cannot apply for more than 25% of the junior hospital posts advertised if he wishes to remain living with his wife. Why should a man have to choose between leaving his wife or pursuing his profession?'[38]

These advocates' arguments circulated around two key points. First, that regardless of whether a surgeon and their spouse lived apart (with the doctor staying on hospital property and the spouse living elsewhere) or if they both lived off-site, either option meant that families would see little of the working parent: 'It is indefensible to expect children to understand why they should have to answer the question, "When did you last see your father?" '[39] Second, both of these options meant that trainee surgeons were not fully embedded within the hospital culture, a distance that might prove pedagogically problematic and curtail future career development. In 1967, 'A

General Practitioner's Wife' wrote to the *BMJ* lamenting the living arrangements she and her husband had been forced to adopt while he completed his hospital training:

> I speak with authority – and bitterness – as we were pushed out of hospital work altogether in order to keep our family together and properly fed and clothed – redeployed into general practice and suburbia after a keen and ambitious start in surgery; frustrated for life, for our temerity in marrying and begetting children.[40]

Instead, she advocated dedicated junior doctor residences, with space for spouse and child: 'If junior doctors had their own flats, and in between dealing with patients 100 hours a week could sit down with their own kids, have coffee made by their own wives, the long hours would irk so much less that they would almost cease to be a problem.'[41] In similar terms, Clarice A. Baker thought that the 'hospital as a whole would benefit greatly', if 'a modest type of married quarters were provided on hospital territory'. This would mean that

> the young houseman's energies could be concentrated on treating his patients, without the need to worry about a pregnant wife or sick baby in a distant flat. The communal property would be better cared for, and … the doctor would not feel obliged to rush off the minute he was officially 'off duty' if home were near by.[42]

This anxiety about trainee surgeons rushing off as soon as the working day was officially over was shared both by those advocating *for* married quarters and those advocating *against*. Doctor John Shepherd wrote to the *BMJ* in 1967:

> Already there is a tendency for a '9 to 5' attitude to prevail, and I believe this is quite contrary to all that is best in surgical … practice. To maintain a high standard of work in hospitals it is imperative that junior staff are trained and encouraged in the idea of continuity of care.[43]

He viewed 'with much disquiet' the trend, as he saw it, 'by which registrars in the major specialties are discouraged from living in hospital except on their emergency nights'.[44] Addressing similar issues, Ronald Macbeth also wrote to the *BMJ* to caution against the introduction of married quarters to hospitals. Like Shepherd he was concerned about the recent tendency of trainees to live in private accommodation, but he was also concerned that the introduction of double beds to hospital residencies might also have pernicious consequences: 'There are two aspects of this matter – duty to one's patients and education of oneself.'[45] Macbeth insisted that duty to one's patients turned 'upon the concept that as a resident one is available to them at all times at a minute's notice'.[46] Commitment to the hospital and its inhabitants must be total, and the line between personal life and professional engagement should be fine and easy to blur: 'It may be argued that this can be achieved if one lives in suitably placed married quarters in hospital. I doubt, however, if engrossment with purely domestic personal matters can always be laid aside as briskly as when one lives bachelor-style in the mess.'[47]

However, the second 'aspect of this matter' – 'the education of oneself' – was more important to Macbeth than the first. And it was here that he emphasised the importance of the firm and demonstrated the value that many mid-century practitioners ascribed to the participation in this social organisation and to an adherence to a certain culture and community. He described the 'educational value' of 'living with the job, even when not actively seeing one's own patients', and advocated for the value of 'being around in the mess for the casual discussion of cases and for consultation at resident level – where, for example, a colleague is uncertain what he should do with a patient sent up to the casualty department'. Macbeth argued that these experiences were 'the stuff whereof the training of a good doctor is made' and that 'one cannot receive this sort of education if one is in the married quarters feeding the baby or washing the nappies'.[48] He was concerned that these distractions were harming the development of surgeons' professionalism: 'It seems to one such that medicine is coming to be regarded more and more as "a job like any other", and less and less as a vocation.'[49] He cautioned young doctors against marriage before they were fully trained, as it might prove distracting. He said that there was no reason for junior doctors to 'prematurely [assume] marital responsibilities' as they must be 'shared with a job which is quite literally full-time'.[50] He concluded his letter with the insistence that 'if people wish to marry young they should not aim to be doctors; they will neglect one or other assignment'.[51] All these writers, whether advocating for or against hospital accommodation for trainee surgeons and their spouses, insisted on the immersive experience of hospital life and attest to the importance of intangible, ephemeral interaction – social or professional – in the construction of identity and workplace cultures.

Social spaces

Eating and drinking was a big part of surgical life. A consultant surgeon I interviewed in 2020 recalled how, when he was training, his consultant would go for tea with the Sister: 'it was very formal, she'd get the best china out'.[52] Dining together was a key way that surgeons bonded with one another and with other members of the hospital workforce. And the 'literally full-time' nature of surgical training was made even more clear by the debates about hospital cafeterias. In 1960, the BMA's Hospital Junior Staffs Group Council received complaints from medical officers at the Dorset County Hospital, 'where a cafeteria-style communal dining-room had recently been established'.[53] This marked a change from tradition. For much of the twentieth century, junior doctors ate, relaxed, and socialised in dedicated spaces on the hospital site – spaces closed off to patients and visitors. The Hospital Junior Staffs Group Council was concerned that a cafeteria, open to both doctors and patients, was a 'retrograde step'.[54] The doctors at Dorset County Hospital had not been consulted beforehand and they thought that the cafeteria system was 'undesirable' because there were 'often matters doctors wanted to discuss among themselves'. Various Group members thought that residents should retain a dining room of their own and many believed that the opportunities for knowledge exchange that these spaces afforded were 'vital for the success of the hospital'.[55] In dedicated dining rooms, doctors could 'discuss their problems' and solicit advice from one another about tricky cases or recalcitrant patients. These spaces also had an educative function. Various interested parties advocated for the traditional practice of trainee surgeons living on the hospital site by insisting on the professional and pedagogical value of the opportunities for informal exchange that being a hospital resident produced. Surgeon Ronald Macbeth particularly emphasised the value of eating together. He wrote to the *BMJ* in 1963, 'Being around in the mess for the casual discussion of cases and for consultation at resident level … these are the stuff whereof the training of a good doctor is made.'[56]

Similar concerns were expressed by A. M. Cantor in his essay on a new hospital, published in 1978. He was troubled by the fact that meals were provided in a 'common dining room for non-medical as well as medical personnel', and that there was 'no dining area allocated specifically to medical staff'. He lamented,

> The usual opportunities for discussion, interchange of ideas and experience, and mutual help, which are such a valuable feature of the doctors' mess, are sacrificed in the interests of 'democracy in hospitals.' This cannot be in the interests of doctors or their patients, and it will be regrettable if this is to be the pattern for hospitals in the future.[57]

Critics of the new and redesigned hospitals that failed to accommodate dining, rest, and relaxation facilities for trainee doctors sometimes framed their complaints in terms of worsening working conditions. In response to A. M. Cantor's lamentation, junior doctors who had, until its recent closure, worked at the Royal Portsmouth Hospital, levied similar critiques at the new Queen Alexandra Hospital in Cosham, into which they were due to move.[58] This new hospital had a mess room, but it was only 14 feet by 24 feet and supposed to house over sixty junior doctors. Even worse, it was located opposite the patients' library, presumably problematic because patients might overhear the staff's discussions of their sensitive cases.[59] The new hospital had 'totally inadequate telephone facilities' in the resident doctors' accommodation, 'no separate dining-room facilities of medical staff', and doctors shared residential blocks with nursing and other staff.[60] The junior doctors concluded their letter with 'we have resolved not to accept the continued decline of our working conditions in this way'.[61]

However, this was not just a problem of adequate working conditions and there was more to the doctors' mess and dining room than just education and the sharing of patient information. They were also places where friendships were made, where professional communities were built, and where the culture of the institution was shaped. Advocates believed that this could only happen in places dedicated to doctors – clinical 'club houses' within hospital walls. The chairman of the Hospital Junior Staffs Group Council believed that it was 'important that a resident should have a mess life'. A 'mess life' implied all those things – friendship, community, and culture, not just work. The chairman also believed that this 'life' had been under threat since 1948 – 'the National Health Service had partly destroyed it' – and the redesign of hospitals was delivering 'the final death blow'. Crucially, hospitals that provided no dedicated space for doctors to eat denigrated their professional exceptionalism, upsetting the conventional hierarchies. The 'final death blow' was to 'treat resident doctors in the same way as resident typists and resident nurses' (who, presumably, had less of a right to a communal, collegiate professional life than their medical or surgical counterparts).[62] A hospital without a mess was just like any other place of ordinary work. In fact, two members of the Hospital Junior Staffs Group Council thought that doctors who were compulsorily resident should not have to pay board and lodging charges at all; instead, they 'should have been thrown in when the NHS came into being, "as in the Army"'.[63]

These references to 'mess life', monasticism, and the army were not coincidental. They underscored the intentional similarities between the post-war British hospital and other places where affluent white men socialised. In cultivating and defending rest, residential, and social spaces for doctors, hospitals and their inhabitants were also cultivating and defending a workplace culture – one that trained young surgeons into a pattern of behaviours and attitudes that served to strengthen connections within the profession and demarcate its boundaries. Surgical culture was created inside the hospital – and maintained as much by the physical buildings as it was by the people who inhabited them. However, this professional culture and community was also made and maintained outside the hospital walls and in other places surgeons frequented with their colleagues.

Away from the hospital

In 1964, Boston surgeon Bentley P. Colcock wrote up his report detailing his recent trip to the United Kingdom in his capacity as one of the James IV Association of Surgeons' 'surgical travellers'. He wrote, 'I have always felt that one of the most interesting aspects of a surgeon's life is the unusual men (and women) he meets in his "surgical world."'[64] Founded in 1957 by a group of British and North American surgeons, the James IV Association of Surgeons was, and continues to be, an international organisation that 'promotes communication among surgeons across the globe'.[65] Since 1961, the Association has funded trips for several 'surgical travellers' each year to encourage 'exchange and camaraderie between surgical communities'.[66] Travellers were required to write up reports of their journeys and exploits for preservation in the Association's archive, and these texts offer unique insight into the social lives, professional identities, and emotional experiences of those 'unusual men (and women)' that populated the 'surgical world' of mid-century Britain.

Much like in the hospital, mealtimes were crucial to the development of platonic and professional connections between surgeons from different countries and were the primary purpose of association-sponsored travels abroad. In his undated report on his trip to the United Kingdom, Ireland, Denmark and Sweden, R. A. Macbeth, from Alberta, Canada, wrote, 'not once did I have lunch alone, nor did Monique [his wife] and I have dinner alone while in Glasgow – and this pace kept up for virtually the entire trip'.[67] Colcock devoted much of his report to a description of the food and alcoholic beverages he consumed while travelling around Britain: 'After stopping at the [Andrew] Kay home to see the children and collect Mrs Kay, we had dinner at a delightful village inn outside the city. The excellent food, fine wine, and much good talk with two wonderful people made it a perfect evening.'[68] Sometimes these descriptions were little more than lists of different drinks: 'The martinis, the burgundy, the scotch, and Drambuie, interspersed with excellent food and the sparkling personality of John Bruce, made it a grand evening.'[69] Here, the food seemed to accompany the drink, rather than the other way around.

The traveller report was an informal genre of writing and surgeons clearly felt comfortable focusing on their social and culinary encounters. Some even described less salubrious experiences: 'I apologize that my account will not be as eloquent as many of those I read. However, I wrote my report each evening during my trip unless the evening festivities resulted in a mild, to occasionally middling, alcoholic haze!'[70] Perhaps unsurprisingly for anyone who has attended professional events in both places, descriptions of alcohol consumption were more frequent in the reports by travellers who visited the United Kingdom than in those who journeyed to North America. Folkert O. Belzer from Wisconsin travelled to England in 1977. He wrote, 'At the hospital, we first had lunch with the entire staff ... We had a delightful lunch including a glass of sherry and a good Bordeaux wine with the meal, a habit we should introduce in the States!'[71] On his later trip to Poland, Belzer continued his forensic exploration of local intoxicants: 'We tasted the local Polish drink, slivovitz, which I must say has a rather potent and delayed action.'[72]

The consumption of food and drink was, of course, always accompanied by conversation and social exchange. The surgical travellers reported on both fine dining and warm hospitality. Writing in 1961, E. G. Muir from London described his trip to Canada and the US: 'My wife and I received everywhere the most charming and generous hospitality, a hospitality indeed which frequently makes the recipient feel quite unworthy of it – but determined to return for more!'[73] In a similar vein, Edward G. Tuckwell described his 1963 travels in Canada: 'From Montreal to Edmonton ... were wonderfully entertained by Walter Mackenzie, Bob Macbeth and Walter Anderson and their wives.'[74] While British surgeons were more likely to lubricate the lunches and dinners of their guests, North Americans were no less welcoming: 'Americans are, of course, famous for their hospitality and the surgical traveller from Ireland was liberally exposed to this delightful phenomenon. My wife and I are most grateful to all those who were so kind to us.'[75] The personality of the various surgeons who different travellers encountered was, therefore, key to their overall impression of their trip.

This emphasis on personalities and social interactions was occasionally made explicit. Bentley P. Colcock described walking back to his hotel with his wife who 'informed me that Sir Arthur [Porritt] had told her that I was "not here to work, but just to meet people" – a delightful assignment!'[76] This distinction between work and pleasure did not, however, usually apply to the surgical career. Much like the surgical community at large, the Association defined pleasure as work and blurred the boundaries between personal and professional lives. The geniality of individuals also blurred with the sociability of the society: 'When he was through, he had his chauffeur take me back to my hotel. This I felt was not just a gesture of respect to the James IV Association, but indicated a natural thoughtfulness in the man.'[77]

While the surgeons who joined the Association were elite members of an already elite faction of medical professional (and many went on to have illustrious careers), when assessing surgeons for potential new membership, the Association relied on social characteristics as much as on clinical aptitude or interest. If potential members had previously entertained past surgical travellers, then they were more likely to be looked upon favourably in assessments of their character. For example, 'Lesley Harold Blumgart ... He has entertained several Surgical Travellers and is an excellent candidate for active membership', and 'Geoffrey R. Giles ... is a strong chap who has entertained previous Travellers and would make an excellent member'.[78] This description of a potential member as a 'strong chap' was a common feature of proposed Association participants. Alan G. Johnson was also 'a very strong chap'.[79] The ways in which surgeons conducted themselves in social interactions became a crucial aspect of the assessment of whether they 'belonged' in the profession. In this way, the Association also served to articulate and draw boundaries around who constituted a surgeon and determined who was allowed entry to the social world of mid-twentieth-century surgery.

In 1975, the full-time salary of a consultant averaged between £7,536 and £10,689 (£57,506.46 to £81,566.69 in 2018).[80] In 1974, the top tax rate on earned income was raised to 83% (the highest permanent rate since the war); however, this only applied to incomes over £20,000 (£204,729 as of 2018).[81] In contrast, the average gross weekly earnings of full-time manual workers in the United Kingdom was £48.63 (an annual salary of approximately £2,500).[82] Surgery was, therefore, a relatively lucrative career. However, it also attracted people from affluent backgrounds – people who already had money. Wealthy families were more likely to send their children to 'good' schools (whether grammars or fee-paying private schools), who were then more likely to attend prestigious universities and medical schools. Surgery was – and to an extent remains – attractive to Britain's elites or those with plenty of disposable income.

And yet, and as with so many things to do with class in Britain, surgery's elite status was not just defined by the financial cost of entry or the salaries earnt by its practitioners. Instead, the relatively closed surgical community upheld an upper-, or at least middle-, class culture. Surgeons were identified as much by their hobbies as by their specialty. These hobbies and leisure activities were, almost invariably, bourgeois exploits and reflected the wealth and social class of mid-twentieth-century medical professionals.

Hugh E. Stephenson visited the United Kingdom and Ireland from his home in Missouri. He described the habits of the surgeons he met: 'Few get involved in community civic work, but many enjoy and pursue their hobbies with great vigour. Professor Charles Wells (Liverpool) and I spent one Saturday afternoon looking over about 1,500 of his young pheasants, which are being readied for the fall shooting.'[83] In Britain, pheasant shooting was a hallmark of upper-class society.[84] Others, like the thoracic and cardiac surgeon Mr Andrew Logan, were 'representative of a sizable number who spend spare time in the serenity and beauty of a garden'.[85] Mr Thomas Wilson, an ophthalmologist from Dublin, was an 'accomplished landscape and portrait artist'.[86] The new president of the RCSEd, Mr J. J. Mason Brown, 'gave … [Stephenson] a lesson in golf (and a sound trouncing) at St Andrews Old Course'.[87] In his prescriptive volume, *The Surgeon's Craft*, published in 1965, Hedley Atkins described the 'typical surgeon': 'He is often good at or fond of games and sports. Amongst my surgical friends, I can call to mind quite readily an Olympic medallist and three international Rugby players.'[88]

Similar accounts of sporting prowess appeared in published obituaries of British surgeons. As an operator, Gordon Irwin was 'a delight to watch'.[89] But much more space was devoted to his hobbies and outdoor pursuits: 'He was a most versatile sportsman, who excelled in all he took up. Fishing and shooting were his great loves, and he will be sadly missed by his friends on the Tweed and on the grouse moors of Northumberland and Durham.'[90] He played hockey and tennis for Northumberland and was a 'keen footballer in his younger days'. Like J. J. Mason Brown, Gordon was 'absorbed and irritated' by golf in his later years, and in 1958 he was 'honoured by being made captain of the Northumberland

Golf Club'.[91] These hobbies made him particularly apt at participating in the surgical cultures and conventions of his era: 'With all this behind him it was natural that Gordon Irwin should be at his best in the verbal badinage of male company, where his culture and wide knowledge of surgery, sport, men and affairs made him the most entertaining of companions.'[92] Similarly, while Mr T. L. Clark was a 'very busy surgeon', he nonetheless found time for 'many other activities both inside and outside his profession'.[93] He was a 'great sportsman' and in his youth he was a 'fine tennis player'. In later years, he was a 'keen fly fisher'. But his favourite activity, and the one he was most proficient at, was 'shot'. Every year, 'even up to the last', he would 'enjoy days on the grouse moors'.[94] These hobbies were either expensive and therefore exclusive, or a part of a culture predicated on the sociability of a certain social class and therefore exclusive. Participating in these leisure activities was a marker of inclusion into the surgical community and they acted as boundary lines between surgeon and non-surgeon. Moreover, many of these activities (shooting and golf) were coded male and therefore doubly exclusionary.

The supportive nature of sociability

There is, of course, nothing inherently wrong with playing golf and going on long, rugged hikes with your colleagues. And few would deny that ease, familiarity, and friendship make working life that much easier and more enjoyable – things that few would want to deny surgeons, who are otherwise required to work incredibly hard, sacrifice a great deal, and deal with profoundly distressing clinical experiences and diagnoses. And there was plenty to commend about mid-century surgical culture. While the firm structured the rigid hierarchy of the clinic and left the experience and advancement of surgical careers in the hands of sometimes capricious authorities, it also offered intangible and emotional benefits. In creating, maintaining, and defending rest, residential, and social spaces for doctors, hospitals and their inhabitants cultivated and shored up a workplace culture – one that inculcated trainee surgeons into a pattern of behaviours and attitudes that served to strengthen connections within the profession and demarcate its boundaries. As we have seen, surgical culture was cultivated inside the hospital – and maintained as much by the physical buildings as it was by the people who inhabited them – and strengthened in the social interactions surgeons had with each other when away from work. As chaplain George Day argued, it was the informal interactions, the intangible exchanges, and the subtle texture of working life that mattered. The various aspects of the surgical community this chapter has discussed so far – the firm, the hospital residence, the doctors' mess – served to bolster the 'things that matter' and produced a cultural homogeneity that helped some participants feel like they belonged.

These things and this sense of belonging also served to protect surgeons from the stresses and strains of surgical life and the excessive temporal commitments their jobs demanded. As Day suggested,

> Many housemen [trainee surgeons and physicians] go through a phase of deep despair; despair that they will ever get on top of their job; that they will ever give satisfaction to their sometimes thoughtless and exacting chiefs; despair that they cannot afford their patients all the unhurried attention they once hoped to be able to give. They often become exhausted in body, mind, and spirit.[95]

His solution to this mental and moral strain was friendship: 'They need befriending. They need to be reassured that they are doing a fine job – as fine a job as anyone could do in the circumstances. They need their spirit renewing within them – to be made to feel worthwhile.'[96]

In similar terms, a paediatric surgeon, interviewed in 2018 about his earlier experiences of surgical life, attested to the supportive nature of this team approach and argued that he could cope with excessive working hours because he was maintained by a sense of comradery. This surgeon was born in 1944 and worked from the 1960s onwards. He described his hospital's structure as 'family-like', and insisted that 'you felt very much like you were part of a firm … Whatever you were doing … you were definitely working within the team and that gave a very strong feeling of belonging and commitment.'[97] He developed close relationships with his colleagues and superiors who could rely on him: 'I think if I look at all the surgical bosses I had, I think I worked well with them because I was sort of around all the time and they got to trust me.'[98] Another urologist I interviewed told me how 'the consultant surgeons took me under their wing', offering a kind of emotional support that he might not have found in a more disparate or individualistic workplace.[99]

Indeed, much of the critique of the redesigned hospitals in the 1970s circulated the damaging effects the loss of dedicated space for rest and relaxation would have on the workplace culture and on the feelings of belonging, commitment, and collegiality experienced by trainees. As A. M. Cantor lamented, 'The most serious fault is in the arrangements for junior medical staff.' There was no provision for a doctors' mess in the original plans and 'the accommodation for junior medical staff [was] haphazardly dispersed in residential blocks which are also used by nursing and other staff'.[100] The residential quarters had 'no doctors' common room' and they were located far from the main hospital building.[101] He noted that 'the effect will be unfortunate because junior staff will be isolated from each other during leisure hours, and they will lose many of the traditional and more pleasant aspects of hospital life'.[102] This sense that ill-conceived hospital architecture could foster isolation and despair was widespread in the letters pages of medical journals and attests to the value doctors ascribed to spending social time together. As Cantor insisted, 'The dining arrangements also militate against the growth of normal working and social relationships among junior (and senior) medical staff.'[103]

No doubt friendship helped mitigate the harmful effects of working all hours, the negative impact of their 'sometimes thoughtless and exacting chiefs', and the frustration of being unable to offer patients the 'unhurried attention' they needed and deserved. And for some, it did more than just mitigate. For those who weathered the storm of intense training, surgery proved a fulfilling career replete with comradery, joy, and professional satisfaction. Obituaries attest to long lives lived fully. And for others, they did not even consider it a storm – just the occasional downpour in a lifetime of sunny days. In other words, even if it caused some people despair – and even if some people did not make it through training, choosing instead an alternative specialty or even career – surgery was appealing. As we will see later in the book, there are many surgeons who look back on their training with affection and some who argue that we should return to these 'halcyon days of yore'. However, the workplace cultures of the firm and the residential hospital were not universally lauded – nor did they provide emotional support and a sense of belonging for everyone who trained or worked as a surgeon in post-war Britain.

The troubling nature of sociability

Throughout the second half of the twentieth century, various people from both within and without the profession critiqued the firm and the surgical cultures it upheld (and in some cases, continues to uphold). These more sceptical voices suggested that the firm was responsible for the routine exploitation of junior doctors and medical students – with those at the bottom of the rung regularly working more than 100-hour weeks (see Chapter 6). They criticised the firm's maintenance of strict hierarchies and individual career progression, the excessive competition between consultants the system encouraged, the lack of credit afforded to other healthcare professions (as opposed to the supposedly more equitable 'multidisciplinary teams' that are now popular), the ubiquity of 'teaching by humiliation', and the lack of structure or consistency to training and education.[104]

In a 1950 article published in the *BMJ*, Donald McI. Johnson was asked to reflect on his clinical training twenty-five years earlier (c.1925). He demurred, 'I have a natural reluctance to make sweeping remarks, particularly when they are damnatory, in a scientific journal.' However, his judgement was uncompromising: 'As regards the hospital part of my education 25 years ago … it was wholly bad. It had certain minor features that might be described as good, but they did not redeem the whole.' Having completed his primary clinical education at Cambridge, he took up his first hospital student appointment as junior dresser in Bart's surgery. He reflected on the emotional costs of the 'sudden and unprepared jump from the cosy realms of theoretical learning to the harsh realities of human pain and suffering', calling it a 'mental shock the effect of which persisted for some time to come'. He recalled how every morning for three months he had 'the experience of seeing and inflicting pain in the Bart's surgery, entirely unaccompanied by any form of teaching'. Johnson's critique of the firm primarily circulated around its entrenched hierarchies and failure to effectively teach its most junior members:

> The 'teaching' part of our day started when … we gathered in the Square to embark on the ward rounds as the least important part of the hierarchy which constituted the 'firm.' Here horror became replaced by boredom as one shambled round on the outer fringe of the cortege accompanying the chief.[105]

This 'education' lasted for six months and 'seemed to lack any guiding principle behind it other than that common to most educational establishments of that day – namely, giving the neophyte a bad time to start with'.[106]

Like others, he compared hospitals to religious orders: 'Who among those educated at one of the older teaching hospitals can doubt that the monastic tradition has descended in strong measure through the hundreds of years from their early foundation?' However, unlike others, his issue with the comparison was not so much a critique of the single-sex nature of hospital accommodation, but rather a critique of the all-encompassing nature of hospital life: 'Who but is conscious of the feeling that, once within these portals, one must acknowledge that the entire universe has contracted itself to the area within these walls, and that one is expected to make the mental surrender to this cosmos.'[107] He implied that the hospital was a kind of 'total institution' and that rather than conferring a sense of belonging and collegiality, the homogeneity and pressures of hospital life were in fact profoundly troubling.[108] He described his own experience of hospital training: 'To the majority this mental surrender perhaps comes easily; it is made temporarily in most cases, permanently in some. In others, however, the reaction is the opposite, and I was one of the others. I became the victim of a wild, tearing claustrophobia.'[109] McI. Johnson's article was not designed as a personal attack: 'In my criticism of the teaching process it has not been my intention in any way to disparage the distinguished gentlemen in whose steps I followed: they were the victims of the system as much as I was.'[110] However, he was uncompromising in his assessment: 'What did I learn from my three years at hospital? The answer is: almost nothing.'[111]

McI. Johnson was not alone in feeling this way, and this experience of hospital life was not confined to pre-NHS days. Like

George Day would go on to do eighteen years later, McI. Johnson also criticised the pressures of hospital life and the peculiar hold it exerted over the minds and emotions of trainee doctors: 'Amour propre, conformity, and tradition make them conceal it. It does not pay to squeal. It would kill their chance of acquiring a good testimonial, which is so necessary for preferment.'[112]

In a 1969 survey of medical staff at Northampton General Hospital, the junior doctors blamed the firm for several of their complaints. Like Day, they lamented the nepotistic nature of promotion decisions and advocated for a new career structure which 'might allow an optional system of staff reporting as used in the Civil Service', because it would 'place more emphasis on the overall record of the doctor when an appointment is being considered and would reduce the influence of a single consultant which is so strong under the present system'.[113] The ideals and practices of patronage and lineage were strong in the firm system. In T. C. Graves' obituary, published in 1964, the first few sentences identify him as 'the grandson of the founder of the firm of Chivers'.[114] For some, the firm connoted prestige and a kind of surgical 'family' – complete with ancestors and descendants; for others, it made career progression and opportunities for promotion dependent on the personality of sometimes capricious individuals. The authors of the survey suggested that the 'traditional concept of the "firm" be replaced by the "department"'. This innovation would 'reduce the isolation of individual units'.[115]

Conclusion

The mid-twentieth-century surgical world was intense and all-encompassing. Whether on the ward, in the operating theatre, or on the golf course, trainees and consultants lived and breathed their work. Indeed, surgeons defined pleasure *as* work and insisted on the professional and pedagogical importance of social interaction. In this way, the social lives and workplace cultures of surgeons were crucial to the development and maintenance of their professional identities and helped to define what it meant to be a surgeon in the first few decades of the NHS. These social lives took place both on and off the hospital wards, and surgeons spent plenty of time with each other at professional events, society dinners, and recreational activities. These various events helped foster social connections, built international networks, and implicitly restricted the conditions of entry to the surgical community along class, race, and gender lines. This chapter has offered, therefore, a cultural history of professionalisation and I have interrogated the ways in which surgeons' social lives – both in and out of hospital – were used to demarcate professional difference and establish who could and could not be included in the community.[116]

However, the 'full-time' nature of surgical work was not, as this chapter has suggested, universally accepted as a good thing. The pressure to spend all your time at the hospital was regularly critiqued and increasingly subjected to scrutiny – particularly as hospital residences began to close and alternative models of living and working emerged. The surgeons in this chapter were more often than not described by their colleagues as affable and attentive – not miles away from the kindly, if paternalistic, ideals put forward in the surgical textbooks in Chapter 1. The surgeons who expressed fondness for their co-workers and the sense of belonging that mid-century hospitals could foster defended their professional lives in emotional terms – just like those who campaigned against the hospital residences because they blurred the boundaries between work and home life or kept trainees away from their families. While they might have had the kind of social lives pursued by Sir Lancelot Spratt, they were hardly aloof or emotionally disconnected from their conditions of labour.

One crucial thing these surgeons and Spratt had in common was their demographic profile – they were all white, socially elite (or at the very least middle class), and male. By this point, there were no structural or legislative barriers to women, medical students from working-class backgrounds, or people of colour becoming surgeons, but that did not mean that there were not plenty of cultural obstacles still in their way. In this chapter I have gestured towards the exclusive nature of surgical social lives and workplace cultures and how they drew boundaries around the profession. In the next two chapters, I will expand on this theme and use oral history interviews and archival material to interrogate the experiences of female surgeons and surgeons from racialised minorities in twentieth- and twenty-first-century Britain.

Notes

1 Agnes Arnold-Forster, 'The Social and Emotional World of Twentieth-Century Anglo-American Surgery: The James IV Association of Surgeons', *Bulletin of the History of Medicine*, 96:1 (2022), 71–101.

2 Hugh Dudley, 'Excerpts from Tributes to Sir John Bruce (1905–1975) by the Hon. David A. Balfour, Adam N. Smith and Professor Hugh Dudley'. Word from the James IV Association of Surgeons, Inc., Spring 1976, Box 1, Folder 2, Minutes, etc. 1971, 1975–1982, James IV Association of Surgeons Records.

3 'Sir James Walton, K.C.V.O., M.S., F.R.C.S.', *British Medical Journal*, 2:4940 (1955), 684.

4 Ibid.

5 Bentley P. Colcock, 'Report to the James IV Association of Surgeons', 1964, James IV Association of Surgeons Records. The Drs. Barry and Bobbi Coller Rare Book Reading Room, New York Academy of Medicine Library.

6 Henry Marsh, 'The Great War's Miracle Worker', *New Statesman*, 13 July 2022, https://www.newstatesman.com/culture/books/2022/07/the-facemaker-review-lindsey-fitzharris-great-war (accessed 7 April 2023).

7 Jackie Clarke, 'Closing Time: Deindustrialization and Nostalgia in Contemporary France', *History Workshop Journal*, 79 (2015), 107–125; Xavier Vigna, Michelle Zancarini-Fournel, and Sian Reynolds, 'Gender History and Labour History', *Clio. Women, Gender, History*, 38 (2013), 176–203.

8 For more on surgeons' professional sociability, see Delia Gavrus, 'Men of Dreams and Men of Actions: Neurologists, Neurosurgeons and the Performance of Professional Identity, 1920–1950', *Bulletin of the History of Medicine*, 85 (2011), 57–92; Peter Kernahan, 'Surgery Becomes a Specialty: Professional Boundaries and Surgery', in Thomas Schlich (ed.), *The Palgrave Handbook of the History of Surgery* (London: Palgrave Macmillan, 2017), 95–113; Thomas Schlich, *Surgery, Science and Industry: A Revolution in Fracture Care, 1950–1990s* (Basingstoke: Palgrave, 2002); Thomas Schlich, 'Degrees of Control: The Spread of Operative Fracture Care with Metal Implants. A Comparative Perspective of Switzerland, East Germany, and the USA, 1950s–1990s', in Jenny Stanton (ed.), *Innovations in Health and Medicine: Diffusion and Resistance in the Twentieth Century* (London: Routledge, 2002), 106–125; and Thomas Schlich, '"One and the Same the World Over": The International Culture of Surgical Exchange in an Age of Globalization, 1870–1914', *Journal of the History of Medicine and Allied Sciences*, 71 (2016), 247–270.

9 Abi Rimmer, 'The Firm: Does it Hold the Answers to Teamworking and Morale?', *BMJ*, 365 (2019), l4104.

10 Agnes Arnold-Forster, 'The Emotional Landscape of the Hospital Residence in Post-war Britain', in Agnes Arnold-Forster and Alison Moulds (eds), *Feelings and Work in Modern History: Emotional Labour and Emotions about Labour* (London: Bloomsbury, 2022), 58–75.

11 Anja Timm, 'The Demise of the Firm: What is Happening to Apprenticeship Learning?', https://bit.ly/2Sb4mZL (accessed 19 May 2021).

12 Rimmer, 'The Firm'.

13 Simon Sinclair, *Making Doctors: An Institutional Apprenticeship* (London: Routledge, 2020).

14 T. N. Bonner, *Becoming a Physician: Medical Education in Great Britain, France, Germany and the United States, 1750–1945* (New York: Johns Hopkins University Press, 1995); Anne Crowther and Marguerite Dupree, *Medical Lives in the Age of Surgical Revolution* (Cambridge: Cambridge University Press, 2007); Laura Kelly, 'Migration and Medical Education: Irish Medical Students at the University of Glasgow, 1859–1900', *Irish Economic and Social History*, 39 (2012), 39–55.

15 L. Rosner, *Medical Education in the Age of Improvement: Edinburgh Students and Apprentices, 1760–1826* (Edinburgh: Edinburgh University Press, 1991).

16 Keir Waddington, 'Mayhem and Medical Students: Image, Conduct and Control in the Victorian and Edwardian London Teaching Hospital', *Social History of Medicine*, 15:1 (2002), 45–64.

17 Sandra V. Kotsis and Kevin C. Chung, 'Application of See One, Do One, Teach One Concept in Surgical Training', *Plastic Reconstructive Surgery*, 131:5 (2013), 1194–1201.

18 Ronald Macbeth, 'Married Quarters in Hospital', *British Medical Journal*, 1:5346 (1963), 1674.

19 W. Arklay Steel, 'Charges for Residence', *British Medical Journal*, 2:4890 (1954), 128–129, 129.

20 Ibid.

21 Ibid.

22 Ibid.

23 Ibid.

24 R. M. Forrester, 'Married Quarters in Hospital', *British Medical Journal*, 2:5348 (1963), 51.

25 'Hospital Junior Staffs Group Council', *British Medical Journal*, 2:5425 (1964), 229–231, 231.
26 Ibid.
27 Ibid.
28 George Day, 'Personal View', *British Medical Journal*, 3:5611 (1968), 182.
29 Ibid.
30 D. W. Dingwall, 'Special Article: Provision of Married-Quarters for House Officers', *British Medical Journal*, 1:5436 (1963), 1664–1665, 1664.
31 Michael Hession, 'Married Quarters in Hospital', *British Medical Journal*, 1:5343 (1963), 1475.
32 Ibid.
33 Dingwall, 'Special Article', 1664.
34 Arklay Steel, 'Charges for Residence', 129.
35 Hession, 'Married Quarters in Hospital', 1475.
36 Ibid.
37 Ibid.
38 P. A. Johnson, 'Married Quarters', *British Medical Journal*, 1:5538 (1967), 505.
39 Cromwell, 'Married Quarters in Hospital', *British Medical Journal*, 2:5348 (1963), 52.
40 A General Practitioner's Wife, 'Married Quarters', *British Medical Journal*, 1:5538 (1967), 505.
41 Ibid.
42 Clarice A. Baker, 'Married Quarters in Hospital', *British Medical Journal*, 2:5348 (1963), 51.
43 John Shepherd, 'Married Quarters', *British Medical Journal*, 1:5538 (1967), 505.
44 Ibid.
45 Macbeth, 'Married Quarters in Hospital', 1674.
46 Ibid.
47 Ibid.
48 Ibid.
49 Ibid.
50 Ibid.
51 Ibid.
52 Interview with male surgeon; interviewed by author, 30 July 2020.
53 'Hospital Junior Staffs Group Council', *British Medical Journal*, 2:5217 (1960), 269–271, 270.
54 Ibid.

55 'Annual Representative Meeting, Swansea 1965', *British Medical Journal*, 2:5454 (1965), 29–68, 60; 'Hospital Junior Staffs Group Council', (1960), 270.
56 Macbeth, 'Married Quarters in Hospital', 1674.
57 A. M. Cantor, 'Personal View', *British Medical Journal*, 2:6146 (1978), 1224.
58 J. H. Tweedie, A. Milosevic, and D. Shuttleworth, 'Facilities for Junior Doctors in New Hospitals', *British Medical Journal*, 2:6150 (1978), 1503.
59 Ibid.
60 Ibid.
61 Ibid.
62 'Hospital Junior Staffs Group Council', (1960), 270.
63 'Hospital Junior Staffs', *British Medical Journal*, 1:5343 (1963), 260–261, 260.
64 Colcock, 'Report to the James IV Association of Surgeons'.
65 James IV Association of Surgeons Records. The Drs. Barry and Bobbi Coller Rare Book Reading Room, New York Academy of Medicine Library.
66 Ibid.
67 R. A. Macbeth, 'Report on the James IV Association of Surgeons Inc. Surgical Travelership to the United Kingdom, Eire, Denmark and Sweden', 1960s, James IV Association of Surgeons Records. The Drs. Barry and Bobbi Coller Rare Book Reading Room, New York Academy of Medicine Library.
68 Colcock, 'Report to the James IV Association of Surgeons'.
69 Ibid.
70 Folkert O. Belzer, 'Report to the James IV Association of Surgeons', Surgical Traveller for 1977 to England, Poland, the Netherlands, and Sweden, James IV Association of Surgeons Records. The Drs. Barry and Bobbi Coller Rare Book Reading Room, New York Academy of Medicine Library.
71 Ibid.
72 Ibid.
73 E. G. Muir, 'Report on a Visit to the United States and Canada as James IV Travelling Professor, 1961', James IV Association of Surgeons Records. The Drs. Barry and Bobbi Coller Rare Book Reading Room, New York Academy of Medicine Library.
74 Edward G. Tuckwell, 'Report of the First Ian Aird Surgical Traveller, United States and Canada 1963', James IV Association of Surgeons Records. The Drs. Barry and Bobbi Coller Rare Book Reading Room, New York Academy of Medicine Library.

75 Terence Kennedy, 'Visit to the USA as James IV Surgical Traveller from Ireland', c. 1964, James IV Association of Surgeons Records. The Drs. Barry and Bobbi Coller Rare Book Reading Room, New York Academy of Medicine Library.

76 Ibid.

77 Ibid.

78 Minutes of the Meeting of the Board of Directors, James IV Association of Surgeons, Inc., September 9, 1983, 'Discussion and Selection of Candidates for Election to Active Membership', James IV Association of Surgeons Records. The Drs. Barry and Bobbi Coller Rare Book Reading Room, New York Academy of Medicine Library.

79 Ibid.

80 Hansard, HC Deb 24 March 1976 vol 908 cc190-1W, https://api.parliament.uk/historic-hansard/written-answers/1976/mar/24/doctors-pay (accessed 19 May 2021).

81 UK Retail Price Index inflation figures are based on data from Gregory Clarke, https://measuringworth.com/datasets/ukearncpi/ (accessed 30 November 2020).

82 Hansard, HC Deb 18 April 1975 vol 890 c176W, https://api.parliament.uk/historic-hansard/written-answers/1975/apr/18/manual-workers-average-wage (accessed 19 May 2021).

83 Hugh E. Stephenson, 'Undergraduate Surgical Teaching in the United Kingdom and Ireland', Reprinted from *Surgery*, 65 (1964), 321–333, James IV Association of Surgeons Records, 324.

84 Mike Huggins, 'Sport and the British Upper Classes c.1500–2000: A Historiographic Overview', *Sport in History*, 28 (2008), 364–388.

85 Stephenson, 'Undergraduate Surgical Teaching in the United Kingdom and Ireland', 324.

86 Ibid.

87 Ibid.

88 Hedley Atkins, *The Surgeon's Craft* (Manchester: Manchester University Press, 1965), 30.

89 'C. G. Irwin, M.B., F.R.C.S.Ed.', *British Medical Journal*, 2:5156 (1959), 889–890, 890.

90 Ibid.

91 Ibid.

92 Ibid.

93 'T. L. Clark, M.D., F.R.C.S.Ed.', *British Medical Journal*, 1:5064 (1958), 225–226, 226.

94 Ibid.

95 Day, 'Personal View'.

96 Ibid.

97 Interview with male surgeon; interviewed by author, 18 January 2018.
98 Ibid.
99 Interview with male surgeon; interviewed by author, 30 July 2020.
100 Cantor, 'Personal View'.
101 Ibid.
102 Ibid.
103 Ibid.
104 Press Association, 'Medical Students "Humiliated by Senior Doctors"', *The Guardian* (1 October 2004), www.theguardian.com/education/2004/oct/01/highereducation.uk1 (accessed 19 May 2021); W. Howieson and D. Cloke, 'The Hidden Curriculum and its Implications for Surgical Specialties: Preventing the Unspoken Academic and Social Messages Taught to Trainees that Lead to Unwanted Behaviours and Results', *Royal College of Surgeons of England Bulletin*, 101:7 (2019), 282–284, 283.
105 Donald McI. Johnson, 'A G.P. On His Clinical Training', *British Medical Journal*, 2:4677 (1950), 493–496, 494.
106 Ibid.
107 Ibid.
108 Erving Goffman, *Asylums: Essays on the Social Situation of Mental Patients and Other Inmates* (New York: Anchor Books, 1961).
109 Johnson, 'A G.P. On His Clinical Training', 494.
110 Ibid., 495.
111 Ibid.
112 Ibid.
113 N. R. Redman, J. P. Toby, and J. B. Peniket, 'Hospital Junior Doctors: Survey at Northampton General Hospital', *British Medical Journal*, 3:5669 (1969), 522–525, 525.
114 'T. C. Graves, B.Sc., M.D., F.R.C.S., M.R.C.V.S.', *British Medical Journal*, 1:5399 (1964), 1711.
115 Redman et al., 'Hospital Junior Doctors', 525.
116 Michael Brown, 'Medicine, Reform and the "End" of Charity in Early Nineteenth-Century England', *English Historical Review*, 124 (2009), 1353–1388.

4

Gender in surgery

You do not have to spend much time with surgeons, or devote many hours to reading about the past and present of the profession, to get a sense of its 'martial, masculine ambience'.[1] The myth of the modern surgeon includes characteristics that are traditionally ascribed to men: 'arrogance, aggressiveness, courage, and the ability to make split-second decisions in the face of life-threatening risks'.[2] These myths persist, even as the actual demographics of surgery have changed. The profession has been open to women since the nineteenth century, and the percentage of female practitioners gradually increased over the second half of the twentieth century.[3]

However, despite decades of gender parity in British medical education, today women remain under-represented in surgery. The results of a survey published in the *BMJ* in 2019 demonstrated that most female surgeons perceive the field as 'male-dominated', and over half had experienced discrimination.[4] Evidence from countries like Australia, and corroborated by my interviews and anecdotes from British practitioners, indicate that female surgeons are also subjected to sexual harassment on an alarmingly regular basis and that gendered language in the workplace is commonplace.[5]

In the previous chapter, I described the workings of the firm. The firm was always more than just a tool for training and education – more than just a way of organising people at work. Instead, it had complex social dynamics. It was a community, even if the relationships within could be fraught. To be a surgeon in the decades immediately following the foundation of the NHS meant that participating in this community and professional success depended on whether people could adhere to the cultural and social requirements. These requirements included excessive temporal commitment, a blurring of boundaries between the personal and professional, complete institutional loyalty, and classed and gendered forms of sociability such as elite and macho sporting pursuits and eating and drinking together. Critics of the firm claimed that these post-war hospital cultures cultivated exploitation, embedded rigid and punitive hierarchies, limited career progression except for a favoured few, impinged on the quality and equity of teaching, and excluded individuals with the 'wrong' personality or interests from participating or succeeding.

Traditional hospital cultures also limited the surgical profession by narrowing the range of people who could be included. The identities and stereotypes developed, maintained, and bolstered in this period – as well as the lived experiences of post-war surgeons – made a lasting impact on the demographic make-up of the profession. Surgeons' social lives were used to demarcate professional difference and establish who could and could not be embraced by the surgical community. The predominance of these activities cultivated a reputation for the profession as male dominated, ethnically homogeneous, and accessible only to those from public schools or who moved in equivalent social circles. In other words, both the stereotypical and real surgeon in mid-twentieth-century Britain tended to be male.

Building on claims made in the first three chapters, in this one I argue that the construction and maintenance of the surgical stereotype as male has had lasting effects on who is allowed access to the profession, what kind of healthcare professionals patients will anticipate or tolerate, and the expectations of appropriate conduct both in and out of the operating theatre. Using written sources as well as oral history interviews, I argue that surgeons in post-war Britain participated in activities open primarily to white, English-speaking men from affluent social backgrounds. While there was plenty of violent and explicit racism and sexism, exclusion was also much more subtle. This chapter is, therefore, an account of individual surgeons' and surgical communities' attempts to implicitly (and sometimes explicitly) restrict the conditions of entry to the surgical profession – a restriction that took place, paradoxically, against the backdrop of increasing diversity within medicine more broadly. Thus, this chapter reveals how a restrictive surgical stereotype persists, even as the demographic reality of the profession has slowly changed.

In what follows, I interrogate the gendered construction of the surgical stereotype, explore the history of sexism, and examine the continued impact of discrimination. Throughout my research, I have heard prompted and unprompted stories of unashamed discrimination, abuse, and harassment.[6] This chapter will tell these tales and examine the individual and structural reasons for the skewed demographic make-up of surgery, both past and present.[7] For the sake of clarity, I have opted to devote this chapter to gender, and the next to the history of race, migration, and ethnicity. At the end of Chapter 5, I address the intersections between race and gender by focusing on the careers of female surgeons of colour.[8] However, by adopting this structure I do not mean to imply that it is possible to anatomise the experience of complex, multifaceted people into different demographic markers. Nor do I want to suggest that women of colour are more defined by their race or ethnicity than by their gender (or, indeed, vice versa).

This chapter travels more or less chronologically through the history of modern British surgery – starting before the foundation of the NHS and coming right up to the present day. Sexism within surgery was, and continues to be, inextricably tied to the social and political context of Britain. Discrimination within surgery has been shaped by the changing politics of 'diversity', female participation in the labour market, gender equality legislation, and shifting cultural norms around things like sexual harassment, as well as parenthood and other caring responsibilities.

Female surgeons before the NHS

Women have been training, qualifying, and working as surgeons since the nineteenth century and continued to do so into the twentieth.[9] Much has been written about women's entry into the recognised medical profession and the earliest pioneers have become household names. Elizabeth Blackwell and Elizabeth Garrett Anderson (who was a surgeon) capitalised on loopholes in the system to become the first women on the Medical Register in the mid-nineteenth century.[10] In the ensuing decades, the campaign for women in medicine developed into a concerted movement. In 1869, Sophia Jex-Blake and several female peers gained admission to a recognised medical degree at the

University of Edinburgh.[11] In 1876, legislation authorised universities to award degrees to women, but did not compel them to do so. A year later, the King's and Queen's College of Physicians of Ireland – then one of Britain's nineteen medical licensing bodies – opened its final examinations to women. By 1892, there were 135 women on the Register.[12] They found work in hospitals and dispensaries for women and children and across the British Empire.

As historians have shown, however, these women encountered staunch resistance from both the public and the profession. There was opposition to their medical education and training (particularly to the prospect of mixed-sex classes), to them taking up public appointments, and becoming members of professional societies. Although Jex-Blake and her peers matriculated at Edinburgh, they were later denied the right to graduate. The British Medical Association did not accept women until 1892 (barring an oversight that led to Garrett Anderson's admission), and in 1895 both the Royal College of Surgeons of England and the Royal College of Physicians of London voted against admitting women – decisions that were not overturned until 1908.[13] However, the number of women on the Register grew more rapidly after 1900. A reduction in male recruitment during the world wars offered more opportunities to medical women, and institutional barriers were gradually removed. In 1910, the Royal Society of Medicine and the Royal College of Surgeons each elected their first women, followed by the RCSEd in 1920, and the RCP in 1934.[14]

By the mid-1930s, 10 per cent of registered practitioners were women and there are many examples of successful female surgeons who worked long, productive careers. In September 1914, Louisa Garrett Anderson described the extent of her surgical role during the First World War: 'We have a lot of surgery: sometimes I am in the theatre from 2 to 9 or 10 at night, and have eight or more operations.'[15] Similarly, an obituary of Maud Mary Chadburn, published in *The Lancet* in 1957, noted that she served as surgeon to the Elizabeth Garrett Anderson Hospital in London for twenty years, with a 'large and successful practice' in general surgery and gynaecology. She managed to combine her career with raising three adopted children. She was described as a 'remarkable woman', with 'quiet persistence'. She was 'indefatigable', and could spend long hours in the operating theatre 'without strain'.[16]

Female surgeons in the early NHS

Despite these early successes, practical and ideological opposition to female doctors persisted. Following the foundation of the NHS in 1948, and amidst wider social pressure to provide equal rights to women, female participation in the labour market expanded. The need to grow the ranks of British-trained doctors was met by an increasing number of women practitioners from the 1960s onwards. Nevertheless, the 'marriage bar' – which curtailed the employment of women after marriage or pregnancy – lasted well into the mid-twentieth century.[17] And, as I suggested in Chapter 2, popular culture often portrayed women as unfit for medical work. One female physician wrote to the *BMJ* in 1958 to complain about the absence of women doctors in the incredibly popular BBC programme *On Call to a Nation*. Despite approximately 15 per cent of the doctors on the medical register being women, she counted just one female practitioner in the programme, and she had a non-speaking role.[18] Even in the 1960s and 1970s – the decades of Women's Liberation – the profession remained implicitly and explicitly hostile to female doctors.

Despite this resistance, women sought medical and surgical education in post-war Britain. According to American surgeon Hugh E. Stephenson, who visited Britain in the 1960s, 'girls' constituted a quarter of medical school students in the UK.[19] When the Universities Central Council on Admissions first measured the proportion of male and female medical applicants in 1963, women comprised around 34 per cent of applicants and 29 per cent of acceptances. However, many female graduates never went on to practice medicine, let alone surgery.[20] In 1967, Jean Lawrie from the Medical Women's Federation wrote to the editor of *The Lancet* to raise the issue of female surgeons. She identified surgery as a peculiarly obstructive speciality for women:

> Comparatively few women today are in training as surgeons. There is some evidence that young women wishing to become surgeons are diverted from their original intent by those who think that it is too difficult and strenuous a career for them, especially if they marry.

And yet, she argued, the training for a gynaecologist or obstetrician, for example, was just as rigorous as that of a general surgeon or other specialist. The challenges came later, when the career intruded 'on leisure and night hours'.[21] As Lawrie observes, there was nothing specific in the requirements or difficulty of surgery that made it a more challenging specialty for women to enter than any other. Instead, and as discussed in the previous three chapters, while the cultures and communities of post-war British surgery were more emotionally nuanced than Sir Lancelot Spratt indicated, the macho surgical stereotype was remarkably powerful and enduring. Even though there were no legal or technical obstacles to women joining the specialty, cultural barriers were strong.

Surgical societies, like the James IV Association, were often the most tangible manifestations of surgery's 'old boys' club'. Their archives offer some answers to the question of why many women left the profession shortly after completing their studies.[22] Mid-twentieth-century surgeons cultivated a masculine culture that coded certain behaviours as appropriate or required. In doing so, they implicitly excluded women from the surgical world. Stephenson described the social and professional pursuits of Professor Sir Charles Illingworth of Glasgow, who was often found 'leading a group of medical students and members of his "firm" on hikes over the rugged west highlands of Scotland'.[23] The week before Stephenson arrived, 'this group had stopped to swim in a cold mountain stream'.[24] As discussed in Chapter 3, much of the socialising undertaken by mid-twentieth-century surgeons took place away from the hospital – on golf courses, grouse moors, and rugged walks – and these were places and pursuits from which women were traditionally excluded.

During the 1970s, the medical school application system became more formalised and merit-based, replacing earlier informal systems which permitted greater class, gender, and ethnicity discrimination. This encouraged more female applicants, who were achieving similar grades to boys in school. Female medical applicants rose to around 40 per cent in 1980 and increased by a further 10 per cent in each subsequent decade.[25] The changing gender composition of the medical workforce was comparable to other professional occupations in the UK. Law followed a similar path, moving from a historically male-dominated workforce that excluded female participation towards near equality. Today, around 46 per cent of legal professionals are women.[26]

However, this sunny picture of progressive change obscures continuing problems in medicine more generally, and surgery specifically. The expansion of female doctors was particularly apparent in primary care, and the overall increase in numbers of GPs can almost solely be attributed to women joining the clinical workforce. From 1988 to 2013, the number of male GPs remained relatively stable, whereas the number of female general practitioners rose from 6,505 to 20,435.[27] Even in this supposedly 'female friendly' medical specialty, however, gender inequalities persist. Despite almost equal numbers of male and female GPs, there are differences in the type of contracts held. Partners of GP practices tend to be men whereas salaried GPs, or contracted employees of a practice, tend to be women.[28] This evidence highlights what sociologists call 'vertical gender segregation' in medicine, which refers to women's reduced likelihood of holding positions of power and prestige within organisations, despite similar levels of skill or expertise.[29]

Surgery is a prestigious specialty, held in high regard by both healthcare professionals and the non-clinical public.[30] It is therefore unsurprising that this 'vertical gender segregation' also applies to women in surgery. While GPs are now roughly equally male and female, the same cannot be said for surgeons, and the pace of change over the past three decades has been remarkably slow. In 1992, a study of women doctors and their careers showed that although almost equal numbers of male and female students qualified from medical school, women held only 15 per cent of consultant posts, only 3 per cent of consultant posts in surgical specialties, and represented just 1 per cent of general surgeons.[31] According to Mend the Gap, the independent review into gender pay gaps in England, surgery today is 'deeply segregated' as a specialty, with women found in lower proportions, and those who are there tend to be younger and more junior.[32] Today, 13.2 per cent of surgical consultants are women. It has taken thirty years to advance ten percentage points.[33]

Progress has been slow despite a range of European and UK policies designed to level the professional playing field. In 1989, the European Commission reported that women remained largely confined to traditionally female occupations, relatively low-level jobs, and atypical forms of work which do not provide the same levels of protection and benefits as traditionally male types of labour.[34] The UK was reluctant to respond by legislating on equality issues. Instead, in 1991 Prime Minister John Major launched 'Opportunity 2000', which was a voluntary scheme without legal or financial compulsion aimed at improving prospects for British women. Prompted by the charity Business in the Community, fourteen of the country's top employers – including the NHS – set out their own ten-year targets to improve women's position in the workforce.[35] As a signatory to 'Opportunity 2000', the NHS Management Executive commissioned a report from the Office for Public Management to profile the 'issues relating to the role of women in the NHS and to build on progress in providing equal opportunities for women'.[36] The report identified four general and pervasive barriers to equality: (1) outmoded attitudes about the role of women; (2) direct and indirect discrimination; (3) the absence of proper childcare provision; (4) and inflexible structures for work and careers.[37] It noted that discrimination could take many forms but was particularly apparent in 'subjective and informal selection procedures; stereotypical assumptions about the ability, character, suitability, and natural role of women; the use of insider, word-of-mouth, and old boys' networks; unnecessary age bars; and excessive mobility requirements'.[38]

Social scientists have come up with concepts that describe these subtler mechanisms of exclusion. While deliberate discrimination – 'first-generation gender bias' – has in Britain been illegal since the 1970s, 'second-generation gender bias' is both harder to spot and more difficult to legislate against.[39] 'Second-generation gender bias' refers to practices that may seem gender neutral, in that they apply to everyone, but nevertheless result in discrimination against a gender (usually women or non-binary people) because they reflect the values of the gender that created the surrounding environment (usually men). This form of bias is often unconscious and unintentional, but no less harmful. It means that even when women have overtly been offered the same opportunities as men, they continue to be under-represented in certain professions and in positions of leadership.[40] As Mary Ann Elston has argued, the 'maleness' of medicine has been a crucial factor in women's experiences of careers in healthcare.[41]

Surgery and parenthood

There were, therefore, multiple cultural obstacles to female participation in the surgical workforce that circulated around the macho mythology of the modern surgeon. But there were other, more material, barriers, and other cultural tropes that aspiring female surgeons had to contend with. The dominant ideal across all classes in early twentieth-century Britain was that of the 'breadwinner family': a household 'headed by a male worker earning a wage large enough to keep his wife and children, typically through secure, skilled work'. While many families deviated from this norm, as Helen McCarthy has observed, 'the family wage retained its ideological power over British society'.[42] And yet, many women in the 1950s sought work outside the home. Between 1931 and 1951 the number of married women who did paid work doubled. One major survey conducted in 1949 found that 45 per cent of married women who worked had children under fifteen, with the overall employment rate among mothers standing at 19 per cent.[43]

Mothers sought work outside the home for a variety of reasons: some due to economic pressures, but others simply because they wanted to and found it meaningful. As the social scientist Gertrude Willoughby argued, 'the work itself is interesting and gives her an opportunity of exercising gifts which are not used in the home circle'.[44] To do so, women had to contend with a key obstacle: the unavailability of childcare. According to one 1951 estimate, there were publicly funded nursery places for just 1 per cent of Britain's under-fives.[45] This reality shaped the career trajectory of many women in this period. In 1965, Alva Myrdal and Viola Klein co-authored *Women's Two Roles*, making the case for women 'having it all', albeit sequentially, becoming first workers, then wives and mothers, and finally re-entering the labour market to become workers again.[46] The 1951 figures on adult women's employment in the United Kingdom indicated what Catherine Hakim has called the two-phase, or bimodal, pattern of female work. After a sharp drop in the economic activity rate in the twenty-four to thirty-four age group, there was a very slight increase for married women aged thirty-five to forty-four. By 1961 the bimodal patterns had emerged clearly, and by 1971 older wives were more likely to be working than younger ones.[47]

As Jane Lewis argues, *Women's Two Roles* was written when the memories of interwar marriage bars in the professions were still fresh, 'in order to promote the idea that educated women need not give up work for ever on marriage'.[48] Myrdal and Klein were not alone in championing women's return to work. Indeed, as Claire Langhamer has argued, the expansion of married women's employment transformed understandings of women's capacity even before the advent of Second-Wave Feminism.[49] However, the problem with the bimodal pattern of female employment was that it did not work for surgeons. Nor did it apply to many women with university degrees and professional qualifications. As such, bodies like the British Federation of University Women and the Medical Women's Federation were anxious to promote women's careers and their 'acquisition of skill and responsibility, and with continuity and progression over time'.[50]

Continuity and career progression were achieved by some medical women. A major study published in 1963 found that nearly two-thirds of female doctors with children under five were still working (17 per cent full time and 46 per cent part time), while four-fifths of medical mothers with school-age children were actively practicing (30 per cent full time and 51 per cent part time). Klein noted that of all professional working mothers, medics were the most likely to pursue their careers continuously rather than take an extended break followed by re-entry to the workplace. However, most medical women achieved this through the 'relative flexibility' of general practice. Less than one in five medical mothers worked in hospital medicine.

While particularly acute for surgeons, the drawbacks of the 'bimodal' pattern of female work was a recognised problem for all women. Against the backdrop of the Women's Liberation Movement in the 1970s, some feminists wanted women to divest themselves from the constraints of domesticity entirely, and these demands became increasingly fraught and politicised. In 1974, feminist Ann Oakley argued for the total abolition of the housewife role and called for women's complete liberation from the home. But critics of this radical movement argued that, in practice, 'seventies feminists [had] simply prescribed a new set of impossible ideals for mothers'. Now, they not only had to be good mothers and partners, but ambitious women with glittering, professional careers. This dual demand became increasingly pressing in the 1980s, accompanied by anti-discrimination and equal opportunities legislation that should have made reconciling family and career easier for women.[51] But the figures suggest otherwise. While the picture for working mothers more broadly had improved, for professional women in traditionally male-dominated industries the rate of progress was slow. By the early 2000s women made up half of Britain's workforce and the participation rate of mothers with dependent children was nearly two-thirds.[52] In contrast, by the 1990s, just 10 per cent of senior civil servants, 14 per cent of barristers, and 7 per cent of university professors were female.[53]

In 1998, American anthropologist Joan Cassell published her book, *The Woman in the Surgeon's Body*. She followed thirty-three female surgeons through hospital corridors, onto the wards, and into the operating theatre, analysing what it was like to be a woman in these environments and explore how she was perceived by colleagues and patients. 'Anybody but the girl! Give me a trained monkey – I'd rather have anybody but the girl!', raged a senior male surgeon when scheduled to have a female trainee assisting him. While many of the elements of American healthcare are very different to the NHS, the book was reviewed favourably in the British medical press, with women on this side of the Atlantic observing similarities between Cassell's observations and their own experiences. As Sarah Creighton observed in the *BMJ*, 'Some difficulties experienced will be familiar to any woman working full time in a busy job either in or out of medicine.'[54]

Cassell's book and Creighton's review both identify many of the same challenges recognised by the Office for Public Management in 1991, including the problems involved in mixing surgery with parenthood. As one of the female surgeons interviewed by Cassell remarked, 'we need a wife' to help blend lengthy working hours with the running of the home, social life, and childcare.[55] Indeed, one of the most well studied and widely acknowledged difficulties about surgery is its inability to accommodate people with caring responsibilities. As one senior surgeon reflected in 2021, 'It used to be that you could be in theatre and then go out for a drink or to a meeting and go home knowing that everything was taken care of [by your wife]. I know it's not like that for many surgeons now.'[56]

Of course, people of all genders can be parents – and many surgeons are in same-sex relationships, where the gender dynamics of their union work differently. One male surgical trainee wrote to the Royal College of Surgeons in 2020 to say, 'I struggled to work part-time … with childcare issues. The Deanery may have pretended to be supportive, but all consultants in this trust were very difficult.'[57] In addition, many women cannot have children, are childfree by choice, and even if they do have kids they are not necessarily the primary care giver at home. With all those crucial caveats in mind, it remains true that women in heterosexual relationships undertake most of their family's reproductive labour, and a key obstacle to them advancing in their surgical careers is how hostile or impenetrable the profession can be to those with these kinds of responsibilities. In a survey of medical graduates conducted in 2017, while having children or wanting to have children had influenced the specialty choice of 59 per cent of women, just 29 per cent of men made a similar calculation.[58]

In 1997, the Labour Party won a landslide victory and brought in a series of NHS reforms. Modernising Medical Careers and the European Working Time Directive not only reduced working hours but also introduced part-time training and work contracts designed to enable more women to participate in the clinical labour force. However, over twenty years later, the challenges involved in combining parenthood and a surgical career remain, and almost every female surgeon I interviewed reflected on the difficulties of fitting family life around their jobs – even if they had not yet had children or were never intending on becoming parents. Male surgeons, on the other hand, only very rarely talked about their children or offered up difficulties they had experienced navigating the tensions between work and family life. While in many ways the gender politics of surgery reflect those of broader society, the profession still lags behind the British workforce as a whole. In 2018, the rate of mothers who participated in the British workforce with dependent children was nearly three-quarters.[59] A survey, also conducted in 2018, found that half of respondents agreed that 'motherhood and childcare commitments' were the greatest obstacles for female surgeons.[60] One female trainee was told that children 'simply [weren't] compatible with a career in surgery'.[61]

This mirrors the experiences of surgeons I interviewed, who brought up various explanations for the gender imbalance in their profession, including the unequal burden shouldered by mothers and fathers. While issues around gender equity pervade many different jobs and are a challenge for pretty much anyone trying to work in Britain, there are also some pressures unique to surgery that make the problem particularly fraught. Female surgeons tend to have their first child later in life, have fewer children, and report more issues with infertility when compared with the general population of women.[62] Most of the medical women who opt to defer parenthood do so because of the perceived threat children pose to their careers.[63]

This perception is, to some extent, accurate (or at least accurately describes how surgery is currently set up) and many of the women I interviewed reflected on how difficult it was to combine a full-time surgical career with parenthood. A female general surgeon, born in 1970, recalled her working experiences in the 1990s. She had a husband and a young baby and 'none of us were coping. The baby was on the ninth centile … I never met any sympathy … I walked out of that job.'[64] When she told her boss that she was pregnant, her line manager responded with, 'Oh well, why don't you just give up.'[65] This was not just a problem for women, but also affected men, even if they had not considered family life when selecting a surgical specialty. I asked a male paediatric oncology surgeon, who was born in 1944, about his experiences of combining a surgical career and parenthood. This was not something he had considered before, but on reflection he determined that perhaps he had not been the best father to his six children. None of them had opted to go into medicine and he thought that perhaps the career he had modelled for them had not been an inspiring or encouraging one. He told me that surgery 'destroys your home life'.[66]

One example of the unique pressures faced by female surgeons – and something that is very much tied to the professions' history – is that until relatively recently, surgical trainees were expected to devote hundreds of hours every week to their work and education. Even though twenty-first-century policies have (in theory) curtailed the duration of hospital doctors' shifts, surgery still requires excessive temporal commitment. Chapter 6 is devoted to this issue of what I call 'surgical time', but briefly, most surgeons acknowledge that their working hours are a considerable obstacle to mothers' participation in the profession. In 2017, just 32 per cent of surgeons surveyed thought that their speciality was 'family-friendly'.[67] For some surgeons, the excessive temporal commitment is an essential and innate feature of the job. It is impossible, they argue, to become a surgeon, acquire and maintain the requisite skills, without putting in the hours. As a result, trainees who are 'distracted' from their day job by children or other caring responsibilities are fundamentally unable to become surgeons, or at least competent ones.

The challenges associated with being a surgeon with caring responsibilities were partly addressed by the introduction of part-time, or less-than-full-time training. In 2009, the RCP commissioned a report in response to the rapid rise in the number of women entering the medical profession. The report, authored by Mary Ann Elston, recommended that NHS workforce planning must consider part-time or other forms of flexible working.[68] However, this route into the surgical profession is not without its criticism and has not been taken up by most of the people entering the field. One of the reasons for the criticism it attracts is that less-than-full-time training supposedly does not provide sufficient time in the operating theatre and so surgeons complete their training with less experience and a depleted skillset. It can also take an incredibly long time for trainee surgeons to become consultants. One trainee surgeon I spoke to, who is training on a less-than-full-time contract, told me that it is going to take her somewhere in the region of seventeen years to become a consultant after beginning her specialty training.[69] However, those who actually pursue this route claim it offers them as much, if not more, time in the operating theatre because they are better equipped or more empowered to prioritise surgical work – as in actually *operating* on patients – over administrative or bureaucratic labour.

It is pretty telling that where it is available, less-than-full-time training is accessed less frequently by surgical trainees compared with doctors in other medical specialties. Just 10 per cent of surgeons reported ever having worked less than full time, compared with almost half (47.7 per cent) of GPs, for example.[70] There was plenty of disagreement among the surgeons I have interviewed over how important time actually is in training or in acquiring the necessary skills to become a proficient surgeon. Some of the practitioners I spoke to insisted that it was crucial to spend as much time as possible in the operating theatre and they lamented the reduced amount of time that all current trainees (whether on part- or full-time contracts) can devote to the acquisition of new surgical skills because of different pressures that exist in the twenty-first-century hospital. There are plenty of surgeons today who critique the current round of trainees for being insufficiently experienced by the time they become consultants. In contrast, other surgeons I spoke to were far more ambivalent about the role of excessive temporal commitment in the acquisition of necessary surgical skill or technique. Rather than advocating for hours spent, these surgeons said that the quality of training and education trainees received was much more important than the time you managed to chalk up in theatre. There is also evidence to suggest that those in less-than-full-time roles are not being set up for success, as they report little logistical support and experience undermining behaviour as a result.[71]

Subspecialty stereotypes

The barriers female surgeons face identified in the 1992 report – outmoded attitudes about the role of women, discrimination, the absence of proper childcare, and inflexible structures for work and careers – all still apply to surgery and are hangovers from past decades, much like the ones I have been describing in this chapter and the previous three. Surgery is a broad church, however, and the issues vary widely from hospital to hospital, person to person, and subspecialty to subspecialty. This final caveat is crucial. When discussing diversity within surgery, the different subspecialities have very different profiles, are associated with different stereotypes, and face different challenges. As one person I interviewed said, plastic and ear, nose, and throat (ENT) surgeons are supposed to be skilled at fine-tuned, detailed work that requires plenty of manual dexterity (and are, as a result, attractive specialities to women with their supposedly more delicate fingers).[72] Cardiothoracic surgeons and neurosurgeons are both thought to have 'god complexes' and are populated by the most arrogant and self-assured practitioners.[73] They are, also, some of the most hostile to female surgeons and are some of the least diverse.

Multiple women I interviewed reported being recommended breast surgery as a particularly 'female friendly' subspecialty. It was also one of the first subspecialities to consider what was then called 'equal opportunities' and to advocate for more female surgeons joining its ranks. There was some research conducted in the 1980s and 1990s that looked at patient preference when it came to their breast surgeon. This research determined that female patients, by and large, would rather be operated on by a woman and so there was a concerted effort to recruit more female surgeons to the subspecialty by altering workplace practices, cultures, and labour conditions.[74] Paediatrics, also, is seen as an appropriate destination for female surgical trainees and has the highest proportion of women among its ranks of any subspecialty.[75]

Patient perception has proven profoundly influential in other aspects of female surgeons' progression, or lack thereof. There is plenty of research that suggests that patients perceive expressions of warmth and emotional connection in a male surgeon as indicating operative competence. In contrast, female surgeons who adopt or express similar emotional styles are assumed to be neither skilled nor capable.[76] Almost all the female surgeons I interviewed talked about being mistaken for a nurse on a regular basis. This was particularly true for the Black and South Asian women I spoke to. Nurses are highly skilled professionals who are equal partners to surgeons in the delivery of healthcare, but it is also a profoundly gendered occupation and practitioners are often dismissed in the public arena (and sometimes in clinical spaces as well) as inferior to doctors. As a result, patients who assume that female surgeons are nurses are indirectly (and probably inadvertently) denigrating their professional status and skill.

The surgical stereotype is not, and has never been, a consistent or homogeneous image, and the supposed differences between subspecialties are constantly re-inscribed by cultural representations and healthcare professionals themselves. In the popular American television drama, *Grey's Anatomy*, Derek Shepherd, aka McDreamy, the neurosurgeon, is reserved, aloof, and arrogant, whereas his female colleague, the paediatric surgeon Arizona Robbins, is bubbly and warm, and zips around the hospital on shoes with inbuilt roller-skate wheels.[77] Similarly, the US ophthalmologist, who goes by 'Dr Glaucomflecken' on social media sites, has become famous from his TikTok videos that send up the different surgical and medical specialities and frequently portrays general surgeons as workaholics unable to maintain relationships with family and friends, vascular surgeons as unfeeling masochists, and orthopaedic surgeons as weight-lifting 'bros'.[78]

Orthopaedics is perhaps – along with cardio- and neurosurgery – the most notoriously male. It is the subspeciality where the 'old boys' club' is supposedly most influential and still has a reputation of being largely populated by public school boys. It is also the subspeciality which seems to have made the most effort to reform its image, particularly through social media campaigns.[79] Orthopaedic surgeons specialise in surgical treatments for problems caused by disease, injury, and trauma to the bones and joints. As one female consultant said to me, there did not used to be so many 'power tools' in orthopaedics, and so a 'kind of physicality' used be to a necessary attribute of orthopaedic surgeons.[80] It is easy to overstate the influence of this obstacle, as women have trained and qualified as orthopaedic surgeons for a century or more – well before the introduction of power tools – but there were also other, subtler cultural barriers. As the same female consultant observed, 'There used to be an absolute stereotype of the orthopaedic surgeon being this grunting gorilla.'[81] Despite her optimistic turn of phrase ('used to be') and the efforts of reforming 'orthopods' (as they are colloquially known), that stereotype persists and change within the subspecialty is painfully slow. In 1995, just 2 per cent of orthopaedic consultants were women, and just 3 per cent of trainees.[82] As Sian Caiach, a female orthopaedic consultant herself, said, 'My own experiences as a trainee would hardly encourage other members of my sex.'[83] When I started this book, only 11 per cent of those in orthopaedics were women and the situation has not improved much since.[84]

These perceptions of different subspecialities – as well as of surgery as a whole – are powerful and continue to dissuade women from selecting the profession. As discussed, stereotypes of the archetypal surgeon often embody masculine traits: competitive, stubborn, and confident. These same traits in a woman are frequently interpreted as aggressive, inflexible, and difficult.[85] Coupled with a lack of senior female role models in surgery, these cultural barriers have proven remarkably enduring. As one female surgeon I interviewed said, 'it's all very well trying to encourage women into surgery', but if there are not any good role models, then it does not seem like an attractive option for trainee surgeons selecting their future careers.[86] A female orthopaedic trainee I interviewed in 2021 said that orthopaedics is 'particularly bad', dominated by 'alpha male', 'golfing' types – a stereotype that was off-putting because she did not want to have to subscribe to a 'certain personality type' just so that she could succeed in her career.[87]

This notion that women must conform to a particular way of being or behaving in order to assimilate is widespread and causes its own problems. Many female surgeons I spoke to talked about the women who had managed to climb the surgical career ladder, but who either possessed or had adopted a personality style that aligned closely with the macho men that they worked with. The female orthopaedic trainee mentioned above described how the women who succeeded in orthopaedic surgery – and particularly members of the previous generation – tended not to have children (either by choice or necessity – or some complex combination of the two) and were completely focused on their careers. These were women who were incredibly successful professionally – talented, senior surgeons – but who had a life that she did not want to emulate.

The subtlety of discrimination

The idea that women who want to succeed in surgery must assimilate into male professional and emotional cultures was also expressed by those who felt they *had* managed to emulate the behaviours and attitudes of their male colleagues. Several female surgeons I spoke to initially denied that they had ever faced discrimination or that their gender had proven problematic in their career, or they minimised the sexism they had experienced. One interviewee said that she had only had 'problems with sexism' on a handful of occasions.[88] However, as our conversation developed, it became clear (to her) that her experience was perhaps more ambivalent than she had first thought. She described how the more time she spent on surgical rotations, the more she had herself 'adhered to the stereotype'. For her, this was a strategic act. The more she behaved 'like a surgeon', the more respect she received from her (mostly male) colleagues.[89]

She was not alone in pursuing this strategy, nor was she alone in identifying other – usually more senior – women as obstacles rather than allies in the workplace. Many female interviewees described how other women, particularly those who had trained in previous decades, could be hostile or ally themselves with male colleagues to defend traditional, even regressive, models of surgical behaviour. This behaviour was often rationalised by the argument that these women from previous generations had had to overcome extreme opposition and discrimination, and that they had often had to make great personal sacrifice for the sake of professional advancement. Trainee surgeons thought that these more senior women felt that because they had survived, even thrived, under these conditions, then all the women who came after them ought to do the same. They were often unwilling to entertain altering the surgical landscape to better accommodate women and other marginalised groups, or saw younger female surgeons as professional rivals seeking to undermine their sometimes-precarious position within the hospital.

These narratives can sometimes be an unintended consequence of internalised misogyny on both sides. Professional success is often hard won by women and those who manage to weather the storm can end up understandably jaded or mistrustful. In addition, the patriarchal structures in which women work are designed to undermine the connections and community that can form between women by stereotyping female professionals as cruel, insensitive, or 'catty'. Moreover, there is an unsaid assumption that there is only enough room in some professional circles for one successful woman at a time, whereas there is infinite space for male surgeons to thrive, however mediocre they might be.

Sexual harassment

In the early decades of the NHS, there were no legal or technical obstacles to women becoming surgeons, but there were also few legal or technical *protections* for female clinicians, and sexual harassment and discrimination were commonplace in mid-twentieth-century surgical communities. The Sex Discrimination Act – which protected men and women from discrimination on the grounds of sex or marital status – was only passed in 1975.[90] Even in the absence of straightforward sex-based discrimination or harassment of individuals, sexual language and conduct permeated hospitals and helped create a culture that was hostile to female professionals. The ABC Club – a society of travelling fellows in orthopaedic surgery from America, Britain, and Canada – recorded the japes and exploits of their members while on tour.[91] The first ever group of fellows who visited North America from Britain in 1948 included one woman, Marion Pearson from Pinderfields, Yorkshire. She, along with the rest of them, visited New York, Boston, Washington DC, Montreal, and Chicago.[92] Her words are absent from the archival accounts of their trip, but there are suggestions that perhaps her position as the only woman put her in uncomfortable situations.

One of the group's American hosts told a version of his 'celebrated "Uncle Fud" story'. Despite a 'pointed suggestion to Marion that she should leave the room', she insisted on remaining. Hugh 'pulled no punches in telling the rather rambling story in full, lurid detail, including dockside language, at the same time doing a striptease so that, by the time the story ended, he was stripped to the waist!' His escapades 'raised some rather prudish English eyebrows'.[93] While there is no reason to think that Marion, as a woman, was any more prudish than any of the men in her company, the raucous, macho behaviour of her male colleagues calls to mind the 'laddish', fundamentally exclusionary behaviour of men in a range of modern and contemporary social and professional settings such as public schools, universities, and gentlemen's clubs.[94] On another occasion, Marion had to suffer through a protracted joke in which another orthopaedic surgeon paraded around 'stark naked'.[95]

Sexual attention was frequently directed towards women in the clinical workplace. Hugh E. Stephenson recorded the tradition of Edinburgh medical students signalling their approval of lectures with 'a stomping of feet'. His 'first encounter with this action' took place prior to the start of a lecture, 'when Sister McLeod, an attractive young nurse in charge of Professor Sir John Bruce's ward, suddenly walked into the classroom accompanied by thunderous stomping of feet'.[96] It is not clear whether the students were applauding Sister McLeod's skill and technical abilities, or whether they were showing their appreciation for her 'attractive' appearance. On his visit to England, Scotland, and Ireland in 1964, Colin C. Ferguson praised the proficiency and professionalism of British and Irish nurses: 'Nursing Sisters in charge of surgical wards occupy a much more responsible position than do their colleagues on this side of the Atlantic.'[97] His praise contained, however, a comment on their looks:

> All of them were extremely competent, pretty, young ladies with a sense of humour which certainly helped them to cope with their numerous clinical problems. They worked long hours, arranged for the admissions and discharges of patients, changed dressings, removed sutures, reassured anxious parents and gave instructions for postoperative home care.[98]

Nurses were often objects of desire in the hospital and they frequently married the surgeons and physicians they worked with. The 1960s witnessed an emerging sexualised stereotype of nurses, partly a product of popular culture like the television series and film *Doctor in the House* and the *Carry On* films.[99] Romance novels were also increasingly featuring doctors and nurses as the heroes and heroines in their narratives of heterosexual love. In the 1962 novel, *Staff Nurses in Love* (written under the pseudonym Hilda Pressley and published by Mills & Boon), the heroine's best friend Brenda says, 'For every one Florence Nightingale in nursing … there are dozens more like me who take up nursing because they think they might be able to hook a famous doctor or surgeon.'[100] This strategy was often successful – and not just in the fictional world of medical romance. Healthcare professionals still tend to marry one another and 40 per cent of doctors today are currently married to other healthcare professionals.[101]

Sexual harassment and bullying are also still relatively common features of the surgical career. While some of the surgeons I interviewed suggested that female colleagues were partly responsible for the challenges they faced in their careers, most identified male surgeons or broader, patriarchal structures for the discrimination they received. One woman who had left the profession said that while she loved operating, all the 'other stuff' made it untenable for her to continue with her surgical career. Giving up medicine was a 'big deal' for her – it was something she had always wanted.[102] But the stereotyping of women she observed was oppressive. She said it was active in every hospital she worked in, and she was surprised at how obvious and explicit it was. Many of the difficulties she experienced were to do with the profoundly hierarchical structure of surgery – this was a world where senior practitioners publicly 'put down' their juniors. She also suggested that 'less emotionally tuned in' personalities were drawn to surgery, and that when on orthopaedic rotations others insisted that she 'really had to be a man' to succeed in the subspeciality.[103]

She described instances of public humiliation where consultants who were supposed to be responsible for her wellbeing and career progression asked her to clean their muddy boots or fill up their water glasses to precise levels. If she erred, even slightly, she was shouted at. None of her more senior male colleagues respected her, and instructed her to undertake menial tasks. Other doctors expressed surprise when she told them she was a surgical trainee and she faced dismissive assumptions about her operating skills. She was not given appropriate opportunities and her efforts were not recognised. She told me how she did not have many female friends who stayed in surgery; instead they left to take up positions in paediatrics or general practice. When I asked her what she thought the root cause of this bullying, discrimination, and harassment was, she said that while 'old white men lead everywhere', in healthcare everyone is bound by hierarchy.[104] Echoing some of the themes of Chapter 3, she described the influence of 'old money' and 'patronage' and suggested that part of the problem was that hospitals did not have robust human resources departments.[105] There was no infrastructure to provide her with support, opportunities for retribution, or sanction her discriminatory colleagues. Unlike the organisations that she worked in since leaving medicine (like information technology companies or government), HR departments in healthcare often have insufficient capacity and insufficient expertise to tackle the embedded nature of gendered discrimination and harassment.[106]

Bullying has recently been recognised as a serious problem in British surgery. In 2015, the NHS Staff Survey for England reported that almost a quarter of all NHS staff experienced harassment, bullying, or abuse from colleagues over the course of the previous twelve months.[107] In response, various professional organisations established web pages and resources for their members designed to reduce the prevalence and impact of these behaviours. As the RCSEd's website acknowledges, 'Not only does this have a devastating impact on individuals and the teams within which they work, but it can have dire consequences for patient care.'[108] Studies in the US have attributed disruptive behaviour in and around the operating theatre to 67 per cent of adverse events, 71 per cent of medical errors, and 27 per cent of perioperative deaths.[109] In the case of the female surgeon described in the previous paragraphs, bullying was one of main the reasons she chose to leave the profession entirely. And she is not alone. Research suggests that bullying costs the NHS in England at least £2.3 billion a year in sickness absences, employee turnover, productivity, and employment relations.[110] While these issues occur across the health service, surgeons acknowledge that they are particularly common within the specialty. One trainee surgeon I interviewed was told to stop holding her scalpels and other tools 'like a girl' and to stop allowing her 'uterus' to control her mind. A female foundation-year doctor was asked in front of a room full of senior surgeons which sexual act she had performed to obtain an MRI in a timely fashion. One woman even told me about a time she was sexually harassed and groped *while operating* on a patient.[111]

Conclusion

In 1980, the then president of the Royal College of Surgeons doubted 'whether surgery is particularly suitable for women'.[112] It is unlikely that someone in a similar position of power and influence would get away with saying something like this today. And there are many male surgeons (including those I have interviewed) who are actively working to dispel harmful gendered stereotypes about the profession, men who are taking it upon themselves to challenge co-workers, structures, and institutions about the way they treat their female colleagues and advocate for lasting change. However, it is important to note that the goodwill of individuals is necessary but not sufficient to change the culture of surgery. While there are plenty of admirable programmes that aim to empower female surgeons and increase the visibility of women in clinical fields, there also needs to be structural transformation and an acknowledgement that female surgeons in positions of prominence can only do so much.

As this chapter has shown, one of the key obstacles facing women in surgery today is workplaces ill-equipped to handle parenthood. Thus, there need to be new efforts to change the anti-social, anti-family, and anti-wellbeing cultures of surgical work (that harm everyone, not just women) such as expanded opportunities for less-than-full-time work, greater support for people in those roles, and increasing acceptance of shared parental leave. Many women working today would recognise the observation made by a female doctor in 1978: 'One has to have a co-operative husband, undemanding children, reliable help at home, limitless mental and physical energy, and enormous determination.'[113] Or, as the women interviewed in Cassell's ethnography suggested, they need 'wives' of their own.

However, we also need to make the men responsible for the stories described above accountable for their cruel and sometimes criminal behaviour. We need to not only empower women to pursue surgical careers, but ensure that they feel confident enough to report the misogynistic behaviour they encounter, safe in the knowledge that the behaviour will be sanctioned appropriately and will not negatively impact their own careers. And finally, we need to not just place the onus on women for their own liberation. Male surgeons need to address their own capacity for sex-based harassment and discrimination and, at the very least, call out their colleagues when they speculate about their female co-worker's deployment of sexual acts in the workplace.

There also needs to be an acknowledgement that while many of the issues female surgeons tackle are challenges faced by women in all sorts of twenty-first-century professions, there is also something particular about surgery that requires tailored attention. Surgery has long been a male-dominated profession, but it is also a profession with deeply felt and widely held assumptions about what a surgeon looks and behaves like. Moreover, those assumptions are held by fellow healthcare professionals, members of the general public, and – crucially – medical students. Indeed, as this chapter has shown, the construction and maintenance of the surgical stereotype as male has had lasting effects on who is allowed access to the profession, what kind of healthcare practitioners patients will anticipate or tolerate, and the expectations of appropriate conduct both in and out of the operating theatre. In the next chapter, I will explore a similar story of discrimination and exclusion, although this time I will focus on race and ethnicity and the enduring construction of the surgeon as not just male, but white, British-born, and English-speaking.

Notes

1 Joan Cassell, 'Doing Gender, Doing Surgery: Women Surgeons in a Man's Profession', *Human Organization*, 56:1 (1997), 47–52, 47.

2 Ibid.

3 See Claire Brock, *British Women Surgeons and their Patients, 1860–1918* (Cambridge: Cambridge University Press, 2017).

4 Maria Irene Bellini et al., 'A Woman's Place is in Theatre: Women's Perceptions and Experiences of Working in Surgery from the Association of Surgeons of Great Britain and Ireland Women in Surgery Working Group', *BMJ Open*, 9 (2019), 1–8.

5 Wendy Crebbin et al., 'Prevalence of Bullying, Discrimination and Sexual Harassment in Surgery in Australia', *Australia and New Zealand Journal of Surgery*, 85 (2015), 905–909.

6 Agnes Arnold-Forster, 'Sexism in Surgery: Little has Changed', *BMJ Opinion* (2018), https://bit.ly/3ozkOPL (accessed 20 May 2021).

7 See Roberta Bivins, 'Picturing Race in the British NHS, 1948–1988', *Twentieth Century British History*, 28:1 (2017), 83–109; Jack Saunders, 'Emotions, Social Practices and the Changing Composition of Class, Race and Gender in the NHS, 1970–79', *History Workshop Journal*, 88 (2019), 204–229.

8 Black feminist scholar Kimberlé Crenshaw coined the term 'intersectionality' and critiques the 'narrow scope' of the concept of discrimination and its 'tendency to marginalize those whose experiences cannot be described within its tightly-drawn parameters'. Kimberlé Crenshaw, 'Demarginalizing the Intersection of Race and Sex: A Black Feminist Critique of Antidiscrimination Doctrine, Feminist Theory and Antiracist Politics', *University of Chicago Legal Forum*, 1:8 (1989), 139–167, 152.

9 Brock, *British Women Surgeons and their Patients, 1860–1918*.

10 Agnes Arnold-Forster and Alison Moulds, 'Medical Women in Popular Fiction', *BMJ Opinion* (2018), https://blogs.bmj.com/bmj/2018/09/26/agnes-arnold-forster-alison-moulds-medical-women-popular-fiction/ (accessed 20 May 2021).

11 Shirley Roberts, 'Sophia Louisa Jex-Blake (1840–1912)', *Oxford Dictionary of National Biography*, www.oxforddnb.com/view/10.1093/ref:odnb/9780198614128.001.0001/odnb-9780198614128-e-34189 (accessed 20 May. 2021).
12 Alison Moulds, 'Medical Women: Perspectives from the Victorian Medical Profession', *Royal College of Surgeons Bulletin* (2017), 255–257, 255.
13 Brock, *British Women Surgeons and their Patients, 1860–1918*, 19.
14 Royal College of Physicians, 'Helen Marion Macpherson Mackay', https://history.rcplondon.ac.uk/inspiring-physicians/helen-marion-macpherson-mackay (accessed 20 May 2021).
15 Quoted in Brock, *British Women Surgeons and their Patients, 1860–1918*, 2.
16 'Maud Mary Chadburn C.B.E., M.D. Lond.', *The Lancet*, 269:6975 (1957), 938–940, 940.
17 'Women, Work and the NHS: Balance for Better', *NHS Voices of Covid-19*, www.nhs70.org.uk/story/women-work-and-nhs-balance-better (accessed 20 May 2021).
18 Evelyn Mary Biske, 'On Call to a Nation', *British Medical Journal*, 2:5105 (1958), 1162.
19 Hugh E. Stephenson, 'Undergraduate Surgical Teaching in the United Kingdom and Ireland'. Reprinted from *Surgery*, 65 (1964), 321–333, James IV Association of Surgeons Records, 326.
20 Ibid.
21 Jean Lawrie, 'Training our Specialists', *The Lancet*, 289:7484 (1967), 74.
22 James IV Association of Surgeons Records. The Drs. Barry and Bobbi Coller Rare Book Reading Room, New York Academy of Medicine Library.
23 Stephenson, 'Undergraduate Surgical Teaching in the United Kingdom and Ireland', 324.
24 Ibid.
25 Laura Jefferson, Karen Bloor, and Alan Maynard, 'Women in Medicine: Historical Perspectives and Recent Trends', *British Medical Bulletin*, 114:1 (2015), 5–15, 8.
26 Ibid.
27 Ibid., 9.
28 Ibid.
29 Ibid.
30 Marie Norredam and Dag Album, 'Prestige and its Significance for Medical Specialities and Diseases', *Scandinavian Journal of Public Health*, 35:6 (2007), 655–668, 657.
31 Peter Forster, 'Equal Opportunities: Progress so Far', *British Medical Journal*, 304:6827 (1992), 630–632, 631.

32 Jennifer Trueland, 'And You Thought Surgery was Hard…', *British Medical Association* (11 June 2021), www.bma.org.uk/news-and-opinion/and-you-thought-surgery-was-hard (accessed 4 August 2022).
33 Royal College of Surgeons, 'Statistics', www.rcseng.ac.uk/careers-in-surgery/women-in-surgery/statistics/ (accessed 20 May 2021).
34 Forster, 'Equal Opportunities: Progress so Far', 630.
35 Ibid.
36 Ibid., 632.
37 Ibid.
38 Ibid.
39 Claire L. Donohoe and H. M. Mohan, 'Pregnancy, Parenthood and Second-Generation Bias: Women in Surgery', *British Journal of Surgery*, 108:1 (2021), 1–2, 1.
40 Ibid.
41 Mary Ann Elston, 'Medicine: Half our Future Doctors?', in Rosalie Silverstone and Audrey Ward (eds), *Careers of Professional Women* (London: Routledge, 1980), 99–139.
42 Helen McCarthy, *Double Lives: A History of Working Motherhood in Modern Britain* (London: Bloomsbury, 2020), 3.
43 Ibid., 201.
44 Quoted in ibid., 212.
45 Ibid., 208.
46 Jane Lewis, 'Myrdal, Klein, *Women's Two Roles* and Postwar Feminism 1945–1960', in Harold L. Smith (ed.), *British Feminism in the Twentieth Century* (Aldershot: Edward Elgar, 1990), 167–188, 167.
47 Ibid., 168.
48 Ibid.
49 Claire Langhamer, 'Feelings, Women and Work in the Long 1950s', *Women's History Review*, 26:1 (2017), 77–92, 79.
50 McCarthy, *Double Lives*, 279.
51 Ibid., 358.
52 Ibid., 4.
53 Ibid., 360.
54 Sarah Creighton, 'Reviewed Work(s): The Woman in the Surgeon's Body by Joan Cassell', *British Medical Journal*, 317:7165 (1998), 1088.
55 Ibid.
56 Royal College of Surgeons of England, 'The Royal College: Our Professional Home. An Independent Review on Diversity and Inclusion for the Royal College of Surgeons of England. An Exciting Call for Radical Change' (March 2021), 30.
57 Ibid.

58 Trevor W. Lambert, Fay Smith, and Michael J. Goldacre, 'Combining Parenthood with a Medical Career: Questionnaire Survey of the UK Medical Graduates of 2002 Covering Some Influences and Experiences', *BMJ Open*, 7:8 (2017), 1–8, 1.
59 McCarthy, *Double Lives*, 4.
60 'More than Half of UK Female Surgeons have Experience of Workplace Discrimination, Poll Suggests', *British Medical Journal* (2018), www.bmj.com/company/newsroom/more-than-half-of-uk-female-surgeons-have-experience-of-workplace-discrimination-poll-suggests/ (accessed 4 August 2022).
61 Trueland, 'And You Thought Surgery was Hard…'.
62 E. A. Phillips et al., 'Does a Surgical Career Affect a Woman's Childbearing and Fertility? A Report on Pregnancy and Fertility Trends Among Female Surgeons', *Journal of the American College of Surgery*, 219 (2014), 944–950.
63 L. L. Willett et al., 'Do Women Residents Delay Childbearing due to Perceived Career Threats?', *Academic Medicine*, 85 (2010), 640–646.
64 Interview with female surgeon; interviewed by author, 12 January 2018.
65 Ibid.
66 Interview with female surgeon; interviewed by author, 18 January 2018.
67 Lambert et al., 'Combining Parenthood with a Medical Career', 1.
68 Mary Ann Elston, *Women and Medicine: The Future* (London: Royal College of Physicians, 2009).
69 Interview with female surgeon; interviewed by author, 18 February 2021.
70 Trueland, 'And You Thought Surgery was Hard…'.
71 R. L. Harries et al., 'Less than Full-Time Training in Surgery: A Cross-Sectional Study Evaluating the Accessibility and Experiences of Flexible Training in the Surgical Trainee Workforce', *BMJ Open*, 6 (2016), e010136.
72 Interview with female surgeon; interviewed by author, 17 February 2021.
73 Ibid.
74 Iona Reid, 'Patients' Preference for Male or Female Breast Surgeons: Questionnaire Study', *British Medical Journal*, 317:7165 (1998), 1051–1060.
75 Nicola P. Smith, Evelyn H. Dykes, George S. Youngson, and Paul D. Losty, 'Is the Grass Greener? A Survey of Female Pediatric Surgeons in the United Kingdom', *Journal of Pediatric Surgery*, 41:11 (2006), 1879–1881, 1880.
76 C. E. Ashton-James, J. M. Tybur, V. Grießer, and D. Costa, 'Stereotypes About Surgeon Warmth and Competence: The Role of Surgeon Gender', *PLoS One*, 14 (2019), e0211890.

77 Deborah Lupton, 'Grey's Anatomy is Unrealistic, But it Might Make Junior Doctors More Compassionate', *The Conversation* (19 February 2018), https://theconversation.com/greys-anatomy-is-unrealistic-but-it-might-make-junior-doctors-more-compassionate-92040 (accessed 20 May 2021).

78 Eleanor Cummins, 'How Dr Glaucomflecken Overcame Death to Get Internet Laughs', *Medscape* (10 March 2021), www.medscape.com/viewarticle/947199 (accessed 20 May 2021).

79 #HammerItOut, https://twitter.com/hammeritoutuk (accessed 20 May 2021).

80 Interview with female surgeon; interviewed by author, 24 November 2017.

81 Ibid.

82 Sian Caiach, 'Training Doctors', *British Medical Journal*, 310:6992 (1995), 1473.

83 Ibid.

84 Tom Moberly, 'A Fifth of England's Surgeons are Women', *British Medical Journal*, 363 (2018), 209.

85 L. A. Rudman and P. Glick, 'Feminized Management and Backlash toward Agentic Women: The Hidden Costs to Women of a Kinder, Gentler Image of Middle Managers', *Journal of Personal and Social Psychology*, 77:5 (1999), 1004–1010.

86 Interview with female surgeon; interviewed by author, 24 February 2021.

87 Interview with female surgeon; interviewed by author, 18 February 2021.

88 Interview with female surgeon; interviewed by author, 11 February 2021.

89 Ibid.

90 Sex Discrimination Act (1975), www.legislation.gov.uk/ukpga/1975/65/pdfs/ukpga_19750065_en.pdf (accessed 20 May 2021), 1–81.

91 F. G. St Clair Strange, *The History of the ABC Club of Travelling Fellows* (London: British Editorial Society of Bone and Joint Surgery, 1998).

92 Ibid., 2.

93 Ibid., 16.

94 University of Sussex, National Union of Students, 'That's What She Said: Women Students' Experiences of "Lad Culture" in Higher Education', http://sro.sussex.ac.uk/id/eprint/49011/1/That's_what_she_said_full_report_Final_web.pdf (accessed 20 May 2021).

95 St Clair Strange, *The History of the ABC Club of Travelling Fellows*, 23.

96 Stephenson, 'Undergraduate Surgical Teaching in the United Kingdom and Ireland', 326.

97 Colin C. Ferguson, 'Summary of a Visit to England, Scotland and Ireland as a James IV Surgical Traveller', 1965, James IV Association of Surgeons Records.

98 Ibid.

99 Malcolm Newby, 'Nursing at the Movies', *Nursing Standard*, 3:32 (1989), 13.

100 Hilda Pressley, *Staff Nurses in Love* (London: Mills & Boon, 1962), 9.

101 AMA Insurance reported in the 2014 'Work/Life Profiles of Today's U.S. Physician' that 40 per cent of doctors marry other doctors or healthcare professionals: www.kevinmd.com/blog/2016/03/doctors-marry-doctors-challenges-face.html (accessed 20 May 2021). The case in the UK is similar: Kathy Oxtoby, 'Love on the Wards: Relationships between Doctors', *British Medical Journal*, 351 (2015).

102 Interview with female surgeon; interviewed by author, 17 February 2021.

103 Ibid.

104 Ibid.

105 Ibid.

106 J. R. L. Wild et al., 'Undermining and Bullying in Surgical Training: A Review and Recommendations by the Association of Surgeons in Training', *International Journal of Surgery*, 23:1 (2015), S5–S9.

107 Sarah Johnson, 'NHS Staff Lay Bare a Bullying Culture', *The Guardian* (26 October 2016), www.theguardian.com/society/2016/oct/26/nhs-staff-bullying-culture-guardian-survey (accessed 20 May 2021).

108 Royal College of Surgeons of Edinburgh, www.rcsed.ac.uk/professional-support-development-resources/anti-bullying-and-undermining-campaign (accessed 20 May 2021).

109 Alan H. Rosenstein and Michelle O'Daniel, 'A Survey of the Impact of Disruptive Behaviors and Communication Defects on Patient Safety', *Joint Commission Journal on Quality and Patient Safety*, 34:8 (2008), 464–471.

110 www.rcsed.ac.uk/professional-support-development-resources/anti-bullying-and-undermining-campaign.

111 Arnold-Forster, 'Sexism in Surgery: Little has Changed'.

112 '"It is Absurd," Says Dr Anne Gruneberg, "That it should be a Handicap in Obstetrics to have had a Baby"', *The Guardian* (7 April 1980), 8.

113 Berenice Beaumont, 'Talking Point: Training and Careers of Women Doctors in the Thames Regions', *British Medical Journal*, 1:6106 (1978), 191–193, 192.

5

Race and ethnicity in surgery

In the wake of the Black Lives Matter movement in summer 2020, Professor Neil Mortensen, president of the Royal College of Surgeons of England, commissioned an independent review into the diversity of the leadership of the surgical profession and of the College. Led by Baroness Helena Kennedy QC, the report concluded that the College was not a 'diverse and inclusive institution' and did not reflect society nor the changing profession of surgery. The report was published in March 2021 and is replete with personal testimonies of racism and discrimination: 'I feel [as a Black surgeon] that I suffer a different level of scrutiny from other surgeons – and have access to much less support – and it can be very frightening.'[1] As shown in the previous chapter, surgery is male-dominated, but it has also – at least historically – been predominantly white.

While the proportion of practitioners from minoritised races has increased since the foundation of the NHS, surgeons of colour continue to report professional discrimination and cite unconscious bias, reduced opportunities, and restricted career progression as obstacles to full participation in the surgical community. Black surgeons in particular are woefully under-represented in the profession.[2] Both overseas doctors and surgeons from minoritised races born in the UK have been subjected to racism by both colleagues and patients. There also does not seem to be an obvious trajectory of improvement, with racist violence and abuse directed at healthcare professionals increasing in recent years.[3] The problem is even more acute for women of colour, who experience a double discrimination and are excluded on grounds of both ethnicity and gender.[4] These various challenges and inequalities are products of surgery's history – as well as the cultural, social, and political dynamics of modern and contemporary Britain.

In this chapter, I explore this facet of surgery's history, tracing the experiences of the surgeons from minoritised races who moved to Britain after the Second World War, as well as those who were born here, educated at UK universities, and trained in the NHS. I set surgery in its historical context and map shifts within the profession against broader political, legislative, and administrative transformations. The story of surgeons of colour is, to some extent, the story of all people of colour in Britain. In other words, the NHS and the surgical profession are both part of British society, and as a result they reflect even its worst aspects. As the RCS's review observed, 'there is no institution in the land that would survive close scrutiny'.[5] But there are some things about surgery – its stereotypes and the way it has been organised and structured – that have made it into a particularly hostile or exclusionary profession.

Since the mid-twentieth century, the language we use to talk about different races and ethnicities has changed and there is still plenty of debate over what works best. Prior to around 2000, most people within surgery talked about 'overseas' or 'foreign' doctors or described people according to their place of birth – 'Indian' or 'Pakistani', for example. Today, the phrase most commonly used to describe surgeons who have moved to the UK for work or training is 'International Medical Graduate' or 'IMG'. In this chapter, and wherever possible, I have been specific about surgeons' ethnic identity and used the terminology they use to describe themselves. I have also avoided defining people by what they are not and stayed away from terms like 'non-white'. However, at various points it has been useful to speak collectively about surgeons from minoritised races. In Britain, the phrase 'Black and Minority Ethnic' – frequently shortened to 'BAME' – has been widespread in government, professional circles, and in common parlance since the beginning of this millennium. Recently, however, it has been criticised for inaccurately homogenising people with very different experiences of life, work, and racism.[6] I have, as a result, opted not to use the phrase, using instead 'minoritised races'. The term 'minoritised', coined by Yasmin Gunaratnum in 2003, provides a 'social constructionist approach' to better encapsulate the variety of ways that people are *actively* minoritised by others.[7] The idea is to emphasise that minoritisation is a social process, 'shaped by power', rather than an accidental, automatic, or natural phenomena. Where appropriate and where possible, I have used more specific terms like Indian, Black, and Asian. I have also joined the Associated Press and the RCS's review in capitalising 'Black' throughout.[8]

Race, migration, and surgery in post-war Britain

The post-war surgical cultures and communities described in Chapter 3 were primarily open to white, English-speaking practitioners. In a range of implicit and explicit ways, race, ethnicity, and language acted as conditions of entry to the surgical profession. This was true even in a country and health service that was becoming increasingly ethnically diverse, and in a profession that prided itself on its global community and on the virtues of an international 'language' of science. As Roberta Bivins has shown, 'race' in the wake of the Second World War was a 'hotly contested and politically sensitive term and concept'. While the notion of fixed biological race was in 'sharp decline', 'race' (or 'colour') remained a key variable and analytic category in medical research, practice, and public health.[9]

Since its inception in 1948, Britain's National Health Service has depended on the talents of its diverse workforce. In the same year, the passengers of HMT *Empire Windrush* disembarked at the Port of Tilbury on the 22nd of June. Throughout its history, the NHS has employed doctors, nurses, and other healthcare practitioners who travelled to Britain from its past or present colonies. These men and women not only brought their substantial skills and expertise, but met a crucial need. By 1955, the Ministry of Health had official recruitment campaigns in sixteen British colonies, both current and former.[10] In his 1964 assessment of undergraduate surgical teaching in the United Kingdom and Ireland, visiting American surgeon Hugh E. Stephenson explained why doctors from India were an essential component of the British health system. While approximately 1,600 students graduated from the twenty-six medical schools each year, 'this total is considered inadequate for providing proper medical care under the National Health Service'. Thus, approximately 4,000 (about 50 per cent) of the residency positions in the British Isles were 'currently filled by graduates from foreign medical schools'. To partially address this shortfall in ‘home-grown’ medical students, ‘two new medical schools are, I understand, in the planning stage and possibly will be located at Southampton and Nottingham’.[11] However, even these institutions would be insufficient to provide the person-power required, and so Britain looked abroad for recruits.

Britain was not the only nation in the Global North dependent on the labour of mostly Asian healthcare professionals, and the situation in the United States was similar. Under the Hart-Celler Immigration and Nationality Act of 1965, the US began to solicit foreign medical graduates largely from South Asian nations. These graduates were granted permanent residency or US citizenship in exchange for medical services in marginalised communities. Although this arrangement was initially conceived of as a temporary solution, and much like in Britain, it soon become a ‘permanent fix’, with foreign doctors now comprising a quarter of the physician labour force.[12] As in Britain, and according to historian Eram Alam, ‘the care provided by foreigners was received as different, an imperfect facsimile of their US counterparts’.[13] Sasha Mullally and David Wright tell a parallel story about the migration of trained health personnel from South Asia to Canada in the mid-twentieth century, which formed part of a large-scale movement of doctors relocating across national borders in the 1960s and 1970s. These international migrations attracted concern, and not just from white British, Canadian, and American surgeons. Alfonso Mejia, chief medical officer of Manpower Systems for the World Health Organisation, noted in 1978 how ‘anxiety evoked by migration was reach[ing] a peak in both major donor and recipient countries’. This ‘brain drain’ was predicated on global economic inequalities and proved profoundly profitable for Britain, Canada, and the United States of America.[14]

Experiences of surgeons from minoritised races in post-war Britain

By 1971, 31 per cent of all doctors in the UK were born and had qualified overseas.[15] It is, however, incredibly difficult to find data on the historic ethnic make-up of British surgeons. This is true of the 1970s, and it is also true of the twenty-first century. While the royal colleges (of England, Edinburgh, and Glasgow) now collect information on the number of women in each subspecialty and in the profession as a whole, they do not collect parallel statistics on the race or ethnicity of surgeons in the United Kingdom. It is tricky, therefore, to make evidenced claims about whether the number of surgeons of colour has increased, decreased, or stayed roughly the same since the foundation of the NHS. Anecdotally, and based on evidence we have about the changing racial and ethnic demographics of the healthcare workforce and the British population more broadly, it seems that the number of surgeons of colour *has* increased, albeit slowly and unevenly. Moreover, that the royal colleges have never collected this data suggests that the racial and ethnic diversity of the surgical workforce has not been a top priority for the profession's leadership.

We do know that as of March 2020, 77.9 per cent of NHS staff identified as white.[16] We also know that as of March 2021, just 19 per cent of the RCS's 'ecosystem' (council members, faculty, surgical tutors, etc.) *did not* identify as white.[17] These statistics do, however, belie substantial variation within broad racial or ethnic categories: 5.2 per cent of NHS medical staff are Black and 2.6 per cent are Chinese (compared to the 30.2 per cent who identify as 'Asian').[18] Similarly, just 1 per cent of the RCS 'ecosystem' are Black African and only 0.2 per cent are Black Caribbean.[19] These statistics suggest an overwhelmingly white industry, profession, and surgical leadership. However, there are plenty of gaps in the information available – particularly for the second half of the twentieth century. The demography of surgery in post-war Britain was a product of the country's social and political context, as well as colonial legacies and international geopolitics. But what happened to these aspiring students or trainee doctors who travelled in the UK looking for work and education? And what about the British-born surgeons from minoritised races who had to navigate a socially conservative and traditional professional community and healthcare system? As discussed, statistics will only get us so far. Instead, to paint a picture of race, ethnicity, and post-war British surgery we need to use personal stories, oral histories, and first-hand accounts.

The doctors who came to Britain after training abroad brought considerable expertise, met a crucial need, and propped up their new healthcare systems. Of course, many white British surgeons acknowledged the value and contributions of overseas doctors, and recognised how much they and their colleagues depended on this new clinical labour. Moreover, many surgeons who came to Britain seeking work and training described positive experiences of working life and professional acceptance. In 2020, I interviewed an eighty-six-year-old plastic surgeon who had been born in Egypt and moved to England in 1961. I asked him what it was like coming to the UK and working in the NHS and he replied, 'I was euphoric. I loved everything, the work in the hospital, the social life.'[20] He was enthusiastic about living in a new country and spent every weekend he was not on call visiting London and 'going places'. He 'loved working in the NHS'.[21] Evidently, while Britain in general, and surgical social life in particular, could be racist or exclusionary, it was possible for overseas doctors and surgeons of colour to feel accepted by their new colleagues.

However, many overseas doctors were not necessarily greeted with the gratitude or enthusiasm they deserved. In Britain, most of the trainee surgeons and physicians who arrived in the early decades of the NHS came from South Asia and other ex-colonies. These overseas doctors – and particularly trainee surgeons from minoritised races – faced substantial abuse, aggression, and discrimination. In 1961, Duncan Macaulay wrote an article in the *BMJ* in which he claimed that the 'majority of the postgraduates now staffing the hospitals of the United Kingdom come from India and Pakistan'.[22] He described how most of those doctors returned to their 'own country' after a period of 'training' (his inverted commas) in the United Kingdom with

> a sense of grievance, because to all intents and purposes the doors of teaching hospitals are closed to them when it is a matter of making appointments to the junior staff ... It is rare even for an Indian to be short-listed for a post in one of these places, whatever his qualifications. It is not difficult to imagine the feelings of an Indian doctor with higher qualifications obtained in Britain when he hears, as they sometimes do, that the first step in compiling a short-list is to exclude all Indians and Pakistanis.[23]

Macaulay called this 'snobbery' an 'ancient British vice', but he could equally have described it as racism or xenophobia.[24] He wrote about how this vice flourished in 'many of our "better" hospitals' – 'teaching hospitals are the worst offenders' – but that it was common everywhere. There were many institutions across the country which seemed to 'pride themselves on never entertaining applications from doctors from these Commonwealth countries'.[25]

According to the self-described Asian doctor, Leslie de Noronha, the British health service was becoming more hostile to foreign practitioners in the post-war period rather than less. In 1961 he wrote in the *BMJ* about the 'nostalgia' he felt for the 'hospitality, cordiality, and what is naturally more important, the training' he had received when he first arrived in the UK in 1953.[26] He described a 'growing resentment against foreign doctors', which he blamed on the 'increasing influx of, for example, Indo-Pakistan medicos', and compared it to the 'hate' against Irish doctors that was expressed in the 'average doctors' mess' in the 1950s.[27] As shown in Chapter 3, the mess was somewhere that could foster a real sense of community and belonging among some surgeons. But these places could equally make practitioners feel uncomfortable, particularly if they came from 'foreign' cultures or countries. In addition, this quotation suggests that one of the ways that doctors cultivated community in the hospital was by bonding over discrimination and finding common adversaries.

De Noronha also suggested that the recent Immigration Bill had 'confused the issue further', or at least led to some 'spirited arguments during "elevenses"'.[28] The Immigration Bill, passed as the Commonwealth Immigrants Act in 1962, controlled the immigration of all Commonwealth passport holders (except those who already held British citizenship).[29] Prospective immigrants now needed to apply for a work voucher, graded according to the applicant's employment prospects. Before the Act was passed, Commonwealth citizens had extensive rights to migrate to the UK, and the question of immigration in general was less fraught. In the 1940s, a 'colour problem' was generally seen as alien to Britain. Racism was seen as not a British problem, but an American one, particularly during the Second World War. BBC audience research on 'Changes in the State of British and Public Opinion on the USA' in 1944 reported that the colour bar, as practised by US forces, was widely condemned: 'The attitude of white American troops to their coloured compatriots was mentioned only to be condemned and used as evidence against the reality of American democracy.'[30]

This characterisation of race within both Britain and the United States has more to do with British narratives of liberalism and tolerance as important national characteristics than the realities of people of colour living in the UK. However, in the 1950s, the legislative landscape and the tenor of the popular debate did shift. There was increasingly widespread opposition to immigration in Britain from a range of political groups, including the Conservative Monday Club whose MPs were vocal in their opposition to 'mass' immigration. The leader of the opposition, Labour MP Hugh Gaitskell, called the act 'cruel and brutal anti-colour legislation'.[31]

The characterisation of Britain as liberal and tolerant, especially in contrast to the United States, is partly reliant on a pervasive amnesia about, and misunderstanding of, the impact of empire. The experience of surgeons of colour, whether born in Britain or trained 'overseas', was profoundly shaped by the vestiges of the colonial order. By the time Enoch Powell gave his infamous 'rivers of blood' speech in Birmingham in 1968, the formal British empire had, with a couple of exceptions, dissolved.[32] But memories persisted and the 'ferocity of emotion' that infused the subject of race in the 1960s and 1970s was in part a product of those recollections.[33] Indeed, as historian Bill Schwarz argues, colonial societies relied on race, and 'the conception of civilization which was diffused by the British throughout the many lands of their empire ... was, for all its liberality, one that was racialized'. And perhaps most crucially, 'racial *whiteness* [my emphasis] ... played a crucial role in empire, both in colony and metropole'. Throughout the empire's lengthy lifespan, 'domestic' British people were encouraged to 'narrate their own lives as imperial men, women, and children', and identifying oneself as white 'functioned as the precondition for these narrative acts'. However, for much of the empire's existence, this identity went unchallenged. The increased immigration of minoritised races into post-war Britain turned something relatively abstract into something much more pressing and much more fraught: 'whiteness became a more intensely immediate phenomenon'.[34]

Against this backdrop, and because of the enduring memories of empire and the perception that white British culture was under threat, the surgical community became increasingly hostile to foreigners. Despite insistence from professional societies like the James IV Association that surgery was a global community that traded on the international 'language' of science, they were broadly uncertain about expanding the geographical and linguistic boundaries of their world. Surgeons from this period frequently used Orientalist and othering language, even if they kept away from explicitly derogatory or discriminatory terms or sentiments. This demarcated racial lines around communities of clinical professionals and cultivated both explicitly and implicitly hostile working environments for surgeons of colour. American surgeon Bentley P. Colcock ruminated on the lofty ideals of surgery and considered the grand designs of the James IV Association: 'Since my experiences as a surgical traveller, I am more than ever convinced that we as physicians have a unique advantage in helping to solve these problems.'[35] This 'unique advantage' was their capacity – 'unlike any other profession in the world' – to speak a 'universal language'. The 'universal language' he referred to was the lingua franca of scientific humanity. In contrast, Anglophone surgical communities were far more specific and restrictive in their determinations of the *actual* language members should use to communicate and connect.

The minutes of a 1979 meeting of the North American members of the James IV Association of Surgery record a discussion of potential destinations of travel:

> The Secretary reported that the question had arisen as to whether a traveller should travel to a country where … the English language is not freely spoken. This came about after one of the recent travellers had gone to China where there is not a James IV Member and interchange was carried out through an interpreter.[36]

The members concluded that this 'did not comply with the original aims of the Association, which were that the travellers would travel to member countries where the English language is freely spoken'. It is unclear why 'interchange carried out through an interpreter' proved so troubling to the Association or why 'embarrassment' might have resulted from 'the Traveller who arranges his own itinerary and makes his own arrangements without consulting the Secretary'.[37] Perhaps the Association was concerned by any potential loss of control over the activities of their members. Moreover, this anxiety was prompted not by travellers' occasional extravagant socialising, but instead by a member who journeyed beyond the Anglosphere. The Association agreed that in the future, all travellers should, 'submit [their] proposed itinerary to the Secretary or Assistant Secretaries for their approval before any definite travel plans are effected'.[38]

While most of the Association's travellers visited Europe and North America, some were permitted to venture further afield. For the Association's purposes, India was considered part of the Anglosphere (English was and continues to be one of the country's official languages). When reflecting on their trips to India, some travellers made Orientalist observations and reaffirmed their commitment to English (rather than science) as the lingua franca of surgery. British surgeon Victor Riddell wrote in his 1963 report,

> I had never been to India. It was therefore with much pleasure that I heard of my good fortune in being nominated as a James IV Surgical Traveller. It seemed desirable that I should promptly refresh and improve my knowledge of this ancient land of 'dusky faces with while silken turbans wreathed' (Milton: *Paradise Regained*, IV, 76).[39]

He went on to praise the pluck and determination of Indian doctors: 'In spite of all the difficulties and obstructions there is still a touching eagerness amongst the young there to seek knowledge overseas. Their motto, very properly seems to be: "Travel is the life blood of medicine."' Finally, he turned his attention to the adoption of English as an official language (in 1950): 'The consequence of this decision in the political field are immeasurable.'[40] He applauded the end of 'the wasteful situation in which scientific books were being translated into Hindu or Urdu' and decried the slow, painstaking, and expensive process that rendered the outputs useless and out of date.[41]

Of course, Riddell's praise of Indian doctors' travel, determination, and use of the English language was not taking place in a vacuum. As discussed, Indian doctors were emigrating to Britain in increasing numbers and playing a crucial role in the new NHS.[42] Despite their services to the welfare state, these doctors were being subjected to sometimes vitriolic attacks about their perceived ability to speak the English language and held to a higher standard of conduct and performance than their white colleagues. The James IV Association was and remains a small, and in many ways unusual, selection of the surgical profession. However, the kind of exclusionary language and behaviour they traded in was common across the community in this period.

As Camilla Schofield has shown in her study of Enoch Powell and his followers in late 1960s and early 1970s Britain, the welfare state played a key role in anti-immigration sentiment, politics, and action.[43] The welfare state was understood and articulated as a reward for wartime sacrifice. While Britain's non-white colonial forces were fundamental to the nation and empire's military success, this sacrifice was 'whitewashed' by Powell and his supporters, who refused Commonwealth migrants' welfare entitlement. This manifested itself in a 'jealously guarded NHS', with immigration law and the welfare state frequently used in tandem.[44] As Grace Redhead has argued, the legal exclusion of Commonwealth migrants in the 1960s and 1970s, marked by increasingly restrictive Commonwealth Immigration Acts, depended on discourses of 'welfare parasitism', a fear that such migrants would 'exploit and overrun the welfare state'.[45] This only continued into the 1970s, when British political regimes were 'in flight from socialist principles and welfare state inclusivity'. To justify their limits on welfare, they used notions of 'strangers and aliens' that were remarkably powerful and salient.[46]

Patients were sometimes the most vociferous opponents of surgeons from minoritised races' incorporation into the NHS workforce. In 1976, Mr P. Harding wrote a letter to the chairman of the Royal Commission on the National Health Service (the report was published in 1979) to complain about the foreignness of some of his healthcare providers: 'I am particularly concerned at the quality of the administrative, financial and personnel staff employed with the NHS.' His understanding of 'quality' was informed by his racism:

> I have a specific question concerning the medical competence and, more significantly, ability to speak the English language of foreign-educated doctors … who escaped the recently imposed set of English tests as they were registered here in the period before the recent crackdown on low grade 'doctors' from abroad.[47]

He referred to two specific doctors in his letter. Despite not being a patient of either, he had serious concerns about their ability to practise, and cast aspersions on their medical credentials: 'I know that on a number of occasions patients … have expressed their difficulty at being able to communicate in English with (1).' He went on, 'I doubt both his English language and medical competence. Just what does one make of MBBS Bihar? Is it up to English standards? In the case of (2) I would also like your view as to the standard of MB Calcutta.'[48]

The rhetoric of scarcity and othering evidently had a profound effect on migrant patients, but also on migrant surgeons. Rajgopalan Menon trained in the southern Indian city of Visakhapatnam and started working for the NHS in 1974. Reflecting on his forty-year career in the NHS, he wrote, 'all non-white staff faced overt racial abuse, but we just had to cope'. He describes how being 'referred to as a "wog" was a regular occurrence', and that patients constantly called him a 'black bastard'.[49] Racial discrimination could also be subtler, but no less damaging to people's lives and careers. In a personal view, published in the *BMJ* in 2000, an anonymous doctor described his experiences of working in the UK as a 'Ugandan Asian with a British passport' in the 1970s. Despite speaking the language 'fluently' and being able to play Bob Dylan 'rather well', his career had been anything but 'plain sailing'.[50] After four years as a rotating senior house officer and registrar, he was summoned by his higher surgical training committee: 'Do you really think that you will become a general surgeon?', they asked. He was twenty-eight, with two fellowships, had written two papers, and was completing a recognised registrar rotation in surgery in a teaching hospital. 'Yes', he replied. The committee responded by saying that he was being 'unrealistic', reminded him that he was Indian, and walked him through the fate of all previous Indian registrars in the city: 'So you see, not one has made it.' The committee deemed him unsuitable for further training because of his ethnicity.[51]

Addressing the 'problem' of overseas doctors

In 1982, Sir David Innes Williams, then director of the British Postgraduate Medical Federation, wrote, 'For many years some overseas doctors have been forced to find employment in the narrower specialties such as ENT surgery, geriatrics, or mental handicap, which are almost always inappropriate to their training requirements.'[52] In 1984, the Overseas Doctors Training Scheme was set up to improve the quality of postgraduate training that overseas doctors received in Britain.[53] The scheme dictated that an agreed proportion of posts approved by the royal colleges, at senior house officer and registrar levels in general medicine, general surgery, and some of their related specialties, were to be made available for trainees on the scheme, with a few at senior registrar level for suitable candidates. Overseas doctors would be appointed to these posts for a maximum of four years and receive structured training relevant to their needs. Ten years later, while the scheme had proven popular, many questioned how far it had achieved its aims.[54]

The Royal College of Surgeons of England started its own version of the scheme soon after 1984, and it quickly attracted many applicants.[55] By 1992, they had had more than 10,000 enquiries and 2,000 formal applications. Overwhelmed, the college had to close its lists for two years and only restarted accepting new applications in spring 1994.[56] In that year, the RCS had 239 overseas trainees in post, most in general surgical jobs. Despite its popularity, however, the scheme failed to deliver for many of the overseas doctors who participated.[57] The Tavistock study of junior doctors showed that those who had come from overseas

> face[d] difficulty at every turn … their remoteness from home and family support, their conflicts with consultants and other members of staff and their failure to get jobs … for which they see themselves qualified … some write many letters of application (one spoke of writing hundreds) but are repeatedly rejected. Others settle for expediency, applying for and getting only those jobs … which they know few other doctors will want … in one sense they form an underclass within the NHS. They are assumed to have been relatively poorly trained in their home countries, and accepted on sufferance.[58]

A journalist for the *BMJ* described the ‘tremendous variation’ in the experiences of overseas doctors. While some were making an ‘excellent job of tailoring suitable training schemes to meet their needs’, many ran into serious professional and personal difficulties.[59] She also noted that few were prepared to publicly voice any criticism of their host country. The same journalist noted that Britain in 1994 seemed to be becoming less and less interested in and accommodating towards overseas doctors.[60] Dr Akram Sayeed, president of the Overseas Doctors Association, wrote, ‘Some hospitals used to provide free board and lodgings to overseas doctors on unpaid clinical attachments, but this practice has been abandoned as hospital budgets have been honed.'[61] Since 1993, overseas doctors have been required to pay £120 a month to simply sit as an observer in casualty or outpatient departments.

Surgeons of colour in contemporary Britain

British-born doctors and surgeons from Black and Asian backgrounds hardly fared better than their 'overseas' counterparts. In 1990, an article was published in the *BMJ* that explored the effects of discrimination by sex and race on the early careers of British medical graduates between 1981 and 1987. The article concluded that there were 'striking differences in career patterns between graduates of native European origin and those of ethnic minority origin'.[62] Graduates from 'ethnic minorities' reported lower success rates and more difficulty in obtaining house officer and registrar posts. They were also more likely to have experienced spells of unemployment while seeking work and to have changed their original choice of career because of difficulty in obtaining suitable posts or undesirable career prospects.[63] Most of this discrimination took place in the process of shortlisting applicants. The article's authors suggested that this might have been based on non-European names, country of birth, and other clues to ethnic origin. They also acknowledged that many posts in England and Wales were filled by 'personal arrangement' rather than open competition.[64] As discussed in the previous two chapters, British surgery operated much like a gentlemen's club with jobs and promotions offered over boozy lunches and at the golf club. The informal nature of surgical career progression not only shaped the class and gender profile of the profession, but its ethnic diversity as well.

Today, the situation for racially minoritised surgeons has improved. Since the mid-twentieth century, attitudes towards discrimination have changed and there is now a whole 'equality, diversity, and inclusion' (EDI) industry (sometimes referred to as 'equality, diversity, and belonging') that has been taken up by the NHS and its constituent institutions – including the royal colleges. EDI has become professionalised, with trained experts called in to assess, critique, and make recommendations for improvement.

A shift in terminology has tracked this development. From the 1960s through to the 1980s, most people spoke in terms of 'race relations' or 'equal opportunities'.[65] 'Diversity' as a term and as a goal only really emerged in the 1990s and has been subjected to substantial critique, particularly its manifestations in the corporate world.[66]

In my interviews with practitioners, it is clear that despite this emergent 'EDI industry', the surgical profession still has far to go. I spoke to one surgeon who was born in India before moving to the UK for training.[67] He went to medical school in the 1990s, before starting his career in the early 2000s. He told me that when he started out, he did not know a single surgeon of colour who had managed to get a training number – and this was even after the Calman Reforms which were supposed to professionalise and streamline the medical and surgical training process and make it less susceptible to nepotism and the subjective preference of consultants. He considered leaving the UK for the US, which he perceived as more open and welcoming, but finally got a number and was shortlisted for six jobs. By the sixth interview, he was 'fed up'. At every new hospital he went to, he came up against the 'old boys' club' described by other surgeons of colour and female practitioners. Finally, he turned up to an interview and was cautiously optimistic to see one Asian consultant on the panel. He was the last to be interviewed, and was eventually offered the job. Afterwards, the Asian consultant came up to him and said, 'we need to support our own', the implication being that solidarity among surgeons of colour was necessary to mitigate the tendency of white consultants to favour *their* own in hiring and career development.[68] This experience is by no means unique. As one surgeon of colour told the RCS Diversity Report, 'Many of us are "good enough," maybe even better, but we are only considered when there isn't a White man available for the job.'[69]

In the RCS Diversity Report's survey, the 'old boys' network' was perceived as the biggest single barrier to achieving leadership roles in the College.[70] One person described the RCS as 'both Masonic and colonial'.[71] Of the respondents who cited this 'old boys' network', 37 per cent said that racial discrimination and a lack of role models in senior leadership positions were barriers.[72] For example, one participant said, 'I have not seen a Black man or woman on the Council, no role models to make me think this is achievable.'[73]

The problem of role-modelling – both within and without the RCS – is pervasive, and works in both directions. As one person quoted in the Report acknowledged, coming from a medical family where you are constantly in the company of people who look like you who have had the success you seek, makes navigating the surgical career much easier: 'My uncles are all surgeons … it definitely helps … I grew up hearing about things that other students might not know about … And I can go to them for help when I need it.'[74] For Black medical students, not only do they struggle to see themselves in senior or leadership roles, the people of colour who have made it to consultant grade do not paint an appealing picture of the process:

> When I [a fourth-year medical student] speak to Black surgeons they emphasise how hard it is … I've never heard a Black surgeon say anything different. It worries me because I think I know how hard you have to work to be a surgeon without having to work even harder because I'm Black.[75]

Surgery is a profession in which senior members have a huge amount of power over students and trainees. While the firm no longer connotes quite the same social and professional community – and despite reforms designed to systematise and depersonalise applications and selection – the process of hiring and enabling career progression is still very dependent on personalities and sometimes-capricious individuals. This can have deeply problematic effects for aspiring surgeons of colour, and means that workplace discrimination can be difficult to address. As one respondent to the RCS's Report said, 'One of the people who said the "N word" is a very senior boss. I can never do anything about that because I want a good job.'[76] This incident also demonstrates the very real limitations to the framing of workplace discrimination along the lines of ethnicity and race using the now-popular phrases 'unconscious/implicit bias' and 'microaggressions'.[77] While much of the racism experienced in operating theatres and on the wards is subtle and couched in such a way as to deny its hurtfulness and harm, there are also plenty of examples of shocking and straightforward racist abuse, and much of that abuse goes unreported, often for very understandable reasons.

One of the pervasive themes that emerges from survey data, personal accounts, and oral history interviews is the notion that surgeons of colour feel the need to hide an aspect of their personality, background, or culture while at work. A surgeon I interviewed told me that being Indian was a very big part of who he was – that he was 'Indian at heart'.[78] However, for much of his career he would not show his 'Indian-ness' at work. He did not take a day off for Diwali, would not wear certain clothing or accessories, and would not speak Hindi either to colleagues or to patients. Only once he became a consultant did he feel comfortable enough to let his 'Asian side' come out to his colleagues. He described how much of the way he chose to behave while at work was a product of racist abuse, harassment, and violence he experienced as a child and teenager growing up in Britain. He told me about frequent episodes of 'Paki bashing' while walking to and from school.[79] While very different in form, content, and history, the experiences of LGBTQ+ surgeons has something in common with this tendency on behalf of surgeons of colour to deny an aspect of their identity while at work. Seventy per cent of LGBTQ+ surgeons reported to the RCS that they had endured harassment or abuse from colleagues, which meant many felt unable to talk about their private life or personhood while at work.[80]

Much like in the 1970s, the challenges faced by surgeons of colour today are not just a result of problematic or harmful colleagues, but the result of racist patients. As one surgeon told the RCS, 'As a Black man, a consultant, it's shocking when a Black patient says I want to see a White surgeon, but it does happen … what can you say?'[81] Experiences like this one came up in almost every interview I conducted with surgeons of colour, both male and female, and reflect an uncomfortable truth about the state of racism in Britain today. While certainly distressing, it might not be all that surprising to hear about instances of racist abuse levied at surgeons of colour by patients in the 1970s, but these issues are not confined to the past. Nor do they seem to be abating with sufficient speed. Instead, in 2020 the proportion of NHS staff who reported being the target of some form of discrimination had risen by a quarter over the previous five years, with 28.5 per cent saying they experienced harassment, bullying, or abuse of some kind. Of those who had been discriminated against, half said it was linked to their 'ethnic background'.[82]

In 1980, Rajan Madhok moved from his home in Delhi to the United Kingdom. He initially trained as an orthopaedic surgeon in the NHS, before switching to public health and he is now medical director of NHS Manchester. In 2010, he reflected on what had changed over the course of the past four decades. He argued that one must 'recognise the need to find a balance between "celebration" and "complacency"'.[83] Progress has been made, but many remain unconvinced and insist that change has been too slow, that there is insufficient momentum, and that the system will drift into complacency unless it is constantly challenged. There are now more racially minoritised medical students than there have ever been – so much so that the 'white male student is in danger of becoming the new minority'.[84] However, throughout the period covered in this book, racially minoritised surgeons have been over-represented in the lower grades of the profession, under-represented in senior managerial positions, and work in the less popular places and subspecialties.[85] There are relatively few consultant surgeons of colour, compared to general practitioners, for example. In addition, and as discussed, the category 'racially minoritised surgeons' collapses distinctions between different ethnicities. While surgeons of Indian descent are comparatively common, Black African or Black Caribbean practitioners are particularly scarce. Also, while the raw data seems to suggest a greater diversity among the clinical professions, that does not mean that the experiences of surgeons of colour has necessarily improved.

Female surgeons of colour

Quantitative and qualitative evidence demonstrates two things about the state of twentieth- and twenty-first-century surgery: one, that women and people of colour have been prevented from entering the profession in the numbers they should have done; and two, that female surgeons and surgeons of colour have all faced either racism or sexism. However, some women are also Black; and some people of colour are also women. As legal scholar Kimberlé Crenshaw argued, gendered, raced, and classed oppressions intersect, and to focus on each alone risks denying the 'multidimensionality' of marginalised subjects' lived experiences.[86] Moreover, not only has recent research shown that intersectionality is crucial if one wants to understand inequalities in health, it is also essential to any analysis of workplace discrimination.[87] Female surgeons of colour have been doubly disadvantaged by gender and ethnicity in relation to career progression and in problem areas such as recruitment, training, research, and awards.

In early 2021, I interviewed a female surgeon who had moved to the UK from Cameroon after completing medical school to train in the NHS. She described the challenges associated with navigating the specialty's 'old boys' club' and we discussed the difficulties of being a Black woman who had trained overseas and who had embarked on her career with young children in tow.[88] She had needed to be at the very 'top of [her] game', and like many people of colour and women I have interviewed, she described how she felt there was no room for error. Whereas her white, male colleagues could afford small mistakes or learning opportunities, she had to maintain perfection in and out of the operating theatre. She moved around a lot, relied heavily on her mother for childcare and support, and lamented the lack of 'Black input' into her training. She told me she had experienced her 'fair share of obstructions' and plenty of racism from her patients. While working in the Midlands, she was regularly on the receiving end of racist slurs and abuse, which abated when she returned to work in and near London. She described these aggressions and 'microaggressions' as part of the 'rich tapestry' of surgical work. She reflected, with remarkable generosity, on her relative power as compared to patients and attributed her confidence in the face of discrimination and harassment to her age, experience, and resilient personality.[89]

Evidently, and despite the obstacles faced by women of colour in the UK, many have succeeded as surgeons over the past seventy years, and particularly more recently. Samantha Tross was born in Georgetown in Guyana in 1968. She qualified in the 1990s, becoming the first Black female orthopaedic surgeon in Britain. She reflected on her achievements: 'I wasn't aware of this [being the first Black female orthopaedic surgeon in the UK] when I was training, so it took a while for the enormity of that to sink in.'[90] While Tross's career is undoubtedly a cause for celebration, that the first Black female orthopaedic surgeon in Britain only qualified in the 1990s is an indictment of the slow progress the profession has made. The president of the British Orthopaedic Trainees Association from 2019 to 2020 was also a Black woman. In an article, she described her experiences. Despite her many achievements, she was 'always the exception, the only one'. 'When you are the only Black person at the table', she said, 'the burden of being the exception is heavy'. Her gender and race intersect:

> We often hear people talking about breaking down the glass ceiling that stands in the way of women. However, it is not the same for me as a Black woman. I don't face a glass ceiling; I face a concrete ceiling. You can see through glass to the level above and you can smash it. You can't see through concrete, there is no role model for me to aspire to, it is tough to break and practically impossible to break by yourself.[91]

However, while the quantitative and qualitative data colludes to evidence a dire picture for female surgeons of colour, many of those I have interviewed painted a more ambivalent picture of racism and sexism in the workplace. I asked one interviewee, 'Has being the daughter of immigrants impacted your career?' She replied, 'I don't think so.'[92] She credited her character and the geographical region in which she lived and worked for this experience: 'I'm not aware of that, I don't know if I'm being naive about it, but I'm not aware of that having impacted it because my personality has carried me through ... I think in London and the South East, I've always been a South East trainee ... and it's not been an issue.'[93]

This kind of insistence that they had not been subject to racial or gender discrimination was widespread among the women of colour I interviewed and among the autobiographies written and published by Black and Asian female surgeons. Shireen McKenzie is a Black surgeon from Leeds, whose story was included in a collective biography:

> When she was 14 years old, an acquaintance of the family, a white male primary physician, gave her career advice. He did not discourage Miss McKenzie from medicine. He did do so for surgery, stating that as a Black woman, she would be better off pursuing a career in gynaecology, rather than surgery. Unknowingly, he probably strengthened her resolve to be a surgeon.[94]

This experience, to me at least, seems discriminatory. McKenzie, however, denied that characterisation, insisting instead that 'during her time as a trainee, all her mentors were white males who gave her their utmost support'. While she had 'heard about toxic environments where people were overlooked because of their race, religion, or gender', that was just not her experience of training or work.

It is not my job as a historian to deny people's experiences or question their own interpretations of their lives. However, it is my job to put those personal narratives into their broader, historical contexts. As historian Roberta Bivins has argued, soon after their arrival in twentieth-century Britain, many migrants encountered another facet of responses to their presence: efforts aimed at their assimilation, integration, and later, under the remit of 'multiculturalism', a more limited – but still normative – agenda of incorporation into a fluid but supposedly singular 'national culture'.[95] Denying experiences of racism or discrimination could, therefore, be part of this assimilation. An unconscious – but sometimes very necessary – effort to 'fit in'.[96]

Surgeons of colour and COVID-19

Inequalities between healthcare professionals of different ethnicities are important to address not just because a more diverse workforce benefits all, but because racism and discrimination have tangible and alarming consequences for people's health and safety – even for the health and safety of otherwise privileged healthcare professionals. The coronavirus pandemic exposed and exacerbated systemic racism within the NHS.[97] Despite the many think-pieces about how viruses do not discriminate, COVID-19 was not an equal opportunity disease. Even as politicians, managers, and UN officials gave pep talks about how everyone was 'in it together', segments of society had vastly different experiences of the pandemic. Rather than proving to be any sort of 'great leveller', coronavirus claimed the lives of the most vulnerable – people from Black and South Asian backgrounds, poor people, disabled people, the old, and the disenfranchised – at a much higher rate than the white and the wealthy. These inequalities also extended to NHS staff. The effect of the novel coronavirus on healthcare workers reflected the injustices baked into the rest of society, with doctors and nurses from Black and South Asian backgrounds with disproportionately high death rates. While people of colour account for approximately 21 per cent of NHS staff, 63 per cent of those who died from COVID-19 in the first half of 2020 were from minoritised races. Perhaps most starkly, 94 per cent of the doctors and surgeons who died were people of colour.[98]

The reasons for this disparity are complex and are yet to be fully researched. But one cause is the class system found in the health service's internal structure and the historical precedent this chapter has delineated. Though it might have been naive to think that the introduction of the NHS in 1948 could have levelled the social and professional playing field, it was certainly an opportunity to flatten some of the hierarchies in hospitals and other healthcare settings that had become increasingly entrenched over the preceding 150 years. Aneurin Bevan wanted the health professions – doctors and nurses alike – to become salaried employees of the state. But, and as argued in the second chapter of this book, surgeons, physicians, and general practitioners resisted, insisting on the historical exceptionalism they had come to value, even despite its relatively recent vintage. They and the institutions they were attached to negotiated a different relationship to the new National Health Service and perpetuated the working cultures they had been accustomed to.

As this chapter and the two before it have shown, hospitals are hierarchical institutions. At the bottom of the pecking order are the non-clinical workers – men and mainly women who tend to be employed on less secure, temporary, and precarious contracts with limited union protection, and who come from already disadvantaged groups with far less social, economic, and political capital than doctors or nurses. Cleaners, porters, and ancillary healthcare workers have also become increasingly likely to be contracted out, paid by companies external to the NHS and not afforded the same labour protections as others hired 'in house'.[99] At no time is this ideal. During the coronavirus pandemic, it meant that they were also at the bottom of the list – the least well protected – when it came to things like the distribution of personal protective equipment.[100] Why, though, did doctors, surgeons, and nurses from minoritised races also die at faster rates than their white counterparts? Presumably they were, at the very least, on parallel contracts and entitled to the same quality and quantity of protective equipment. Could it be that good education, good salaries – even being one of our nation's 'heroes' – are also not the great levellers we have so often taken them to be? We know that racism permeates British society. It permeates the NHS too.

Conclusion

The subjects analysed in this chapter are live issues, and became particularly pressing in 2020 when the pandemic ripped through the global population and has now killed at least 210,000 British citizens. The pandemic levied extra burdens on women, who undertook most of the reproductive and emotional labour as much of the workforce moved online. As shown, coronavirus also revealed and made worse existing health and social inequalities, killing racially minoritised people at a disproportionate rate.[101] This unequal distribution of death and ill health also affected surgeons, which demonstrates (just in case any further evidence is needed) the tangible consequences of racism and inequality in the clinical workplace.[102]

Until the publication of the RCS's Diversity Report in March 2021, there was not only scant data on the ethnic diversity of British surgery available to researchers and policymakers, but there was little explicit or public acknowledgement of the role racism plays in contemporary surgical life. While there has been a much longer tradition of evidence gathering on the proportion of male and female surgeons in both the profession as a whole and in individual subspecialities, surgery as a community has been relatively slow to tackle the pervasive problems of racism and sexism in operating theatres and on hospital wards. As discussed in this chapter and in Chapter 4, part of the explanation for surgery's demographic make-up and the negative experiences of people who do not quite fit the Sir Lancelot Spratt mould can be found in the profession's cultural history and the enduring nature of surgical stereotypes. Once again, the problem remains that certain aspects of this image and identity work well for those it serves. The 'old boys' club' suits the 'old boys', even if it excludes women, people from working-class backgrounds, and people of colour. The informal nature of applications, interviews, career progression, and training was ripe for abuse, but meant that if you had worked in the right places, knew the right people, or were the right kind of person yourself, then your passage through surgical life could be relatively smooth sailing.

Surgery has, however, changed. As the next two chapters will show, the second half of the twentieth century witnessed profound policy transformations that affected not just the structures and experiences of the profession, but the dynamics of the NHS as a whole. While many of these transformations were designed not just to diversify the speciality and improve the lot for individual practitioners, their impact on the nature and conditions of surgical work was uneven and frequently a target for vehement critique and dissatisfaction. However, and as Chapter 6 will show, some of these transformations received push-back precisely because they disrupted or contravened powerfully felt notions of surgical identity, and contradicted elements of the surgical stereotype many people held dear.

Notes

1 Royal College of Surgeons of England, 'The Royal College: Our Professional Home. An Independent Review on Diversity and Inclusion for the Royal College of Surgeons of England. An Exciting Call for Radical Change' (March 2021), 9.
2 Royal College of Surgeons of England, 'Black Surgeons Past and Present' (27 October 2020), www.rcseng.ac.uk/news-and-events/news/archive/black-surgeons-past-present/ (accessed 21 May 2021).
3 Ashley Tan, 'Racism on the Frontline: Britain's Asian Healthcare Workers', *Al Jazeera* (27 April 2021), www.aljazeera.com/features/2021/4/27/under-fire-on-the-frontline-britains-asian-healthcare-workers (accessed 21 May 2021).
4 Malika Sharma and Shail Rawal, 'Intersections of Race and Gender in Surgical Training', *JAMA Surgery*, 156:5 (2021), 498.
5 Royal College of Surgeons of England, 'The Royal College: Our Professional Home', 2.
6 Kamlesh Khunti et al., 'The Language of Ethnicity', *British Medical Journal*, 371 (2020), m4493; Peter J. Aspinall, 'Ethnic/Racial Terminology as a Form of Representation: A Critical Review of the Lexicon of Collective and Specific Terms in Use in Britain', *Genealogy*, 4:87 (2020), 1–4.

7 Yasmin Gunaratnam, *Researching Race and Ethnicity* (London: SAGE, 2003); Adrienne Milner and Sandra Jumbe, 'Using the Right Words to Address Racial Disparities in COVID-19', *The Lancet*, 5 (2020), e419–e420, e419.

8 Royal College of Surgeons of England, 'The Royal College: Our Professional Home', 6.

9 Roberta Bivins, *Contagious Communities: Medicine, Migration, and the NHS in Post War Britain* (Oxford: Oxford University Press, 2015), 7.

10 Stephanie Snow and Emma Jones, 'Immigration and the National Health Service: Putting History to the Forefront', *History & Policy* (8 March 2011), www.historyandpolicy.org/policy-papers/papers/immigration-and-the-national-health-service-putting-history-to-the-forefron (accessed 21 May 2021).

11 Hugh E. Stephenson, 'Undergraduate Surgical Teaching in the United Kingdom and Ireland'. Reprinted from *Surgery*, 65 (1964), 321–333, 322. For more information on the structures and experience of South Asian doctors in twentieth-century Britain, see Joanna Bornat, Parvati Raghuram, and Leroi Henri, '"Without Racism There Would be no Geriatrics": South Asian Overseas-trained Doctors and the Development of Geriatric Medicine in the UK, 1950–2000'; and Julian M. Simpson, Stephanie J. Snow, and Aneez Esmail, 'Providing "Special" Types of Labour and Exerting Agency: How Migrant Doctors Have Shaped the UK's National Health Service', both in Laurence Monnais and David Wright (eds), *Doctors Beyond Borders: The Transnational Migration of Physicians in the Twentieth Century* (Toronto: University of Toronto Press, 2016); and Julian M. Simpson, *Migrant Architects of the NHS: South Asian Doctors and the Reinvention of British General Practice (1940s–1980s)* (Manchester: Manchester University Press, 2018).

12 Eram Alam, 'Cold War Crises: Foreign Medical Graduates Respond to US Doctor Shortages, 1965–1975', *Social History of Medicine*, 33 (2018), 132–151, 136.

13 Eram Alam, 'The Care of Foreigners: A History of South Asian Physicians in the United States, 1965–2016' (2016). Publicly Accessible Penn Dissertations, https://repository.upenn.edu/edissertations/2161, 3.

14 Sasha Mullally and David Wright, 'Connecting to Canada: Experiences of the South Asian Medical Diaspora during the 1960s and 1970s', in Laurence Monnais and David Wright (eds) *Doctors Beyond Borders: The Transnational Migration of Physicians in the Twentieth Century* (Toronto: University of Toronto Press, 2016), 230–256, 231.

15 Snow and Jones, 'Immigration and the National Health Service'.
16 UK Government, www.ethnicity-facts-figures.service.gov.uk/workforce-and-business/workforce-diversity/nhs-workforce/latest (accessed 21 March 2021).
17 Royal College of Surgeons of England, 'The Royal College: Our Professional Home', 42.
18 www.ethnicity-facts-figures.service.gov.uk/workforce-and-business/workforce-diversity/nhs-workforce/latest.
19 Royal College of Surgeons of England, 'The Royal College: Our Professional Home', 42.
20 Interview with male surgeon; interviewed by author, 31 March 2020.
21 Ibid.
22 Duncan Macaulay, 'Nationalities of Junior Staff', *British Medical Journal*, 2:5269 (1961), 1777–1778.
23 Ibid.
24 Ibid.
25 Ibid.
26 Leslie de Noronha, 'Nationalities of Junior Staff', *British Medical Journal*, 2:5269 (1961), 1777–1778, 1778.
27 Ibid.
28 Ibid.
29 Commonwealth Immigrants Act (1962), 1–24.
30 Quoted in Wendy Webster, *Englishness and Empire 1939–1965* (Oxford: Oxford University Press, 2005), 150.
31 Mark Pitchford, *The Conservative Party and the Extreme Right 1945–1975* (Manchester: Manchester University Press, 2011); Gary Younge, 'In these Bleak Times, Imagine a World Where you can Thrive', *The Guardian* (10 January 2020), www.theguardian.com/commentisfree/2020/jan/10/bleak-times-thrive-last-column-guardian (accessed 21 May 2021).
32 Bill Schwarz, *The White Man's World* (Oxford: Oxford University Press, 2013), 5.
33 Ibid., 6.
34 Ibid., 9–10.
35 Bentley P. Colcock, 'Report to the James IV Association of Surgeons', 1964, James IV Association of Surgeons Records. The Drs. Barry and Bobbi Coller Rare Book Reading Room, New York Academy of Medicine Library.
36 Minutes of an Interim Meeting of the North American Members, James IV Association of Surgeons, Inc. October 23, 1979, James IV Association of Surgeons Records. The Drs. Barry and Bobbi Coller Rare Book Reading Room, New York Academy of Medicine Library.

37 Ibid.
38 Ibid.
39 Victor Riddell, 'Visit to India as James IV Surgical Traveller 1963', James IV Association of Surgeons Records. The Drs. Barry and Bobbi Coller Rare Book Reading Room, New York Academy of Medicine Library.
40 Ibid.
41 Ibid.
42 Simpson et al., 'Providing "Special" Types of Labour and Exerting Agency'.
43 Camilla Schofield, *Enoch Powell and the Making of Postcolonial Britain* (Cambridge: Cambridge University Press, 2013).
44 Grace Redhead, '"A British Problem Affecting British People": Sickle Cell Anaemia, Medical Activism and Race in the National Health Service, 1975–1993', *Twentieth Century British History*, 32:2 (2021), 189–211, 192.
45 Ibid.
46 Ibid.
47 The National Archive, BS6/10, Letter from Mr P. Harding to A. Merrison, 21 March 1976.
48 Ibid.
49 Rajgopalan Menon, 'The NHS Owes Doctors Who Trained Abroad an Apology for Racism', *British Medical Journal*, 361 (2018), https://doi.org/10.1136/bmj.k2360.
50 'Trying to Overcome Racism in the NHS', *British Medical Journal*, 320:7235 (2004), 657.
51 Ibid.
52 Quoted in Tessa Richards, 'The Overseas Doctors Training Scheme: Failing Expectations', *British Medical Journal*, 308:6944 (1994), 1627–1631, 1628.
53 Tessa Richards, 'The Overseas Doctors Training Scheme', 1628.
54 Ibid.
55 Ibid.
56 Ibid.
57 Ibid.
58 R. Hale and L. Hudson, 'The Tavistock Study of Young Doctors: Report of the Pilot Phase', *British Journal of Hospital Medicine*, 47:6 (1990), 452–464.
59 Richards, 'The Overseas Doctors Training Scheme', 1630.
60 Ibid.
61 Quoted in ibid.
62 P. M. McKeigue, J. D. Richards, and P. Richards, 'Effects of Discrimination by Sex and Race on the Early Careers of British

Medical Graduates During 1981–7', *British Medical Journal*, 301 (1990), 961–964, 961.

63 Ibid.

64 Ibid., 964.

65 Frank Dobbin, *Inventing Equal Opportunity* (Princeton, NJ: Princeton University Press, 2011).

66 Sara Ahmed, *On Being Included: Racism and Diversity in Institutional Life* (Durham, NC: Duke University Press, 2012); Ellen Berrey, 'Diversity is for White People: The Big Lie Behind a Well-Intended Word', *Salon* (26 October 2015), www.salon.com/2015/10/26/diversity_is_for_white_people_the_big_lie_behind_a_well_intended_word/ (accessed 21 May 2021); Kira Lussier, 'What the History of Diversity Training Reveals About its Future', *The Conversation* (7 September 2020), https://theconversation.com/what-the-history-of-diversity-training-reveals-about-its-future-143984 (accessed 21 May 2021).

67 Interview with male surgeon; interviewed by author, 22 February 2020.

68 Ibid.

69 Royal College of Surgeons of England, 'The Royal College: Our Professional Home', 10.

70 Ibid., 35.

71 Ibid., 28.

72 Ibid., 35.

73 Ibid., 22.

74 Ibid., 25.

75 Ibid., 26.

76 Ibid.

77 Nao Hagiwara, Frederick W. Kron, Mark W. Scerbo, and Ginger S. Watson, 'A Call for Grounding Implicit Bias Training in Clinical and Translational Frameworks', *The Lancet*, 2:395 (2020), 1457–1460.

78 Interview with male surgeon; interviewed by author, 22 February 2020.

79 Ibid.

80 Royal College of Surgeons of England, 'The Royal College: Our Professional Home', 17.

81 Ibid., 31.

82 Milo Boyd, 'NHS Staff can now Refuse to Treat People who are Racist or Sexist Towards Them', *Mirror* (18 February 2020), www.mirror.co.uk/news/uk-news/nhs-staff-now-refuse-treat-21523570) (accessed 21 May 2021).

83 Rajan Madhok, 'Foreword', in Emma L. Jones and Stephanie J. Snow, *Against the Odds: Black and Minority Ethnic Clinicians and Manchester, 1948 to 2009* (Manchester: Manchester NHS Primary

Care Trust, in association with the Centre for the History of Science, Technology and Medicine, University of Manchester, 2010).

84 Ibid.

85 Emmeline Lagunes Cordoba et al., 'Time to Get Serious about Distributed Leadership: Lessons to Learn for Promoting Leadership Development for Non-Consultant Career Grade Doctors in the UK', *BMJ Leader*, http://dx.doi.org/10.1136/leader-2020-000395 (accessed 21 May 2021).

86 Kimberlé Crenshaw, 'Demarginalizing the Intersection of Race and Sex: A Black Feminist Critique of Antidiscrimination Doctrine, Feminist Theory, and Antiracist Politics', *University of Chicago Legal Forum*, 1:8 (1989), 139–167, 139.

87 Amy J. Schulz and Leigh Mullings (eds), *Gender, Race, Class, and Health: Intersectional Approaches* (San Francisco: Jossey-Bass, 2006); Cecily Jones '"Human Weeds, Not Fit to Breed?": African Caribbean Women and Reproductive Disparities in Britain', *Critical Public Health*, 23:1 (2013), 49–61.

88 Interview with female surgeon; interviewed by author, 15 February 2021.

89 Ibid.

90 Moya Lothian-McLean, 'How to Become an Orthopaedic Surgeon, By the Woman who was First in her Field', *Stylist*, https://bit.ly/3f8NADV (accessed 21 May 2021).

91 Tricia Campbell, 'You Can't Have Diversity without Inclusion', *British Orthopaedic Association* (15 July 2020), www.boa.ac.uk/resources/knowledge-hub/you-can-t-have-diversity-without-inclusion.html (accessed 21 May 2021).

92 Interview with female surgeon; interviewed by author, 24 November 2017.

93 Ibid.

94 Praise Matemavi, *Passion and Purpose: Black Female Surgeons* (Deleon Springs, FL: A 2 Z Press, 2020).

95 Bivins, *Contagious Communities*, 9.

96 Ibid.

97 Agnes Arnold-Forster, Caitjan Gainty, and Lucas Camino, 'Covid-19 and Health Inequality', *History Workshop Online* (8 June 2020), www.historyworkshop.org.uk/covid-19-and-health-inequality/ (accessed 21 May 2021).

98 T. Cook, E. Kursumovic, and S. Lennane, 'Exclusive: Deaths of NHS Staff from Covid-19 Analysed', *Health Service Journal* (21 June 2020), www.hsj.co.uk/exclusive-deaths-of-nhs-staff-from-covid-19-analysed/7027471.article (accessed 21 May 2021).

99 Shimaa Elkomy, Graham Cookson, and Simon Jones, 'Cheap and Dirty: The Effect of Contracting Out Cleaning on Efficiency and Effectiveness', *Public Administration Review*, 79:2 (2019), 193–202.

100 Robert Booth, 'Residential Homes "Desperate" for PPE, As Two Care Workers Die', *The Guardian* (6 April 2020), www.theguardian.com/society/2020/apr/06/residential-homes-desperate-for-ppe-as-two-care-workers-die (accessed 21 May 2021).

101 Mohammad S Razai et al., 'Mitigating Ethnic Disparities in Covid-19 and Beyond', *British Medical Journal*, 372 (2021), 1–14.

102 Cook et al., 'Exclusive: Deaths of NHS Staff from Covid-19 Analysed'.

6

Surgical time

In 2018, I interviewed a consultant general surgeon who began her training in the early 1990s. As a 'houseman', she was on call one out of every three nights. The previous generation had been on call more like one in every two, but as she pointed out, back then there were fewer patients and relatively speaking more doctors. She described how she would start her job on Friday morning at 7:30am. She would finish on Monday afternoon, perhaps Monday evening, and the nurses did not even know that she was doing night shifts:

> So you'd see a night nurse and then the following night, they would be there and they would not know you've never been home. They'd been home, been asleep, seen their kids, eaten, and come back and you could have not eaten, not drunk. And they will make each other tea and toast but they never offered it to you because they just said they considered you just, you know, an irritating person who was never there because they kept bleeping you.[1]

As she wryly acknowledged, 'you get quite crap when you're tired'.[2] While it might seem extreme, this surgeon's experience of working life in the late twentieth century was by no means unique. Excessive working hours; lengthy stretches spent in the operating theatre or on the ward with no time off or opportunities to rest, relax, eat, or drink; and intense fatigue were the norm, not the exception.

These experiences or demands were not just because surgery is a difficult job that requires real dedication: surgeons' relationship with time was – and continues to be – a product of their professional identity. And, over the course of the twentieth century, time's role in the self-made myths of modern surgery became increasingly fraught and increasingly prominent. After the Second World War, time was both a crucial resource for surgical workers and a rhetorical device used to articulate distinct strands of the surgical image and identity. This period witnessed increasing debate over the relationship between time, professional devotion, and surgical vocation.

Key to the mythology of the modern surgeon, since at least the late nineteenth century, is the notion that surgical work is in some way distinct from other kinds of labour or employment. Unlike other jobs, surgery and related professions are understood as 'vocations' or 'callings'. This myth of surgical exceptionalism was used to justify and rationalise excessive temporal commitment on behalf of practitioners. Rejecting what he saw as the slow creep of a 'nine to five' attitude towards work on the part of some of his colleagues, one surgeon said in a 1963 letter to the *BMJ*, 'It seems to one such that medicine is coming to be regarded more and more as "a job like any other," and less and less as a vocation.'[3] Not only were surgeons expected to devote substantial quantities of time to their professional lives, but – and continuing the arguments of Chapter 3 – they were required to maintain blurred boundaries between their working and leisure hours, and between their personal and professional selves.

The 1970s was a decade of profound change in the NHS. Inheriting plans from the Conservative predecessors in government, in 1974 Labour implemented the first major reorganisation of the health service. The reorganisation created a new system of 'area' and 'district' health authorities, and marked a new era of ongoing debate about the shape and structure of the NHS, its priorities, and inequalities. These administrative and managerial changes profoundly impacted the way that doctors and nurses worked – transforming the nature and conditions of surgical labour. It prompted practitioners to think not just about the *amount* of time they dedicated to their work, but what they could use that time for. Reorganisation brought with it the spectre and reality of increased bureaucracy. With the introduction of the internal market under Margaret Thatcher's government in the 1980s and early 1990s, new management practices and ideologies intervened in the availability of surgical work time, and shaped its allocation.[4] Managerialism also offered a new way of conceptualising time, and in doing so, became itself something new for surgeons to both rail against and profit from.

For many of the surgeons I met during my research, the past looms large. They spend a lot of time reflecting on their own professional histories and drawing comparisons between how it once was and how it is now. Many surgeons are preoccupied with the differences between what they see as the 'traditional' styles of surgical work and the managed, bureaucratic, and individualistic experiences they have on wards today. While there is some debate over when the shift from 'traditional' to today occurred, the managerialism introduced by the 1974 reorganisation and its crystallisation under Margaret Thatcher in the 1980s is frequently targeted as the culprit. These comparisons between then and now are nostalgic in tone.

Throughout the NHS's history, there have been periodic complaints about the untenable hours that surgeons are expected to work. However, in my oral history interviews, practitioners also frequently expressed anxiety about the implications for surgical professionalism of managerialism, 'modernisation', and new European Union policies designed to limit doctors' working hours.[5] These men and women (although mostly men) connected long hours to commitment and saw working overtime as a heroic contribution to both patients and the profession. This connection is, of course, not confined to medical labour, and scholars of management, industry, and capitalism have acknowledged efforts on behalf of employers to convince workers of the value of long hours and their contribution to corporate success. Nonetheless, NHS policy transformations in the second half of the twentieth century were perceived as changing the surgical rota and therefore the surgical identity, and not necessarily for the better. Commercialisation, financial incentives, conflicts of interest, challenges to occupational autonomy, a measurable loss of public trust in medicine, a decline in deference and the social standing of surgeons, and an increase in 'patient-centred' medicine have all emerged to jeopardise surgery's traditional self-image. How has the surgical stereotype responded to the reshaping of working time and its meanings in the managed healthcare bureaucracies of late twentieth-century Britain? How have so-called 'neoliberal' notions of clinical labour interacted with older visions of surgical vocation? And how does nostalgia figure in the narration of surgical lives and in critiques of changing workplace practices and meanings?

Excessive temporal commitment

Surgeons training in the new NHS had to progress through a standard series of jobs before becoming consultants. Once they had passed their final medical school examinations and received their degrees, they could start work at a hospital as a pre-registration house officer, often known as a houseman or just house officer. Newly qualified doctors were only allowed provisional registration with the General Medical Council and they spent the first year of their clinical careers in this hinterland between graduation and full registration. Being a house officer usually involved two six-month jobs, one with general surgery (a house surgeon) and one in general medicine (a house physician). As a result, pretty much all doctors in Britain spent at least six months doing surgery and training as a surgeon. House officers occupied the lowest rung in the medical hierarchy of qualified doctors, and they were most often called on by nursing staff to see patients on hospital wards and worked the longest and least sociable hours. It was usual for junior medical and surgical staff to work 80 to 120 hours a week, doing a major part of the ward, outpatient, and much of the routine operating work and almost all the out-of-hours emergencies in British hospitals.[6]

From the foundation of the NHS onwards, there was an increasingly vibrant debate about the value, and potential harm, of this excessive temporal commitment. In 1968, surgeon Neville Stidolph wrote, 'It has been generally accepted for many years that the staffing structure of the NHS is urgently in need of revision. Professional bodies, politicians, the national press, and individuals ... have kept up a continuous pressure for review of working condition.'[7] These discussions were taking place in a broader social, cultural, and political context that was shifting the nature and meaning of labour in Britain. Attesting to these changes, in 1966 doctor N. G. Sanerkin from Cardiff wrote,

> In a society in which the 9 a.m. to 5 p.m. day and the 40-hour week are the accepted norm for all workers, both manual and professional, and in which leisure has come to be a most highly valued commodity, it is unreasonable to expect a body of highly skilled and devoted workers to be on duty or on call for up to 100 hours a week on the present meagre basic pay.[8]

These debates and the relative merits of long working hours circulated around several key themes.

First, anxieties about the damage to doctors' physical and emotional health were increasingly aired in the pages of the medical and mainstream press. Second, concerns were raised about the impact of these excessive hours on the quality of patient care and ideas about the damaging effects of fatigue on capability entered the professional lexicon. Third, lengthy shifts were increasingly raised as barriers to female surgeons' career development and to all surgeons' ability to spend quality time with their families. Fourth, various writers and doctors pushed back against these critiques of excessive temporal commitment, arguing for the necessity of long working hours to adequately train junior surgeons and allow them enough time in the operating theatre to progress and practice safely. Fifth, push-back also critiqued the supposed erosion of surgical 'vocation'.

Many of those distressed by the working hours of junior doctors complained about the demands placed on them by their employers. An article published in the *BMJ* reported on the 'deadened voice of one doctor who had worked over 100 hours a week for the past eight months'. Disillusioned, this doctor had been asking herself: 'Am I sacrificing too much just for a job?'[9] Medical staff were not alone in newly considering the deleterious effects excessive hours might have on the health and wellbeing of workers. In 1954, the *British Journal of Industrial Medicine* published the proceedings of the first conference of the British Occupational Hygiene Society. While they were primarily preoccupied with the health of manual and factory labourers, and particularly miners, they reflected broadly on the damage done to workers by fatigue and consistently lengthy shifts.[10] Indeed, as Vicky Long and Victoria Brown have observed, the labour market changed after the Second World War, and the demise of the industrial sector in the UK saw a corresponding decline in physical illnesses and disabilities linked to work.[11] At the same time, there was a surge in mental health issues associated with the rise of the service sector and changing workplace cultures, such as longer working hours, zero-hour contracts, and a blurring of boundaries between home and work.[12] In the middle decades of the twentieth century, social scientists, healthcare professionals, and the popular press were increasingly preoccupied with stress, particularly in the context of post-industrial labour.[13]

By the 1960s, healthcare professionals, policymakers, and the public had turned their attention to medical practitioners and the excessive hours they were called upon to work. The British Medical Association took a particular interest in the negative effects overwork could have on junior staff members' social, emotional, and physical health. They acknowledged, too, the damaging effect working hours were having on recruitment. In 1961, Dr H. L. Matthews from Sheffield said that it was 'beginning to be recognised in some quarters that peripheral posts were not being filled because people did not want to work endlessly'.[14] In 1970, the BMA debated the advisability of extra-duty payments. Dr W. J. Appleyard said that the hours junior doctors were being expected to work were still too high: 'No doctor should be required to work such hours.' He did, however, grudgingly approve of extra-duty payments, if only because they 'went some way to compensate junior doctors for the severe encroachment into their personal life', and that they had 'focused the attention of the public on the quite unacceptably long hours of work expected of the junior hospital doctors by the Health Department'.[15] Dr G. T. Walker argued that 'all juniors … [should] get off-duty to enjoy recreation, study, and, above all, to get a good night's sleep'.[16]

The question of sleep and the deleterious impact of fatigue on the physical and emotional health of shift workers was increasingly taken up by mid-century researchers, including those interested in hospital surgeons and physicians.[17] In a write-up of the BMA's Annual Representative Meeting in 1973, Dr D. Lynch from South Middlesex declared that 'fatigue was a bodily state well known to the medical profession, which resulted in both physical and mental clumsiness – and in its turn to accident proneness and faulty decisions'. He observed that medical advice had prompted statutory rest periods being imposed on pilots, coach-drivers, and truck drivers. However, the same solutions had not been offered to medical practitioners: 'Apparently doctors were exempt from fatigue, because the Government had given the consultants an open-ended contract, with one for junior doctors up to 100 hours a week.'[18]

Articles in the medical press increasingly attested to the importance of a rounded social and professional life, one that had time for both work and play. In a reflective piece, M. J. Evans recalled his days of training: 'Reality dawned – 120 hours plus. No time to do the washing, visit the bank, to lead a social life or more importantly study for part one of the membership examination of the Royal College.' He lamented, 'Why is it that the caring profession finds it so hard to look after its own junior doctors?' However, he identified other issues, not just excessive temporal commitment. He cited the 'constant search for training posts, the need to move on, never able to make friends'.[19] Surgeons in training deserved a rounded social and professional life, but they also needed time for family and parenthood.

As argued in Chapter 4, surgery was and remains an overwhelmingly male profession. There were very few female surgeons working in mid-century Britain. Of the ninety-six women who graduated from the University of Birmingham between 1959 and 1963, not one went on to become a surgeon.[20] Chapter 4 was devoted to analysing the many and various reasons for this. However, one additional reason was the excessive temporal commitment demanded of trainees. In a society and culture in which women were called upon to perform the majority of reproductive labour, including housework and homemaking, more-than-100-hour working weeks made motherhood and surgery almost entirely incompatible.[21] Of course, many women managed to combine both roles, and many others opted not to have children at all, but these women were in the minority. Surgery was, therefore, a profoundly exclusionary profession. However, the excessive temporal commitment demanded of trainees also had negative consequences for men who had little time for their wives and children.

Throughout the 1960s and 1970s, medical leaders expressed anxiety about the impact of working hours and conditions on male surgeons' family life. As shown in Chapter 3, these junior surgeons frequently lived on site, and debates about the value of, and the harm done by, hospital residences frequently circulated around anxieties about excessive temporal commitment. As 'A General Practitioner's Wife' argued in 1967, 'If junior doctors had their own flats, and in between dealing with patients 100 hours a week could sit down with their own kids, have coffee made by their own wives, the long hours would irk so much less that they would almost cease to be a problem.'[22] It is no surprise, therefore, that many doctors advised their junior colleagues against marriage before qualification, or before settling on a more permanent location.[23] In 1968, surgeon Neville Stidolph reflected that the surgeon might well be 'in his early forties before he becomes a consultant'. Becoming a consultant was the culmination of a training period of twenty years, 'during which he has for several years had to seek a new appointment each six months, to uproot his family from home and school with equal frequency, and to spend the years of his early married life in grinding work'.[24]

However, while many railed against the excessive working hours demanded of junior hospital staff, many others critiqued efforts to impose limits on shifts and temporal commitments. These proponents of the 100-hour working week justified their arguments in various ways. Some suggested that the lengthy working week was essential to ensure that surgeons received adequate training. Doctor John Shepherd wrote to the *BMJ* in 1967, 'To maintain a high standard of work in hospitals it is imperative that junior staff are trained and encouraged in the idea of continuity of care'.[25] When interviewed in 2020, urology consultant Ian Eardley reflected fondly on his training in the 1980s and on the hours he was expected to devote to hospital life: 'we were busy, we were expected to run the hospitals'. He praised the steep learning curve he travelled as a result of this business. He attested to the amount he learnt, the quantity of surgery he performed, and the degree to which he acquired knowledge by 'trial and error'. However, it is worth noting that some surgeons were sceptical of the 100-hour working week, not because it damaged their emotional and physical health, but because the constant and relentless drudgery of labour left them little time for thought and reflection:

> Doctors who engross themselves in work for 100 hours a week have little time to speculate on more philosophical concepts ... selection of the brightest and most able sixth-form students leads to the production of medical graduates who, for the most part, form a grey and uninspiring picture of competent mediocrity.[26]

Too much time spent at work could also be detrimental to the development of a good and thoughtful surgeon or physician.

The most fervent push-back against efforts to reduce the number of hours trainee surgeons worked came from those anxious about the supposedly declining degree of a sense of vocation in the profession. This was an issue that came up in the debates about hospital residences, when doctor John Shepherd wrote in 1967, 'Already there is a tendency for a "9 to 5" attitude to prevail, and I believe this is quite contrary to all that is best in surgical or medical practice.'[27] Since at least the nineteenth century surgeons had been articulating their profession in terms of a 'calling' or a special devotion to the plight of humankind. This notion of a surgical commitment was deployed in debates over the foundation of the NHS, when various medical practitioners expressed anxiety over the encroachment of the state into their clinical autonomy. It appeared again in the late 1960s and early 1970s, when groups like the BMA began arguing against excessive temporal commitment and campaigning for a more structured and regulated approach to surgical training. Various writers attempted to cleave sharp distinctions between surgery and other types of work.

In 1961, Dr Knight from South-East Scotland argued against the Junior Staffs Group Council determining what a 'reasonable' amount of off-duty time should be for a resident house officer. He lamented that the 'somewhat curious relationship between the houseman and his chief' had been 'lost sight of'. He argued that the house officer was not 'an appointment for a certain salary', but the 'beginning of a career'. It was an important 'period of service', and he ventured that at that stage of one's career, 'the missing of an odd hour or two off-duty was a good investment'.[28] Indeed, while many were broadly in favour of reducing the intensity of trainee surgeons' working hours, they were also wary of introducing regulations or fixed standards to manage workloads. H. S. Howie Wood from the Isle of Wight backed the general notion of extra payments for excessive hours, but thought that 'using a yardstick such as 100 or 105 hours to decide when over-time pay came into operation' was 'lowering the dignity of the profession'.[29] This rejection of standardised or quantifiable regulations and the rhetorical recourse to ideas about professional 'dignity' or autonomy was common in 1960s and 1970s debates about surgeons' working hours. Even those in favour of more humane working conditions were averse to homogeneous guidance applied nationwide, for example.

However, not all surgeons were expected to work long hours. In this early period, consultants were required to 'consult' on cases, offer advice and guidance to their more junior colleagues, and have overall responsibility for patients and the operating theatre. One of the rewards for the excessive temporal commitment expected of junior doctors was the promise of a consultant post that came with increased autonomy, better pay, and fewer hours spent at the hospital. It was in this period that the 'golfing consultant' stereotype really took flight. This notion that consultants were brief and only periodic visitors to the hospital ward and spent most of their spare time pursuing sports and other hobbies was pervasive and continued into the 1980s. One surgeon I interviewed in 2020 told me about a consultant at the hospital where he trained who came in after playing tennis and did the ward rounds in his kit.[30] However, from the 1970s onwards, new contracts for both junior and senior surgeons, along with NHS management and administrative restructuring and reform, increasingly altered the working patterns and behaviours of hospital doctors.

The 1974 reorganisation of the NHS

The 1970s was a transformative decade in the history of the NHS. It witnessed the first major reorganisation of the service in 1974, the first junior doctors strikes in 1975, and the 1979 Royal Commission on the NHS. Together, these events exposed and altered the working conditions and emotional landscape of the British hospital. Specifically, they exacerbated and revealed new tensions about surgical time. Not only did they expose the excessive hours that hospital doctors worked but they added new anxieties about *how* surgeons spent their time while at hospital.

Following a change of government and a change of secretary of state, the white paper on National Health Service reorganisation was published in August 1972. The NHS Reorganisation Act received royal assent on 5 July 1973, and came into effect in 1974.[31] It represented a significant structural and administrative reform of the health service and outlined plans to unify the existing tripartite health system (comprising primary care, hospitals, and community services, established by the NHS Act in 1946) with a unitary, integrated system. It brought general practice and secondary and local healthcare under new authorities and district management teams.[32] Due to the reforms, regional, area, and district authorities replaced regional hospital boards, taking over public health and other services from local authorities in the process.[33] The 1974 reorganisation is a key watershed moment in the history of the NHS.[34] However, in general, it does not have a great reputation among policymakers, health professionals, or historians. The *BMJ* lamented in 1977, 'Any future historian looking at the National Health Service is likely to see the 1970s as the decade of the decline of the hospital service.'[35]

In many ways, and for many observers, this was an accurate assessment of the decade. The middle of the 1970s saw increased tensions between doctors – both junior and senior – and the government. Since the foundation of the NHS, many hospital consultants had combined working in NHS hospitals and treating NHS patients with working in private hospitals and treating private patients (as well as treating private patients in NHS hospitals). Under Harold Wilson (prime minister from 1964 to 1970), Labour had reduced the number of private beds in NHS hospitals. During that period, consultants had begun to develop a model called 'geographical full time', meaning that they pledged to do all of their private work on site, which would give the hospital consultant availability twenty-four hours a day rather than them seeing patients away from NHS property at private hospitals. Consultants stood to lose some of their considerable private practice income through this scheme of work, but insisted that they were prepared to concede for the greater good of the hospital. While in opposition in 1973, Labour pledged to phase out pay or private beds entirely. These plans faced stiff resistance, culminating in hospital consultants suspending all 'goodwill activities' between January and April of 1975, when consultants stuck rigidly to their NHS contract hours.[36] The industrial action was called off only when the health secretary Barbara Castle relented. She allowed part-time consultants to continue private practice and her battle against pay beds had limited success. Only a quarter of pay beds were phased out by 1979, when Margaret Thatcher's election victory brought Castle's plans to an 'abrupt end'.[37] The impact of this was long term and deeply damaging. These disputes weakened the bonds between consultants and their hospitals, compromising the next generation's sense of loyalty to the NHS and their employers.

Junior doctors also took strike action in 1975, walking out over long hours and inadequate pay for extra time. This was the first time in British history that doctors had officially gone on strike and it was largely in response to the kind of excessive temporal commitment described.[38] Prior to 1975, junior doctors had been paid extra whenever they worked above 80 hours a week, clocking 85.6 hours on average. Recognising this workload to be excessive, the Independent Review Body on Doctors' and Dentists' Remuneration (which had been given control over doctors' pay by the government in 1962) proposed to reduce standard hours to forty-four and offered additional pay for any overtime.[39] Initially, some in the BMA were in favour of the new contract as it left doctors 'better able to plan their lives'. However, with the Labour government looking to restrain public-sector pay, no new money was made available and the scheme proposed instead reduced the bonus level for each additional hour by two-thirds. Thus, rather than increasing their salaries, junior doctors claimed that this new contract would instead cut their pay and do little to curb excessive hours. Calling for no wage cuts and a forty-hour standard week, in October thousands of junior doctors organised bans on non-emergency work and various other kinds of collective action in different parts of the country.[40]

In the 1970s, junior doctors framed their collective action in terms of living standards, working conditions, and the emotional costs of excessive temporal commitment.[41] Their strikes took place against a new intellectual backdrop that was increasingly emphasising the damage done by work to mental health and wellbeing. In the 1970s, sociologists began paying greater attention to stress on the job, and particularly to the strains associated with working in large, complex organisations. In 1978, Cary L. Cooper and Roy Payne published an edited volume called *Stress at Work*. They situated themselves within a 'determined effort by social scientists' – that had taken place over the previous ten to fifteen years – to 'consider more systematically the sources of management and organisational stress'.[42] In both Britain and the United States, wellbeing advocates attended to the dehumanisation of doctors – through sleep-deprivation, abuse, and harassment – and advocated balance and recuperation. This marked a major shift in the way that people thought about surgeons' and physicians' wellbeing – from seeing anxious, depressed, or suicidal doctors as impaired or faulty to seeing them as products of their working environment.[43]

Advocates, particularly in the US, championed new risk-based tools, which emphasised prevention. If hospitals and other healthcare institutions could allay doctors' stress, there would be less risk of 'burnout' (a term coined in 1974, referring to human/service workers).[44] These efforts were not just taking place outside organised medicine (although the UK was slightly slower on the uptake than their North American counterparts). The pioneering manual, *Beyond Survival* (1979), was co-written by leaders in the American Medical Association resident section, which was formed in part from the house staff (junior doctor) unionisation movement in the USA.[45] Activist-thinkers like John Henry Pfifferling, a medical anthropologist turned healthcare worker wellbeing advocate, founded the Center for Wellbeing of Health Professionals, an important early organisation in combating these issues.[46]

In 1970s Britain, the junior doctors' industrial action dragged on for months of 'go-slows', partial strikes, and walkouts, continuing until the government found a further £2.3 million (somewhere down the back of the sofa, it seems) to fund their overtime and made concessions over hours. They finally resumed normal working in January 1976. Later that year, the Royal Commission on the NHS called on professional organisations, trade unions, clinical institutions, healthcare workers, patients, and members of the interested public to submit evidence about their experience of the services and their views on its recent history. Many of those submitting evidence – particularly members of the healthcare workforce – discussed pay beds, the junior doctors' strike, and referred to what they saw as the debilitating effects of reorganisation. Chaired by Sir Alec Merrison, the Commission covered England, Scotland, Wales, and Northern Ireland. The report was published in 1979, after the Commission had been 'appointed at a time when there was widespread concern about the NHS' following the first major reorganisation of the service throughout the UK in 1973 and 1974, 'which few had greeted as an unqualified success'.[47]

Dr F. A. Lodge wrote in on 8 December 1975: 'At a time when the average working week is 35 hours, junior hospital doctors are being grudgingly offered an 80 hour week.'[48] He posed a question: 'How did the scheme manage to work, apparently successfully, for so many years if it has always been so badly underfinanced?' He responded: 'The answer is distressingly simple: "By exploitation of those who worked in the Service".'[49] While Lodge was clearly sympathetic to the junior doctors' position, the submissions of evidence also reflected a widespread concern about the regulation of working hours and how that might impede on surgeons' sense of vocation. A surgeon who signed himself Mr Vellacott FRCS wrote to Sir Alec Merrison on 29 May 1976 and said, 'The Government and the Hospital Doctors have to decide whether Medicine is to remain a profession with ethics or to become an industry with strictly regulated hours of work.'[50] Here, he drew a distinction between a profession – governed by 'ethics' – and an industry – governed by regulations. He critiqued the industrial action doctors had been participating in, arguing that the withdrawal of services would 'make nonsense eventually of any idea of Vocation', something which he described as 'over and above job satisfaction and one of the chief prerogatives of the profession'.[51] He argued that 'the element of vocation' is difficult to 'define or evaluate' and described surgeons as having a 'calling' – and that it was 'something personal'. He contrasted this calling against 'job satisfaction', which could be achieved whenever 'the skill and effort employed yield reward'. Anyone could achieve job satisfaction, but surgeons' sense of vocation was different. And it was this sense of vocation that was under attack by regulations designed to limit the hours they worked. In a similar vein, Philip Hugh-Jones from King's College Hospital wrote in to say that in his view the junior hospital staff 'very unwisely acted alone in arranging pay for overtime'. His concern was not so much that their strategies had been ineffective, but that it had 'immediately put the doctors on a par with the trade union and other workers'.[52]

This relationship between vocation and excessive temporal commitment has a long history. However, something new was happening in the 1970s. Much like the pages of the medical press in the 1950s and 1960s, the submissions of evidence to the 1979 Royal Commission were full of complaints about the hours junior medical and surgical staff were expected to work. However, these complaints had acquired new resonance in the climate of increased bureaucracy and regulation, not least because complaints of this kind could now be seen as a push-back against capitalist or managerial conceptualisations of time in the hospital workplace.

The most common complaint in evidence about the reorganisation was that it had added an extra and unnecessary tier or management level. Hospital administrator Keith Mallinson wrote a letter to the Royal Commission on 7 May 1976. He said,

> I see around me a great deal of dedicated service, given by the doctors and nurses and other staff within the hospital, however, one thing which is more than apparent is the excessive bureaucracy. It seems that since reorganisation our hospitals have become over administered, and this is a cause of unrest among staff.

He argued that reorganisation had created a 'cumbersome, expensive, and unwieldy administrative machine'.[53] For surgeons, reorganisation had introduced a new concern. Practitioners in the 1970s were not just concerned by how much time they had at their disposal, but what that time had to be used for. They had to contend with a new debate over what kind of tasks were allocated to a surgeon in the hospital ecosystem. To a new extent, bureaucracy drew surgeons out of the operating theatre and away from their primary professional function. This had painful and lasting effects on their professional identity, notions of exceptionalism, and sense of self.

These new concerns were accompanied or exacerbated by a new, multifactorial conceptualisation of workplace management and workplace stress. As Professor James Parkhouse noted in 1976,

> Merely to have 'enough' doctors is not an answer to the problems of medical manpower. There are three critical questions of distribution: between regions, specialties and grades. All need solving in order to have the right number of doctors available in the right places to do the right kinds of work at the right times.[54]

Similarly, in their volume on stress, Cooper and Payne acknowledged that there was more to emotional distress in large, complex organisations than simply excessive temporal commitment:

> Stress can be caused by too much or too little work, time pressures and deadlines, having too many decisions … fatigue from the physical strains of the work environment …, excessive travel, long hours,

> having to cope with changes at work and the expenses (monetary and career) of making mistakes.[55]

In other words, satisfaction at work was not just associated with *how much* time people spent at their jobs, but *what* they were using that time for.

Letters from staff to the Commission that addressed reorganisation as a key source for their distress were common. As Merrison put it in his report, 'There were allegations in our evidence about the swollen number of administrators, their poor quality and the diversion of clinical staff to administrative duties. Some of these were strongly worded.' As I have mentioned, reorganisation was repeatedly criticised for the Byzantine bureaucratic structure it introduced and the deleterious effect that structure had on staff morale. Merrison quoted a Mr A. J. N. Phair who had written in to the Commission to say,

> Bureaucracy used to be a term to define the most efficient office procedures now in the NHS it can only be used in its pejorative sense of red tape, buck passing and considerable inexcusable delays which is partly caused by administrators shying away from their responsibilities and receding into the management structure cocoon.[56]

One impact of this new bureaucratic web was the increased sense that time was a valuable, and quantifiable, resource in the NHS. The aphorism 'time is money' first appeared in the eighteenth century in an emerging capitalist society.[57] This ascribing of time with a monetary value gained new significance in the second half of the twentieth century, and workers in the welfare state increasingly referred to time as a commodity, a medium for exchange, and a way to measure work, productivity, and value. Nurse Miss E. M. Henslow wrote to the Commission on 2 June 1976 to make this configuration of time explicit: 'Theft of all types of TIME is yet another contributing factor to the continued loss of money.'[58] The 1974 reorganisation was regularly blamed for this kind of theft, or waste:

> Regional Health Authorities … are an unnecessary tier of administration. They try to interfere in the Area Authority functions and produce much ill feeling between Area and Region. The waste of time and money produced by these authorities and their numerous self-perpetuating committees must be enormous.[59]

Time became an increasingly scarce resource for surgeons in the 1970s, but not because they had more operations to perform or because their working hours increased. Instead, it became perceived as limited because they were now also expected to undertake administrative and bureaucratic work on a new, unprecedented scale.

Towards the end of the twentieth century, Sir George Godber, Chief Medical Officer from 1960 to 1973, made a series of observations about the ill effects of 1970s NHS reform. In the notes for an article entitled 'History and Origins of the NHS', he wrote, 'The unique quality of the British is their power of self-deception', and suggested that in 1966 he had 'no doubt that the British National Health Service was the finest in the world' and that he would have rather been a patient in this country than in any of the many he had visited.[60] However, he identified two hazards: 'Ministers (i.e. politicians) and Civil Servants (i.e. bureaucrats)'.[61] He decried, 'what they have done in the last ten years has been greatly to the detriment of the service to the sick'.[62]

As discussed in the introduction, he lamented the new administrative and bureaucratic burden shouldered by hospital workers after reorganisation: 'The best nurses no longer attend the sick. They walk around the hospital corridors clutching sheafs of papers and demanding coffee from the overworked ward sister', and lambasted the amount of 'office work' clinical staff now had to do.[63] The new bureaucracy had negatively affected the emotional health of the hospital workforce: 'Not surprisingly morale amongst doctors and nurses has dropped. Requests for new developments have to go through at least three bodies. Not only does this waste time, but communications are paralysed and decisions cannot be taken.'[64]

Margaret Thatcher and the introduction of the internal market

Anxieties about working time continued into the 1980s, but as with the 1970s, new and altered concerns also appeared in response to a rapidly changing political climate. In the 1980s, Thatcherism represented a systematic, decisive rejection and reversal of the post-war consensus, whereby the major political parties largely agreed on the central themes of Keynesianism, the welfare state, nationalised industry, public housing, and close regulation of the economy. There was one major exception: the National Health Service, which was widely popular (as demonstrated by the 1979 Royal Commission) and had broad support in the Conservative Party. In 1982, Thatcher promised that the NHS was 'safe in our hands'. Despite these assurances, Thatcher set about introducing a range of reforms that fundamentally altered the nature of work in the NHS.[65] At the time, many critiqued these reforms, arguing that they set the service on a downwards trajectory. And Thatcher's approach to the NHS has been repeatedly identified as a key contributing factor in health service decline, particularly by commentators on the political left. In the 1980s, modern management processes were introduced in the NHS to replace the previous system of consensus management. Outlined in the Griffiths Report of 1983, this involved the recommendation of the appointment of general managers in the NHS with whom ultimate responsibility should lie. The report also recommended that clinicians – particularly hospital consultants – should be more involved in management.[66]

In 1988, Thatcher announced a review of the NHS. In 1989, two white papers 'Working for Patients' and 'Caring for People' were produced. These outlined the introduction of what was termed the 'internal market', which was to reshape and restructure the health services for much of the next decade and beyond.[67] Despite intensive opposition from the BMA, who wanted a pilot study of the reforms initially confined to one region, the internal market went ahead. In 1990, the National Health Service and Community Care Act (in England) defined this 'internal market', whereby health authorities ceased to run hospitals but 'purchased' care from their own or other authorities' hospitals.[68] The 'providers' became NHS trusts, which encouraged competition but also increased local differences. Doctors' relationship with the government deteriorated during the 1980s. The advance of managerialism under Griffiths irritated many doctors, previously accustomed to a dominant role in NHS governance. Godber described the situation in the 1970s and 1980s: 'Keith Joseph, the last Conservative Minister, had had some business experience and was determined that the management of the NHS should be professional. To this end he recruited professional management consultants, McKinsey & Co.'[69] Godber argued that these changes had had ill-effects on doctors' happiness: 'The frustration which every doctor has experienced seeing the service of which he was so proud being destroyed by ministerial and administrative unwisdom has had its effect on morale.'[70]

However, while there was plenty of change afoot in the 1980s, and despite concessions made by the Labour government in 1975 over doctors' working hours, trainee surgeons continued to work more than 100 hours a week, and the medical and mainstream press continued to cover the deleterious effects of this temporal commitment on medical professionals' wellbeing. In 1981, the *Daily Mail* published an article entitled 'The price of a surgeon's devotion to work'. The author described the breakdown of consultant surgeon Clive Orton's marriage to his wife Sue. He quoted one of Orton's colleagues: 'Unfortunately, break-ups are a common hazard for dedicated specialists. There seems no hope of a cure. Wives just have to accept that family life takes second place.'[71] Another doctor relayed his working schedule to a journalist. Every other weekend he would start work at 9:00am on Friday, and then he would not stop or sleep until 5:00pm on Monday. The senior house officer reflected, 'The argument has always been that it's a good toughening-up process but, obviously, patient care must suffer when doctors have been on their feet for virtually 24 hours.'[72] According to the BMA, in 1981 70 per cent of junior doctors were still working more than eighty-four hours in a week: 'In general it is a story of broken marriages, strain and stress.'[73] In 1989, the Health Minister David Mellor infuriated doctors with an off-the-cuff remark comparing their stories of hours worked to 'fishermen's tales'. It only took a week for the minister to row back on his previous comments, insisting that he was committed to ending the 'unacceptable' hours worked by junior doctors.[74] Just seven days after that, the health secretary Kenneth Clarke committed to a seventy-two-hour working week for junior doctors, although he wanted to get there by negotiation, not legislation.[75]

However, much like in the 1970s, the issue was not so much the number of hours worked by surgeons, but what they had to do in that time and how much autonomy they felt they had over their professional lives. In 2020 I interviewed a senior urologist who had begun his working life in the 1980s. He saw – and still sees – his work as a 'vocation', not just a job. Since beginning his career, however, the professional landscape of surgery had shifted. New management structures, imposed 'by the system', had altered the way he and his colleagues were supposed to think about and organise their working time: 'Now my contract [dictates that] I work so many hours a week and there's a job plan that says I'm doing this on this day and that on that day.'[76] He described how his organisation now managed his time in a 'far more pro-active way' and that this change had eroded his 'professional independence'. He lamented the ways in which his colleagues were 'complicit' in this new system and that he no longer saw the kind of temporal or emotional commitment that was so common when he began his career in the early 1980s: 'You work when you're contracted to work and you don't when you're not contracted to work.'[77]

He argued that it was partly a product of changing managerial and administrative norms, but also down to a 'generational shift': 'Younger colleagues don't want that continuing responsibility for their patients and they want to be able to walk away when they want to.'[78] He suggested that this change was not just down to transformations internal to healthcare, but that you see it in 'all walks of life': 'When I started, everyone lived in order to work nowadays people work in order to live. It's a job and ideally you make enough money to have a nice life.' When asked whether he saw any benefits to this new way of managing surgical time, he responded with an emphatic no: 'From the doctor's perspective it's an error.' He argued that there were now fewer 'dedicated professionals' who were available '24/7' for their patients.[79]

He reflected on the changes he had witnessed over the course of the 1980s and into the 1990s. He argued that the policies and practices introduced by Thatcher's Conservative government – including pledges to reduce working hours – had altered his professional status and negatively impacted surgeons' sense of vocation: 'When I was appointed I effectively had a professional contract. I was appointed to provide urological care to the patients who came in under me.' He argued that he had a 'professional obligation' and that he would 'routinely go into hospital on a Saturday morning or even a Sunday' to see his patients even if he was not on duty.[80] As discussed, the 1980s was a period of increased managerial intervention and oversight, which makes his reflections on the relative freedom of that period in his surgical career particularly intriguing.

From a twenty-first-century gaze, he could reflect on the decade as a time of professional autonomy, even if that decade witnessed some of the most dramatic alterations in hospital governance. It may well be true that surgeons working in the 1980s, despite Thatcher's reforms, still had greater autonomy than practitioners today. Or this could be an example of one of the challenges of oral history interviewing, whereby participants project back current complaints or persuasive narratives that they have used to construct their personal and professional selves. The surgeon's mention of generation provides added weight to this second explanation, suggesting that nostalgia inflected his recollections.

The European Working Time Directive

The long 1990s saw further far-reaching political and NHS policy change. In 1997, Tony Blair won a landslide general election for Labour and the party's manifesto included an intention to abolish the internal market initiated by Thatcher's government. Labour issued interim guidelines instructing trusts and health authorities to co-operate rather than compete, and discussions about a new wave of reforms started, culminating in the White Paper, 'The New NHS: Modern. Dependable', published in 1998.[81] This White Paper contained various suggestions for reform; however, in many respects it represented an evolution, rather than revolution, in the management of the NHS initiated by restructuring in the 1970s and the 'Working for Patients' White Paper published in 1989. Despite a rejection of the competitive ethos of the internal market, the fundamental purchaser–provider split – which separated planning of healthcare from its delivery – was retained. It also continued to strengthen the role of managers in the NHS. Not only accountable for financial performance, boards were now responsible for the quality of care. Moreover, the Labour government continued to use Private Finance Initiatives (PFI) as a way of creating 'public-private partnerships' (PPPs), where private firms were contracted to complete and manage public projects. PFI was implemented in 1992 by John Major and was attacked by the Labour Party while in opposition. However, the use of PFI was limited until 1997, when they were expanded by the NHS (Private Finance) Act, resulting in criticism from many trade unions, elements of the Labour Party, and other political factions.[82]

'The New NHS: Modern. Dependable' did, however, transform the way surgeons and other hospital doctors worked. It included a new contract for consultants which aimed at increasing their accountability and restricting their freedom to work in the private sector. It ushered in a new emphasis on the provision of twenty-four-hour, consultant-led care across all subspecialties. It also recognised the need to continue to reduce the working hours of junior doctors and to 'break down the old hierarchical ways of working'.[83] Developments included the Calman Reforms of medical postgraduate training that introduced shorter, more intensive training programmes; consultants were required to take a more active role in training their juniors (reducing the time available for treating patients); there was greater specialisation, necessitating new arrangements to ensure that hospitals had appropriate and comprehensive medical cover; and they proposed a new consideration of European Union directives restricting the working hours of doctors.[84] The European Working Time Directive (EWTD) forty-eight-hour working week entered law in European Union countries in 1998 and a phased approach to implementation was agreed for doctors in training in the UK, which steadily reduced working hours to fifty-eight in 2004, fifty-six in 2007, and forty-eight in 2009.[85] A key component of the EWTD was that the maximum period of work for a resident without rest is thirteen hours.

'The New NHS: Modern. Dependable' had a self-consciously historical dynamic and situated itself as a turning point in British healthcare policy. It announced proposals for 'far reaching change across the NHS' with 'radical' transformations planned at 'every level'.[86] The rhetoric of NHS modernisation was part of a broader late-1990s trend towards 'rubbishing the past', a past that was characterised by 'old fashioned demarcations between staff and barriers between services, a lack of clear incentives ... over-centralization and disempowered patients'.[87] At the end of the millennium, NHS modernisation required hospital consultants to abandon many of their 'old, outdated' ways of working and to submit themselves to much greater control and scrutiny in order to 'develop a health service fit for the twenty first century'.[88] However, this portrayal of the 'old' ways of medical practice and the vision for a new modern NHS was neither readily accepted nor acquiesced to by surgeons.

The EWTD was a subject of particularly fraught controversy and high feeling. Even twenty years after its final implementation, almost all the surgeons I have interviewed hark back to an era before the introduction of the EWTD. The changing shape of surgical training and work was a thread that ran through all the interviews, intersecting with a range of issues, including professional development, 'work–life' balance, gender, and their experience of adverse or traumatic events. As discussed in Chapter 3, prior to the introduction of the EWTD and Modernising Medical Careers in 2006, surgeons trained as part of a firm – a hierarchical structure of senior and less-senior practitioners. Many of those interviewed attested to the supportive nature of this team approach – and argued that they could cope with excessive temporal commitment because they were maintained by a sense of comradery and mutual understanding. One male plastic surgeon, born in 1946, said, 'The firm system was you knew where you stood. You were working in a small group of people where everybody knew you and you knew all your patients.'[89] Surgeons lamented the loss of the 'family-like' structure of the NHS in days gone by.

This same plastic surgeon was explicit about the source of the current malaise: 'The thing that changed everything for the worst is the European Working Time Directive … That's why I am the hardest of hard Brexiteers. The EU has done so much damage to medicine.'[90] He lamented the changes brought in by the policy:

> All surgical trainees are now on rotas whereas in my day there was no such thing as a rota apart from casualty. This means that the person in charge of the surgical ward changes twice a day. They waste a lot of time on the handovers and the bond between a surgical trainee and the patient is broken because they don't know everything about them. The European Working Time Directive firstly destroyed continuity of care and the second thing they did was that they weren't working long enough hours to learn the skills. If you don't put in the hours you don't learn the skills.[91]

He was convinced that the working cultures and practices of the past made for better surgeons: 'The dangers of working long hours have been greatly exaggerated. It's much more dangerous to be inexperienced. If you've seen it all before, done it all before, then you're confident.'[92]

One male paediatric oncology surgeon, born in 1944, described his past working life and emphasised long working hours, informality and collegiality on the ward, and professional autonomy in the operating theatre. As for so many of his colleagues, when he first qualified in the late 1960s and early 1970s, more-than-100-hour working weeks were 'normal'.[93] In his first job, he had no official time off and leave was arranged on an ad hoc basis with his consultant. The consultant would usually say yes, unless 'things were very busy' or he had 'some very sick patients'; then he 'would just have to stay there until things were under control'.[94] I asked him whether there were any positives to his working life then. He said, 'I got loads of experience … you just do more'. He reflected on how 'very different' this experience was to 'how it's become now' – contrasting his operative independence then to how it became after the introduction of the EWTD: 'In the forty-eight-hour weeks we have now it's just more difficult for trainees to get the necessary experience.'[95]

He framed this shift negatively and reflected nostalgically on his past working life. He said that he was 'quite happy that I lived through that old era'. Key to this happiness was a sense of professional comradery. In the 'old system … you felt very much like you were part of a firm … Whatever you were doing … you were definitely working within the team and that gave a very strong feeling of belonging and commitment.'[96] He developed close relationships with his colleagues and superiors who could rely on him: 'I think if I look at all the surgical bosses I had, I think I worked well with them because I was sort of around all the time and they got to trust me.'[97] In contrast, towards the end of his consultant career in the late 1990s and early 2000s, he 'did get a bit irritated at the restrictions placed on our trainees and felt they weren't around when they should have been … Nowadays people are on rotas and you don't get that continuity.'[98] He argued that these new rotas – brought in by the EWTD – negatively affected the quality of teaching and training: 'Sometimes you hardly know your trainees and it's very difficult to impart a philosophy of practice if you hardly see them.' He finished by saying, 'I think I was lucky to have been brought up in that era … I'm a supporter of how it was than how it is now and I think a lot of old people feel that way.'[99]

His assessment of the majority view was correct. Most of those interviewed had fond memories of the past and made unfavourable comparisons with current and proposed practices and ways of working. Their assessments orbited around the late 1990s and early 2000s as a watershed in the recent history of hospital working cultures. Surgeons were particularly critical of the EWTD, which they argued negatively affected both their own emotional health and wellbeing and patient safety. When interviewed, surgeons denied that long working hours were inherently worse than shorter shifts, suggesting that a sense of community and positive relationships with colleagues and patients made excessive temporal commitment easier to bear. Almost all the surgeons interviewed commented on how informal support networks within the profession and the hospital had, over the past forty years, collapsed. In an article entitled 'Has humanity disappeared from the NHS?' published in the *BMJ*, one doctor wrote, 'It was Monday 27 December 1999 … it was to be the busiest day of the year … Paradoxically, I enjoyed the 24-hour period, unencumbered by the usual other clinical commitments. It was like the "good old days".'[100]

These 'good old days' were also frequently characterised as an era when resources were more plentiful, staff turnover was lower, and work was more enjoyable. One consultant surgeon interviewed as part of a piece of social science research said, 'There was never the same sort of shortage of beds. As a junior doctor, I didn't have to spend anywhere near as much time as my trainees do now juggling around trying to find beds for patients.'[101] Another argued that junior doctors and the consultant contract were the 'big problems associated with institutional change in the NHS … because again people would work for shorter periods of time … and so overall ownership of problems would be lost, because you lose the continuity in terms of the handovers'.[102] Due to junior doctors' restricted hours – a product of the EWTD – consultant surgeons had more work to do without more time to do it in: 'More and more we are having to sift through sometimes big piles of notes to get information ready, whereas years ago the house officer would have done it and would just have alerted us to any problems, but that doesn't happen anymore.'[103] Echoing complaints from the 1970s, the implication here is that surgeons now have less time for operative work because they spend too much time doing administrative labour.

Many surgeons were also nostalgic about a different management culture and landscape. In the past, they say, the specialist knowledge and skills possessed by doctors – which allowed for the smooth running and high quality of service provision – were acknowledged by managers who acted in a supportive role to medical professionals. One surgeon reflected, 'The process in which I grew up in the early days was one whereby the medical profession … had a lot more of a say in running the hospital.'[104] A reduction in autonomy was also key to nostalgic reflections about surgeons' professional pasts. One surgeon said in emotive terms,

> In spite of the pressures in the 1980s and 1990s, a sense of being in control of one's own destiny mitigated against much of the stress. I have lived through thirty-five years of erosion of autonomy and a burgeoning weight of governance, that, in turn, contributes to a sense of jeopardy and peril.[105]

As I have demonstrated, this idea that surgeons should possess unusual autonomy and embody individualism in their work has a long history.[106]

The experiences of those in my sample reflect the outcomes of more wide-ranging research conducted into the impact of the EWTD on the working lives of hospital doctors. Survey data published in the *BMJ* in 2014 demonstrated that policies increased tensions between junior doctors and their senior colleagues, and some consultants indicated that they felt 'beleaguered by carrying some of the workload which used, in the pre-EWTD era, to be undertaken by their junior doctors'.[107] Moreover, some of the senior doctors surveyed were found to be concerned that rotas introduced to comply with working time restrictions had eroded the professionalism of junior doctors and promoted a 'clocking off' attitude – conflicting with expectations that clinical labour is not just 'work', but a vocation.[108] However, it was not just senior doctors that had complaints about their junior counterparts; criticism was levelled in both directions. One junior doctor in the study commented, '[My] main issue is consultants still believing that it should be like the "good old days – 120-hour working weeks", not understanding the difference in patient load, non-ward-based work, new on-call systems.'[109] In this survey, surgeons and clinical oncologists were the specialists most likely to disagree that the changing rules had benefited senior and junior doctors, suggesting that surgeons have an unusual relationship with the past and present of their professional status.[110]

A sense of history – 'the past' – has long been part of medical, and particularly surgical, identities. Since the nineteenth century, practitioners have made use of a clinical chronology and expressed a professional past, present, and future in the construction of their self-image. Christopher Lawrence has delineated a phenomenon whereby surgeons habitually boosted their own era by denigrating former regimes as barbaric or inadequate.[111] They decry their predecessors' 'barbarity', and narrate a 'rags to riches' tale from miserable butchery to scientific surgery.[112] The era before the 1860s (with the gradual introduction and adoption of anaesthetics and antiseptic surgery) was stigmatised as a dismal surgical dark age. The American surgeon J. Ewing Mears averred that the surgeon had climbed from being 'bleeder and barber' to being 'pathologist [and] diagnostician' and was now 'crowned above all as the refined and cultured gentleman'.[113] Thus, for much of surgery's history its practitioners have invoked what sociologist Tim Strangleman calls 'nostophobia' and denigrated their professional forebears for their inability to comprehend 'modern' or recent tools and techniques.[114] In the twentieth century, however, things changed. The dominant discourse moved from a progressive narrative about improvements in surgical knowledge and surgical technique to a set of nostalgic reflections about the nature of surgical work. As Svetlana Boym has observed, this shift tracks a general history of twentieth-century Europe: 'the twentieth century began with a futuristic utopia and ended with nostalgia'.[115]

What, then, are we to conclude from twenty-first-century surgeons' nostalgia? It implies a longing for a by-gone era. For many people, however, working in that era was an unpleasant experience. Indeed, some oral histories and contemporaneous accounts of surgery and hospital care in the 'halcyon days' of the 1960s and 1970s reveal a hierarchical, male-dominated, and exhausting system that relied on nepotism and wives who performed the household labour and childcare that allowed their husbands to work uninterrupted. The 'firm' system, while lauded by many, was also critiqued by several surgeons I interviewed and particularly by female practitioners who argued that it cultivated a macho culture with little time or space for emotional reflection, women, or family life.

Indeed, when junior doctors were surveyed over ten years before the introduction of the EWTD, many reported having carried out intensive work over long hours. Some made vivid comments about fatigue-related stress.[116] To compound these lived experiences, surveys of the literature also reveal a recurring pattern of initiatives to try and improve the working cultures and expand the emotional resources available to practitioners – solutions to problems perceived as widespread. From the foundation of the NHS onwards, articles published in the medical press repeatedly call for the preservation of social spaces in the hospital dedicated to doctors, the protection of surgeons' lunch hours and annual leave, and the provision of psychoanalytic and therapeutic support for staff.[117] As this chapter has also shown, there have been repeated attempts to limit the hours surgeons spend at work and frequent emotionally fraught debates about temporal commitment in the medical and mainstream press.

Nostalgic expression in the clinical workplace does, therefore, obscure negative experiences and memories. This obfuscation could be interpreted as a deliberate process – one designed to denigrate the changing demographic make-up of surgeons and physicians and lament the diversification of NHS staff. For example, Maria Tsouroufli et al. describe nostalgia in hospital medicine as a 'gendered form of othering'.[118] They argue that nostalgic expressions about long working hours in days gone by are subversive practices of resistance, 'with implications for women's career and identity experiences'.[119] The New Labour reforms, such as Modernising Medical Careers and the EWTD, not only reduced working hours but introduced part-time training and work to enable more women to participate in the clinical workforce. In this respect, the reforms were partially successful. Women now make up 40 per cent of all doctors and as of 2015, 54.4 per cent of general practitioners. However, this success has not been mirrored in hospitals, where only 28 per cent of doctors are women. As chapters 3 and 4 have demonstrated, women are still underrepresented in specialties with the most acute and unpredictable workloads such as surgery (only 13 per cent of consultant surgeons in the UK are female). Tsouroufli et al. see nostalgia as 'a mechanism for … resisting change of gender order in the profession at a time of modernisation and numerical feminisation of the NHS'.[120] This is a critique not confined to nostalgia in the NHS, as commentators have drawn attention to various political nostalgic expressions that appeal to an 'old era' that is imagined as predominantly white and predominantly male.[121]

However, it is also possible to see nostalgia in different terms, and there is a small but growing literature that provides a more nuanced consideration, one in which those invoking the feeling are 'neither dupes or disturbed melancholics'.[122] Indeed, while the sociologist Fred Davis defined nostalgia as a 'positively toned evocation of a lived past', he saw it as a productive emotion with the capacity to generate individual, social, and political change.[123] It is 'one of the means ... at our disposal of the never-ending work of constructing, maintaining and reconstructing our identities.'[124] The sociology of organisations in particular seeks to reinterpret nostalgia. Rather than seeing it as a fundamentally (small 'c') conservative emotion, these studies instead suggest that nostalgia represents a 'discursive recourse' that can be selectively deployed as a 'weapon in the armoury of those seeking to drive through ... changes'.[125]

I want to argue, therefore, that nostalgia is not just a rose-tinted vision of a static past that ignores the realities of the twenty-first-century world and workforce, but also a creative tool deployed as part of a broad arsenal of professional identify formation, maintenance, and workplace reform. Svetlana Boym suggests that nostalgia even has a 'utopian dimension' and that while nostalgia and progress are 'like Jekyll and Hyde: alter egos', they are two sides of the same coin.[126] She suggests that 'nostalgia is not always about the past; it can be retrospective but also prospective'.[127] Indeed, surgeons and other hospital doctors often reject the idea that their invocation of the past in their critiques of the present are a static or conservative form of nostalgia,

> I don't think we are fossilized in a particular mode but ... I think cultural change has got to be sensible ... processes are becoming much more complicated and the doctors are having less say in how that process takes place, so you feel that the thing is running away with you and you have less control over it and at the same time you feel somewhat disenfranchised from the process itself.[128]

Sociologist Tim Strangleman describes nostalgia as a tool used to redefine the past and win support for change.[129] Surgeons speak of the past as a place of learning and transformation, resisting the characterisation by NHS managers and in government policy documents of the medical profession as staid, rigid, and in need of dramatic change for the sake of 'modernisation'.

In line with these more revisionist scholars, I am less interested in the accuracy of nostalgic reflections about the NHS than in what they can tell us about the workplace feelings of surgeons in Britain today. The periodic emergence of nostalgic expression prompts us to see the emotion as a way for surgeons to manifest their discontent at the realities of modern working life – what they see as an affront to their professional identity and special social status. Indeed, and as argued elsewhere in this book, the notion that surgical work is in some way distinct from other kinds of work or employment is key to this image and identity. And this notion is particularly acute in the context of the NHS and its quasi-mythic status in British society. Doctors and particularly surgeons tend to have a high opinion of their own profession and see clinical work as exceptional.[130] As I have suggested, medicine and related professions are perceived and described as a 'vocation' or a 'calling', not a career like any other.

Reflecting on the 1990s, surgeons frequently expressed anxiety about the implications of modernisation for medical professionalism and the length of time practitioners expected to be at work:

> We never used to have doctors complain about the amount of time they spent working ... An old boss of mine said 'a professional workman is a professional who always finishes the job' and essentially it didn't matter how much time you took, you started a job and you finished it ... now doctors are starting to feel like workmen, they just come in 9.00am until 5.00pm and any extra work is resented ... I find that sentiment upsetting really because I think that it should be a vocation.[131]

These medical practitioners connect long hours to commitment and see working overtime as a heroic contribution to both patients and the profession. One senior hospital doctor said,

> Current trainees are thinking as a 9–5 cleric rather than someone who is dedicated to the profession, which is not only a profession ... Now I get so annoyed when I ring trainees outside normal hours and they don't like it. Some of these people should be in a different profession.[132]

The relationship between vocation and excessive temporal commitment is not unique to healthcare, and employers across a range of sectors have made similar attempts to link long hours to professional commitment. Nonetheless, NHS policy transformations in the second half of the twentieth century were perceived as reshaping the surgical identity, and not necessarily for the better.

Conclusion

However, the practitioners I interviewed were nostalgic not just for longer working hours, better trained juniors, less bureaucracy, and limited managerial control, but for a different kind of emotional community, one that offered the support, care, and comradery required in a pressurised and sometimes traumatic workplace.[133] Surgeons argued that the shorter sessions of work mandated by the EWTD led to complex rotas and frequent handovers with implications for patient safety and professional wellbeing alike. In contrast, interviewees reflected on an age of long working hours made bearable by the emotional support provided by their colleagues and the compassionate connections they could form with their patients when they were able to maintain some form of continuity of care. These surgeons were nostalgic for a sense of professional comradery, 'a very strong feeling of belonging and commitment'.[134] In the absence of counselling services or mental health support, practitioners filled that space with their own ad hoc and informal versions of care and sought comfort from friends, family, and colleagues. According to these doctors, the introduction of the EWTD delivered the final blow to this sustaining network and emotional community. Moreover, as these informal support systems disintegrated, they were not replaced by any formal or systematic counselling or mental health services.

Nostalgia among surgeons is, therefore, a tool to express profound discontent at the changing nature of their working lives. This nostalgic 'methodology' is perhaps particularly useful for surgeons who tend to avoid explicitly political engagement with the conditions of their labour. Demands to 'take politics out of nursing and medicine'[135] were frequent in submissions of evidence to the 1979 Royal Commission: 'In response to the general dissatisfaction with the state of the NHS, Parliamentary politics should be taken out of the Service.'[136] While junior doctors went on strike in the 1970s and in 2012, and again in 2023, many surgeons find industrial action unappealing in part because it sits uneasily with claims they make about their devotion to their vocation. One hospital staff member wrote to the Royal Commission in 1976 to complain about her 'sorrow at the changed attitude of a great number of staff, who quite definitely considered their own wellbeing to be of greater importance than the welfare of the patients. Reference to the record of some of the strikes … can be taken as evidence of what I am saying.'[137]

This apolitical tendency was partly responsible for a new way of thinking and talking about surgeons, their working conditions, and their wellbeing that emerged in the early twenty-first century. Translated from business, management, and the military, resilience rhetoric relied on a changing hospital culture and a long-standing tradition of using military metaphors to articulate and understand the surgical identity. Chapter 7 will describe the nineteenth- and twentieth-century history of this tradition, before outlining the development of the notion of resilience as a kind of emotional armour that surgeons possess or should acquire. As this chapter has shown, throughout the second half of the twentieth century, some surgeons and other healthcare professionals attempted to curtail their working hours and reconfigure their working conditions via protest and policy change. In contrast, resilience rhetoric is much more individualistic and identifies the internal workings of the psyche as both source and solution to distress.

Notes

1 Interview with female surgeon; interviewed by author, 12 January 2018.
2 Ibid.
3 Ronald Macbeth, 'Married Quarters in Hospital', *British Medical Journal*, 1:5346 (1963), 1673–1674, 1674.
4 Alex Mold, 'Making the Patient-Consumer in Margaret Thatcher's Britain', *Historical Journal*, 54:2 (2011), 509–528, 509.
5 Richard Canter, 'Impact of Reduced Working Time on Surgical Training in the United Kingdom and Ireland', *The Surgeon*, 9 (2011), 6–7.
6 'The Week in Dundee', *British Medical Journal (Clinical Research Edition)*, 287:6385 (1983), 139–155, 143.

7 Neville Stidolph, 'Training of Surgeons', *British Medical Journal*, 4:5627 (1968), 379–383, 379.

8 N. G. Sanerkin, 'Hospital Junior Staff', *British Medical Journal*, 2:5514 (1966), 646.

9 Jenny Firth Cozens, 'Medicine and the Media', *British Medical Journal (Clinical Research Edition)*, 295:6607 (1987), 1199–1200, 1200.

10 Thomas Bedford, S. A. Roach, D. G. Harvey, and J. E. Braham, 'First Conference of the British Occupational Hygiene Society', *British Journal of Industrial Medicine*, 11:1 (1954), 49–62, 51.

11 Vicky Long and Victoria Brown, 'Conceptualizing Work-Related Mental Distress in the British Coalfields (c.1900–1950)', *Palgrave Communications*, 4 (2018), 1–10.

12 Ibid.

13 See Mark Jackson, *The Age of Stress: Science and the Search for Stability* (Oxford: Oxford University Press, 2013); Jill Kirby, *Feeling the Strain: A Cultural History of Stress in Twentieth-century Britain* (Manchester: Manchester University Press, 2019).

14 'Hospital Junior Staffs Group Council', *British Medical Journal*, 1:5240 (1961), 294–297, 297.

15 'Annual Representative Meeting', *British Medical Journal*, 3:5714 (1970), 41–54, 43.

16 Ibid., 44.

17 G. S. Tune, 'Sleep and Wakefulness in a Group of Shift Workers', *British Journal of Industrial Medicine*, 26 (1969), 54–58, 54. See also Natasha Feiner, 'Pilot Fatigue and the Regulation of Airline Schedules in Post-war Britain', in Mark Jackson and Martin D. Moore (eds), *Balancing the Self: Medicine, Politics, and the Regulation of Health in the Twentieth Century* (Manchester: Manchester University Press, 2020), 190–215.

18 'Annual Representative Meeting, Folkestone, 1973', *British Medical Journal*, 2:5868 (1973), 138–155, 142.

19 M. J. Evans, 'Sacrificed to an Archaic Training System', *British Medical Journal*, 303:6793 (1991), 65.

20 A. G. W. Whitfield, 'Women Medical Graduates of the University of Birmingham 1959–63', *British Medical Journal*, 3:5661 (1969), 44–46, 45.

21 Mignon Duffy, 'Doing the Dirty Work: Gender, Race, and Reproductive Labor in Historical Perspective', *Gender & Society*, 21:3 (2007), 313–336.

22 A General Practitioner's Wife, 'Married Quarters', *British Medical Journal*, 1:5538 (1967), 505.

23 J. G. Taylor, 'Encouraging Recruits to Medicine', *British Medical Journal*, 2:5752 (1971), 51.
24 Stidolph, 'Training of Surgeons', 379.
25 John Shepherd, 'Married Quarters', *British Medical Journal*, 1:5538 (1967), 505.
26 Richard Lewis, 'Personal View', *British Medical Journal (Clinical Research Edition)*, 284:6332 (1982), 1867
27 Shepherd, 'Married Quarters'.
28 'Hospital Junior Staffs Group Council' (1961), 297.
29 'Annual Representative Meeting', 45.
30 Interview with male surgeon; interviewed by author, 31 July 2020.
31 Philip Begley and Sally Sheard, 'McKinsey and the "Tripartite Monster": The Role of Management Consultants in the 1974 NHS Reorganisation', *Medical History*, 63:4 (2019), 390–410, 390.
32 National Health Service Reorganisation Act (1973), www.legislation.gov.uk/ukpga/1973/32/enacted.
33 Begley and Sheard, 'McKinsey and the "Tripartite Monster"', 392.
34 Charles Webster, *The Health Services Since the War, Volume II. Government and Health Care: The National Health Service 1958–79* (London: Stationery Office, 1996); Geoffrey Rivett, *From Cradle to Grave: Fifty Years of the NHS* (London: King's Fund, 1998); Rudolf Klein, *The New Politics of the NHS: From Creation to Reinvention* (London: Radcliffe, 2013).
35 'Appeasement 1977 Style', *British Medical Journal*, 2:6103 (1977), 1619–1620, 1619.
36 Jack Saunders, 'When do Doctors' Strikes End? A Perspective from 1975', *People's History of the NHS* (8 February 2016), https://peopleshistorynhs.org/when-do-doctors-strikes-end-a-perspective-from-1975/ (accessed 22 May 2021).
37 Cal Flyn, 'NHS Strikes and the Decades of Discontent', *Wellcome Collection Stories* (12 July 2018), https://wellcomecollection.org/articles/WyjRuCcAACvGno__ (accessed 23 May 2021).
38 Saunders, 'When do Doctors' Strikes End?'.
39 Ibid.
40 Ibid.
41 Jack Saunders, 'The Junior Doctors' Strike: What's Really New About it?', *The Guardian* (6 January 2016), www.theguardian.com/science/the-h-word/2016/jan/06/nhs-junior-doctors-strike-whats-really-new-about-it (accessed 22 May 2021).
42 Cary L. Cooper and Roy Payne, *Stress at Work* (London: John Wiley & Sons, 1978), 82.
43 Agnes Arnold-Forster and Sam Schotland, 'Covid-19 Only Exacerbated a Longer Pattern of Health-Care Worker Stress', *Washington Post* (29

April 2021), www.washingtonpost.com/outlook/2021/04/29/covid-19-only-exacerbated-longer-pattern-healthcare-worker-stress/#click=https://t.co/81YIkeqjZX (accessed 20 May 2021).

44 Matthew J. Hoffarth, 'The Making of Burnout: From Social Change to Self-Awareness in the Postwar United States, 1970–82', *History of the Human Sciences*, 30:5 (2017), 30–45. See also Jackson, *The Age of Stress*.

45 J. Pat Tokarz, William Bremer, and Ken Peters, *Beyond Survival: The Challenge of the Impaired Student* (American Medical Association: Workgroup on Physician Well-Being, Resident Physicians Section, 1979).

46 Ibid.

47 Alec Merrison, *Royal Commission on the National Health Service: Report* (London, 1979), 1.

48 Letter from Dr F. A. Lodge to Dr Summerskill, 8 December 1975, BS6/44.

49 Ibid.

50 Letter from Mr Vellacott FRCS to A. Merrison, 29 May 1976, BS6/79.

51 Ibid.

52 Letter from Philip Hugh-Jones to Mr de Peyer (The Secretary), 5 January 1976, BS6/211.

53 Letter from Keith A. Mallinson to A. Merrison, 7 May 1976, BS6/12.

54 Comments to Royal Commission on the National Health Service, Professor James Parkhouse, December 1976, BS6/5.

55 Cooper and Payne, *Stress at Work*, 82.

56 Merrison, *Royal Commission on the National Health Service: Report*, 31.

57 Benjamin Franklin, 'Advice to a Young Tradesman' (21 July 1748), Founders Online, National Archives, https://founders.archives.gov/documents/Franklin/01-03-02-0130 (accessed 28 February 2023).

58 Letter from Miss E. M. Henslow SRN SCM to A. Merrison, 2 June 1976, BS6/80.

59 Letter from The Somerset Local Pharmaceutical Committee to Sir Alec Merrison, 22 June 1976, BS6/272.

60 Wellcome Library, History and Origins of the NHS, GC/201/A/1/63.

61 Ibid.

62 Ibid.

63 Ibid.

64 Ibid.

65 Martin Gorsky, '"Searching for the People in Charge": Appraising the 1983 Griffiths NHS Management Inquiry', *Medical History*, 57:1 (2013), 87–107.

66 Ibid., 89.
67 Charles Webster, *The National Health Service: A Political History* (Oxford: Oxford University Press, 2002), 174.
68 David Hughes, 'The Reorganisation of the National Health Service: The Rhetoric and Reality of the Internal Market', *Modern Law Review*, 54:1 (1991), 88–103, 88.
69 Wellcome Library, History and Origins of the NHS.
70 Ibid.
71 Ian Fletcher, 'The Price of a Surgeon's Devotion to Work', *Daily Mail* (9 January 1981).
72 'Sleep If and When You Can', *Daily Mail* (7 October 1981).
73 Ibid.
74 'I Will Help to Cut These Hospital Hours, says Mellor', *Daily Mail* (3 January 1989).
75 'Clarke "To Act on Doctors' Hours" ', *Daily Mail* (10 January 1989).
76 Interview with male surgeon; interviewed by author, 30 July 2020.
77 Ibid.
78 Ibid.
79 Ibid.
80 Ibid.
81 Secretary of State for Health, 'The New NHS: Modern. Dependable' (Department of Health and Social Care, 1997), https://assets.publishing.service.gov.uk/government/uploads/system/uploads/attachment_data/file/266003/newnhs.pdf.
82 Geoffrey Rivett, '1998–2007: Labour's Decade', Nuffield Trust, www.nuffieldtrust.org.uk/chapter/1998-2007-labour-s-decade (accessed 22 May 2021).
83 Secretary of State for Health, 'The New NHS: Modern. Dependable'.
84 Ibid.
85 Canter, 'Impact of Reduced Working Time on Surgical Training'.
86 Secretary of State for Health, 'The New NHS: Modern. Dependable'.
87 Ibid.
88 Ibid. See also Stephen Harrison, 'New Labour, Modernisation and the Medical Labour Process', *Journal of Social Policy*, 31:3 (2002), 465–485.
89 Interview with male surgeon; interviewed by author, 23 March 2018.
90 Ibid.
91 Ibid.
92 Ibid.
93 Interview with male surgeon; interviewed by author, 18 January 2018.
94 Ibid.
95 Ibid.

96 Ibid.
97 Ibid.
98 Ibid.
99 Ibid.
100 Anthony Toft, 'Has Humanity Disappeared from the NHS?', *British Medical Journal*, 320:7247 (2000), 1483.
101 Quoted in Ruth McDonald, Justin Waring, and Stephen Harrison, 'At the Cutting Edge? Modernization and Nostalgia in a Hospital Operating Theatre Department', *Sociology*, 40:6 (2006), 1097–1115, 1103.
102 Ibid.
103 Ibid.
104 Ibid.
105 Correspondence with author, 4 February 2019.
106 Christopher Lawrence, 'Democratic, Divine and Heroic: The History and Historiography of Surgery', in Christopher Lawrence (ed.), *Medical Theory, Surgical Practice: Essays in the History of Surgery* (London: Routledge, 1992).
107 Abi Rimmer, 'Working Time Restrictions May Have Increased Tensions Between Trainees and Consultants, Studies Find', *British Medical Journal*, 348 (2014).
108 Ibid.
109 Ibid.
110 Ibid.
111 Christopher Lawrence, 'Democratic, Divine and Heroic'.
112 Ibid.
113 Ibid., 9.
114 Tim Strangleman, 'The Nostalgia of Organisations and the Organisation of Nostalgia: Past and Present in the Contemporary Railway Industry', *Sociology*, 33:4 (1999), 725–746.
115 Svetlana Boym, *The Future of Nostalgia* (New York: Basic, 2001), xiv.
116 Rimmer, 'Working Time Restrictions May Have Increased Tensions'.
117 J. H. Tweedie et al., 'Facilities for Junior Doctors in New Hospitals', *British Medical Journal*, 2:6150 (1978), 1503; J. F. Murray, 'Improving the Hospital Service', *British Medical Journal*, 1:6008 (1976), 507–508; 'The Orthopaedic Surgeon', *British Medical Journal* , 1:5698 (1970), 748–749; Neville Davis and H. Stephen Pasmore, 'Anxious Patient and Worried Doctor', *British Medical Journal*, 1:5061 (1958), 40.
118 Maria Tsouroufli et al., 'Gendered Forms of Othering in UK Hospital Medicine: Nostalgia as Resistance Against the Modern Doctor', *Equality, Diversity and Inclusion: An International Journal*, 30:6 (2011), 489–509.

119 Ibid.
120 Ibid.
121 For a general and illuminating account of the role played by nostalgia in British history, politics, and identity, see Hannah Rose Woods, *Rule, Nostalgia: A Backwards History of Britain* (London: Ebury, 2022).
122 Tim Strangleman and Ian Roberts, 'Looking Through the Window of Opportunity: The Cultural Cleansing of Workplace Identity', *Sociology*, 33:1 (1999), 47–67.
123 Fred Davis, 'Nostalgia, Identity and the Current Nostalgia Wave', *Journal of Popular Culture*, 11: 2 (1977), 414–424, 420.
124 Fred Davis, *Yearning for Yesterday: A Sociology of Nostalgia* (New York: Free Press, 1979).
125 McDonald et al., 'At the Cutting Edge?', 1098.
126 Boym, *The Future of Nostalgia*, xvi.
127 Ibid.
128 Quoted in McDonald et al., 'At the Cutting Edge?', 1098.
129 Strangleman, 'The Nostalgia of Organisations and the Organisation of Nostalgia'.
130 Late Victorians and Edwardians identified surgery with exploration and engineering as being among the great accomplishments of fin de siècle civilisation. Lawrence, 'Democratic, Divine and Heroic'.
131 Quoted in McDonald et al., 'At the Cutting Edge?', 1103.
132 Ibid.
133 The idea that feeling cultures have different binding effects is well established in the emotions history literature. See William M. Reddy, *The Navigation of Feeling* (Cambridge: Cambridge University Press, 2001); Barbara H. Rosenwein, 'Worrying about Emotions in History', *American Historical Review*, 107:3 (2002), 821–845.
134 Interview with male surgeon; interviewed by author, 18 January 2018.
135 Letter from Miss M. Williams to A. Merrison, 26 May 1976, BS6/75.
136 Letter from R. D. D. Henderson to A. Merrison, 19 May 1976, BS6/16.
137 Letter to A. Merrison, 25 May 1976, BS6/59.

7

Military myths and metaphors

Warfare, conflict, and violence have been part of society for centuries, if not millennia.[1] It is not that surprising, therefore, that military metaphors have 'invaded' many other aspects of human society, including surgery and medicine. Thomas Sydenham, one of the most famous physicians of the seventeenth century, suffused his medical writing with military language. He declared a 'murderous array of disease has to be fought against, and the battle is not a battle for the sluggard'. He endeavoured to investigate ill health, understand its character, and 'proceed straight ahead, and in full confidence, towards its annihilation'.[2] In the nineteenth century, doctors, public health practitioners, and laboratory scientists promoted bellicose metaphors of disease, hastened by the rising prominence of germ theories.[3] Patients were now allegorical battlefields – their bodies sites of conflict between modern medicine and enemy disease agents. The close connections between medicine and war also meant that various traits associated with victories on the battlefield – including 'determination', 'courage', and 'perseverance' – were transferred onto healthcare professionals.

In the aftermath of the two world wars, in which surgeons played crucial, strategic roles, the idea that clinicians and military personnel shared similar characteristics became increasingly pervasive. The surgeons of the 1940s and 1950s were 'only too happy to become the soldiers of the post-war era'.[4] This period also witnessed an increasing number of abstract 'wars' against disease. Think, for example, of President Richard Nixon's still yet-to-be-won war on cancer, first declared in 1971. In these instances, the battlefield is not just the human body, but society itself.

The twentieth century also witnessed military metaphors become more expansive and malleable, and infiltrate more dimensions of medicine. For example, first recorded in the Earl of Orrery's 1677 *A Treatise of the Art of War*, the phrase 'front line' refers to the part of the army at the front – the section closest to the enemy.[5] Embedded into the British national psyche by the First World War, the bellicose term has come to signify not only a war against disease, but a conflict between doctors and those seeking clinical care. Maybe not literally – patients are not the enemy – but healthcare professionals frequently conceptualise themselves as under siege. And the opponent they are protecting themselves against is not always a malevolent disease agent, but instead they are besieged by excessive workloads, inflexible managers, and demanding healthcare 'consumers'. In 2020, however, a malevolent disease agent did 'declare war' on the British public and its health service. In response to the emergence of the COVID-19 virus, a new national tradition arose. Every Thursday at 8pm, citizens emerged from their homes to applaud those on the 'front line' of the pandemic. Language that drew analogy between healthcare professionals working closely with potentially infectious patients and soldiers embedded in trench warfare existed before the pandemic, but acquired a heightened significance over the course of this more recent crisis.

The language of war has perhaps been particularly salient in Britain because, over the course of the twentieth century, the country created and commanded a 'military-industrial-scientific complex' that was 'second to none'.[6] While some histories of Britain portray the country's military prowess as in decline – especially after its empire had begun to diminish in size and influence – in his revisionist account, David Edgerton insists that even after the Second World War, rather than being the West's 'weary titan' and 'effete declining power', it was instead 'the pioneer of modern, technologically focused warfare'. Britain was for a long time the leading exporter of arms, bureaucratically and technically proficient, and it saw itself as a 'global, liberal power, as a world political-economic policeman, an arbiter of the fate of nations'.[7] Post-war Britain was always awash with militarism, if militarism is 'a veneration of military values and appearances in excess of what is strictly necessary for effective defence'.[8]

Over the past five centuries, we have internalised these military metaphors, so much so that we are often unaware of how much they influence us, and may not even recognise them as references to bloody conflict. Doctors 'monitor for insidious disease', 'destroy rogue cells', 'search for silver bullets', and 'use all weapons at our disposal.'[9] In the 1970s, writer Susan Sontag waged her own battle against the use of military metaphors in the case of cancer, lamenting the way both medical and mainstream culture framed her illness in terms of a battle with both winners and losers.[10] Her critiques could equally be applied to the very public fall-out of American Senator John McCain's glioblastoma diagnosis and eventual death in 2018.[11] McCain received messages of support and sympathy from across the political spectrum, many of which drew on this ingrained language and traded on an adversarial model of the cancer experience.[12] Then-president Barack Obama tweeted, 'John McCain is an American hero & one of the bravest fighters I've ever known. Cancer doesn't know what it's up against. Give it hell, John.'[13] Obama was, of course, not alone in drawing on McCain's military background, weaving his martial history into his medical present and positioning cancer as an identifiable and malevolent foe.

Military metaphors are, therefore, everywhere in medicine. One American study from 2010 found that physicians use metaphors in almost two-thirds of their conversations with patients who have serious illnesses.[14] Metaphors and analogies are a fundamental mechanism through which we conceptualise and comprehend the world around us, especially in the face of complexity and dread. But evidence suggests they do more than explain similarities – they can invent them where they do not exist, and blur the lines between the literal and the figurative.[15] In other words, while military metaphors are everywhere in medicine, they have the capacity to do harm – to patients, but also to healthcare professionals. In this chapter, I chart the changing use of military metaphors in surgical discussion and debate. I use oral history interviews alongside articles in the medical press to interrogate the shifting cultural script of the surgical identity and investigate how the experience and representations of surgical work have altered alongside developments in organisational ideologies and broad social, cultural, and political shifts.

Starting with a longer history of military metaphors in nineteenth-century medical texts, I look at the language of surgeons' descriptions of operative practice and their attempts to improve patient health and at the increasingly prevalent tendency among healthcare professionals to conceptualise their ward work as unrelenting warfare. This tendency has also had unintended and often problematic consequences. For example, since c. 2000, there has been an increased debate about the importance of 'resilience' in surgery. The logic of this new terminology and set of emotional requirements is that if surgeons are working on the 'front line' of a protected battle, then they must possess some of the attributes of real-life soldiers. Thus, this chapter ends with an exploration of the twenty-first-century emergence of resilience rhetoric in British surgery and interrogates the now widespread notion that resilience is something surgeons should possess or learn.[16]

Building on the claims of the previous chapter about the reshaping of working time and its meanings in the managed healthcare bureaucracies of contemporary Britain, I argue that resilience developed as a popular and pervasive concept in surgery just as the emotional landscape of the British hospital was undergoing a profound transformation. Moreover, despite being framed as a way to ameliorate surgeons' emotional distress and frustration, resilience rhetoric has proven damaging. Current notions of resilience as 'emotional armour' are simplistic, individualistic, and identify the internal workings of the psyche as both source and solution to distress. Finally, and perhaps most troublingly, debates over this addition to the myth of the modern surgeon frequently take the place of vital, politicised, and structural critiques and interventions designed to ameliorate the working cultures and practices of the twenty-first-century NHS hospital.

Military metaphors

The relationship between surgery and warfare has a long history. In the nineteenth century, members of the medical profession exploited and elaborated 'visions of masculinity framed by war, heroism, and self-sacrifice'.[17] As Michael Brown has shown, this rhetorical habit and process of identity formation drew on a range of different threads interwoven through Victorian society and culture. Nineteenth-century Britain witnessed a 'veritable obsession' with heroes and heroism.[18] As explored in chapters 1 and 6, the modern surgical stereotype involves the abnegation of the self and personal sacrifice for the greater good. By the mid-twentieth century, this self-sacrifice took the form of excessive temporal commitment and the denial of a life beyond the hospital's four walls, but in Victorian permutations of the trope, heroes paid little heed to the dangers they put themselves in for the sake of the nation and empire. There was also a clear gendered dimension to notions of heroism. Heroic men were 'intrepid and courageous' – charging straight at danger, rather than passively enduring risk or avoiding it all together.[19]

This obsession with heroism – and the increased availability of martial metaphors for surgeons defining their own professional identities – was partly due to the changing social and cultural role of the military in nineteenth-century Britain. While the Napoleonic wars might have been good 'public relations' for the military, the post-war period 'witnessed a significant decline in the army's popularity', as it was increasingly associated with events like the 1819 Peterloo Massacre and other authoritarian and aggressive suppressions of crowds and protests.[20] However, various historians have argued that the army again became popular among the public in the middle decades of the century onwards. This transformation was down to popular imperialism, the Christianisation of the military, expanded ceremony and spectacle, and various colonial conflicts that took place in the 1850s.[21] Together, these various cultural and political machinations served to create a more positive vision of the British army. And, by the second half of the century, the 'soldier hero' acted as an alluring archetype for middle-class perceptions and performances of masculinity.[22]

This archetype was taken up by surgeons in a variety of ways. They used military metaphors in their description of their efforts against disease and they used them when talking about surgery's supposedly inexorable progress. There was also plenty of coverage in newspapers, magazines, and the medical press of surgeons participating in Britain's various global conflicts. A Dr Smith wrote to *The Lancet* to praise the assistant-surgeons Brady and Phelps of the 57th Regiment for, during the Crimean war, 'coolly and zealously attending to the wounded under the enemy's fire in the advanced trench ... to the great relief of the men who were struck down'.[23] Warfare offered surgeons an opportunity to demonstrate some of their emerging, manly characteristics – stoicism and calm under pressure.

Thinking about clinical practice as a form of warfare against a malevolent enemy was also common throughout the nineteenth century. Military metaphors were used to refer both to the activities of germs, parasites, and cancerous tumours, and to the actions of medical professionals.[24] Robert Koch articulated his efforts against disease as an 'offensive': 'in the past one took a more defensive attitude, we have now moved away from this defensive point of view and have seized the offensive ... We must be prepared, first, to detect the infectious material early and with certainty, and second, to destroy it.'[25] Conceptualising germs as invading entities was commonplace. A French writer in 1885 characterised infection as 'coming from outside, penetrating the organism like a horde of Sudanese, ravaging it for the right of invasion and conquest'.[26] Terms like 'invasion' and 'infiltration' (especially when racialised in this way) characterised late nineteenth-century bacteriology and parasitology, but were also used in discussions of diseases that were very much in the surgeon's wheelhouse like cancer. The surgeon to the Cancer Investigation Committee of the Middlesex Hospital in London, J. Bland-Sutton, wrote in 1907, 'When the breast is attacked by cancer the cells implicate the lymphatics in the underlying fascia and slowly invade them.'[27] Just a year later, Charles Ryall, Surgeon to the Cancer Hospital (now the Royal Marsden) described how malignant cells 'infect and invade the surrounding tissues'.[28] Cancer surgery was, therefore, a war of attrition against a malevolent foe and the profession was 'noble, from its many victories in the eternal warfare it wages against disease and death'.[29]

The military metaphor worked, therefore, on multiple levels. Surgeons were, just like soldiers, bold, brave, and unflappable under pressure. They were also waging war against new and age-old foes – everything from cholera to cancer. They were also part of a society-wide conflict between life and death, cures and killers, progress and stagnation or atavism. In 1900, Surgeon-Extraordinary to the Queen, Frederick Treves, spoke at the annual meeting of the British Medical Association in Ipswich, Suffolk. He gave an address entitled, 'The surgeon in the nineteenth-century', and concluded with a flourish, reflecting on the future of surgery in a passage suffused with military language: 'So as one great surgeon after another drops out of the ranks his place is rapidly and imperceptibly filled, and the advancing line goes on with still the same solid and unbroken front.'[30]

There were, however, some obvious tensions between surgeons and the military archetype. Soldiers were required to kill, and while surgeons and other medical professionals might have represented disease as an enemy to fight – and pictured themselves as a steadily advancing army – the 'essential medical mission remained humanitarian rather than destructive'.[31] This produced an internal conflict within medical rhetoric, with practitioners frequently 'oscillating between religious and warlike imagery and between both feminised and masculinised visions of medicine'.[32] As a result, and as Michael Brown has shown, the surgical identity in nineteenth-century Britain was complex and in constant flux.[33]

The mythologies of surgery – and the place of the military within them – shifted over the course of the century. Surgeons of the early decades were more emotionally expressive and drew on the sentimental cultures of Romanticism in their cultivation of their image and identity.[34] They were inclined to express pity, sadness, and regret and were attuned to the sufferings of their patients. This co-existed with more martial models of medical masculinity and both could be embodied or expressed by a single practitioner. As the century progressed, however, the development of 'Christian militarism' and 'muscular Christianity' served to ease some of those tensions, 'elaborating a vision of war that was compatible with moral and spiritual rectitude'.[35] As a result, and as discussed in Chapter 1, surgeons increasingly adopted a more stoic form of professional identity. As the twentieth century dawned, the self-image of the surgical profession had come to be more focused on its social mission and national contribution than on the interpersonal and emotional qualities of health and wellbeing. This shift was also partly a product of increasingly easy and effective anaesthetics, which reduced the amount of emotional management surgeons had to perform before and during operations. In addition, surgery became more and more effective – it increasingly saved lives and its public reputation benefited as a result.[36]

Wartime surgery

The relationship between surgery and the military was not only metaphorical. One of the reasons for the profession's persistent military associations was that throughout the nineteenth century, and in the twentieth-century's two world wars, surgeons participated in the war effort, engaging both on the literal front line and back home, in military hospitals. As the *BMJ* recorded at the beginning of the First World War:

> In every war in which our army has taken part – in the Peninsula, in the Maratha, Afghan, and Sikh wars, in the Crimea, in the Mutiny – the members of the medical department have freely given their lives in the performance of their duty and in the service of their country.[37]

Thus, and despite broad transformations in the way that surgery was practiced and perceived, the profession's military associations persisted into the post-war period.

Individual surgeons and their innovations were credited with successes on the battlefield. Joseph Lister, 'a great surgeon', developed techniques for antiseptic surgery in the late nineteenth century. As the twentieth century dawned, his methods were used less frequently in civil surgery, but in the trench warfare of the First World War, his principles had 'again come much to the fore'.[38] The popular press was full of accounts of surgical heroism in times of conflict. In 1915, *The Observer* published one story of the 'heroic deeds' of a surgeon in Gallipoli: 'He was badly wounded in both legs. For hours he lay in pain. A great part of that waiting he employed in crawling from one wounded man to another and ministering to their hurts.'[39] Even in moments of intense physical suffering, surgeons were capable of extreme self-sacrifice, serving the needs of their fellow men.

Thus, stoicism and the ability to bear substantial injury was a common feature of newspaper coverage of military surgeons and their exploits in the First World War. In 1914, the *Manchester Guardian* reported on the case of a surgeon major who not only 'begged to remain unnamed', but survived and endured ninety-seven wounds:

> I had just finished attending to my last case, and was about to mount my horse, when it seemed to me as though a clap of thunder burst immediately over my head, and I found myself in a circle of flame.

> A shell had just burst over me. My poor horse was killed on the spot, riddled with shrapnel.[40]

He was picked up by a man in his regiment, and carried over two kilometres on his back: 'To describe what I suffered upon that journey would be impossible.' He finished his tale with a brave statement of national pride: 'But here I am. Have you a cigarette? Thank you! After all, the German shells are not up to much!'[41] This 'gallant surgeon major' had been on the fighting line since the beginning of the war.

However, gallantry and stoicism were not the only behaviours or emotions performed and experienced by surgeons on the front line. In 1914, a surgeon at the front contributed some notes to the *BMJ* on the emotion of fear in battle. His musings were covered in *The Observer*. He drew a distinction between 'terror' and 'funk'. Terror was like 'the unreasoning terror of a child frightened by the dark' and did not abate once the person had reached safety. Funk 'abates in a place of safety' and is 'essentially a reasoning process'.[42] This period saw an increasing medicalisation of the emotional turmoil caused by military conflict and the emergence of terms like 'shell shock'.[43] 'Funk' seems to have something in common with the panic, distress, and wakefulness identified as pathological responses to the intensity of bombardment and hand-to-hand combat during the first and second world wars.

During both world wars, the surgeon was seen as crucial to military and strategic success. As one sociologist put it in 1941, 'we must turn for hope to military sanitation, pharmacy, medicine, and surgery. It is their job to prevent unnecessary human waste and return a larger percentage of us to the firing line.'[44] In addition, there was increasing coverage in the press of surgery's general social utility and the improvements to surgical practice and technique that had come about due to surgeons' participation in military conflict. A 1943 headline trumpeted: 'War-time surgery reveals fresh marvels.'[45] Indeed, the Second World War hastened various developments in a range of specialties including anaesthesia, vascular surgery, and plastic surgery. As the war came to a close, there was a widespread acknowledgement in the surgical field that the conflict had refashioned the professional landscape. Not just by altering operative practice, but by changing the dynamics of the hospital and its workforce.

Thus, while the Second World War ended in 1945, military metaphors did not disappear from the surgical vocabulary, and analogies to the battlefield continued to be used in discussions about surgeons 'conflicts' with individual diseases, in narratives about the 'heroism' of the profession and their 'heroic' interventions, and – perhaps most famously – in the 'war' on cancer. Military metaphors, as well as literal discussions of surgery in times of war, also continued due to Britain's participation in other battles, such as the conflict in Northern Ireland, which lasted for much of the second half of the twentieth century.

Bellicose language in the post-war period

In 1953, The British Empire Cancer Campaign made a fundraising film called *Onwards to Victory*, which interspersed black-and-white footage of laboratories, radiotherapy, and cancer surgery with shots of fighter jets, code breakers, and submarines. They made a similar film in 1958 called *The Modern Crusaders*. Both attempted to use the metaphor of science and technology's contribution to Britain's military victory over Nazi Germany to persuade the public to give generously in support of the campaign to defeat cancer, a 'peacetime menace'.[46] While made most famous by the US's National Cancer Act of 1971, military metaphors for cancer had been common in British surgical communities since at least the nineteenth century and became ubiquitous in the post-war period.[47]

In 1966, *The Lancet* considered whether Britain's research into cancer was progressing too slowly. Referencing the Second World War, they quoted the British Empire Cancer Campaign for Research's 1965 report: 'In the war against cancer it is still only 1940 and the real fight is yet to come.'[48] In 1966, Wilfred Kark published a book called *A Synopsis of Cancer* in which he discussed the profession's long-running conflict against the 'dread disease': 'Conquest in the war against cancer has an attraction and fascination, and promises far greater reward and booty than any other war in human history.'[49] In this protracted battle, surgery had a key role to play. If identified quickly, surgeons might remove a tumour before it had the opportunity to spread. This was the 'ultimate advantage in waging war on cancer'.[50] Other illnesses were not immune to this rhetorical treatment. In a discussion of treatment and prevention of cardiovascular disease from 1979, the authors of the study also argued for early intervention so that the disease could be 'arrested at, or before its onset'. In this way, surgeons could avoid 'battling the ... complications in its terminal stages'.[51]

As the NHS aged into adulthood, the use of military metaphors in surgical debate became more expansive and diffuse. Beyond just applying to the conflict between medicine and disease – with the human body as the battlefield – the hospital and the health service became new sites of 'trench warfare'. Increasingly, surgeons used military metaphors to describe their, often negative, experiences of working in the NHS. As discussed in Chapter 3, trainee surgeons frequently thought about their work in terms of military service and described their hospital accommodation as barracks. Similarly, surgeons frequently talked about their time as house officers using the language of the 'trenches'. This became more common after the reforms of the 1970s and with the increased managerialism of the 1980s. In a 1987 *BMJ* article, the author discussed overly interventionist hospital management and NHS cuts under Margaret Thatcher. He described a colleague who was planning to join the British Medical Association: 'My surgical friend is no medico-political ostrich ... He has always taken an informed interest in NHS management and finance, does more than his fair stint on local professional committees, and speaks with long experience of the district surgical trenches.'[52] Working in hospitals, and particularly in district hospitals, was akin to battling on the proverbial front line. The enemy, however, was not disease; but over-zealous administrators and Conservative Party politicians.

In a 1989 article about the importance of consultants being available on call to ensure that trainees were supervised during complex cases, the author reflected on the challenges of achieving that goal: 'There is ... a feeling within the system that once a person has done his or her "tour in the trenches" and is appointed consultant he or she should not have to take night duty again.'[53] As mentioned in the previous chapter, not all surgeons were expected to work long hours. In this period, consultants were called to 'consult' on cases and rarely were required on site overnight. This was partly because once junior doctors had completed their training 'tour', and the excessive temporal commitment it required, they were supposed to be 'rewarded' with increased autonomy, better pay, and fewer hours spent at the hospital. As discussed, it was in this period that the 'golfing consultant' stereotype took flight.

The language of 'the trenches' became increasingly prevalent towards the end of the twentieth century and was used to articulate several different aspects of the surgical identity. For example, surgeons talked about the context of warfare as a way of demonstrating the difference between theory and practice: 'In the trenches, unexpected factors emerge which were not considered in this or that research study, and individual choices still need to be made.' While plenty of planning might go into a battle or operation, both surgery and warfare were arts as well as sciences, and so while careful preparation was essential, both surgeons and soldiers had to be able to adapt to changing circumstances or unpredictable events. Along similar lines, military metaphors were frequently deployed to indicate the autonomy and professional expertise of surgeons who, like soldiers, had acquired plenty of experience on the 'front line' and so should be able to make decisions without undue intervention from people unfamiliar with the peculiarities of warfare:

> We as professionals, and as … surgeons in particular, have been asked to solve social ills through medical or surgical means. This is not possible, and we should all stand up and proclaim so, rather than meekly accepting what interested parties, particularly some patients, their unions, and attorneys, dictate to us. For those of us who have been in these trenches long, this is a depressing change in how we practice.

Military metaphors conveyed the independence and autonomy surgeons thought they deserved, and demonstrated their belief in the unique power of experience. Warfare, like surgery, was an unusual, if not unique, situation that few people had direct encounters with. As such, only those with the relevant experience should be allowed to pontificate about good practice or legislate for or against certain behaviours.

The front line

Alongside the increasingly prevalent use of 'trenches', the late twentieth century witnessed a new metaphorical phenomenon. People – healthcare workers and members of the public alike – began to refer to working in the NHS as being on the 'front line'. 'Front line' served many of the same needs as 'trenches', by configuring healthcare and the NHS as a conflict zone – not just between health and ill health, but between several interested parties like doctors, surgeons, nurses, patients, politicians, and managers. In 2016, the then editor-in-chief of the *BMJ* called the debate over a seven-day NHS a 'battleground'.[54] She framed it as a conflict between government and the medical profession, accused the health secretary Jeremy Hunt of 'misusing data to beat up on doctors', and insisted that he had 'pitted himself against' frontline workers.[55]

While this tendency to talk about the NHS in these terms existed well before the coronavirus pandemic, bellicose language framing the efforts of the health service and its constituent professionals as participating in dangerous and protracted warfare reached fever pitch in the spring and summer of 2020. In April, Ross Kemp, one-time star of *EastEnders*, thanked every NHS worker for 'the incredible sacrifice they are making on the frontline every day'.[56] The Royal College of Surgeons started a blog series called 'Covid-19: Views from the NHS Frontline', and headlines appeared across the news media comparing the nation's coronavirus effort to warfare. *The Times* published an article called 'The Frontline NHS Staff Battling to Keep Britain Safe During Coronavirus', with this as the standfirst: 'One surgeon likens it to Dunkirk as he helps out with intensive care.'[57] In May, the BMA conducted a survey of 'frontline doctors' and reported on the results using typically militaristic language: 'Under fire on the front line – doctors share their experiences of work during the Covid-19 crisis.'[58]

As other researchers have observed, the war-like imagery that suffused public debate about the COVID-19 pandemic in Britain was not confined to discussions of the health service and its staff. In the queen's live address to the nation, she called to mind the Second World War. She drew comparisons between social distancing and the 'painful sense of separation from loved ones' that was produced by the child evacuation programme in the 1940s. She ended her speech with 'We will meet again', a nod to Vera Lynn's 1939 song, 'We'll Meet Again', which served as the backing track to Second World War soldiers' leaving loved ones behind as they travelled to the trenches. 'We'll Meet Again' was recorded as a charity single in support of the NHS by Vera Lynn and Katherine

Jenkins. As Franziska E. Kohlt has pointed out, the fundraisers for the NHS that gained the widest public recognition and press coverage, like Captain Tom Moore, were those with 'apparent military connections'.[59] Representations, popular understandings, and individual experiences of the NHS remain, as Roberta Bivins has observed, 'haunted by … the language of the military crisis that had preceded it' in 1948. She argues that through this 'warlike language', the British public felt 'duty-bound' to support their health service. This language framed and continues to frame the NHS as a 'site for continued patriotic effort and even sacrifice'.[60]

The pandemic-era prime minister, Boris Johnson, particularly relied on military metaphors in his speaking and writing about COVID-19. In November 2020, he quoted the 1960s classic, *The Great Escape*, and urged the nation to hold tight and prepare for a slow return to normality: 'We are so nearly out of our captivity. We can see the sunlit upland pastures ahead … But if we try to jump the fence now, we will simply tangle ourselves in the last barbed wire, with disastrous consequences for the NHS.'[61] He also likened the development of effective vaccines to the 'morale-boosting bugle-blasting excitement of Wellington's Prussian allies coming through the woods on the afternoon of Waterloo'.

While Johnson made frequent recourse to patriotic language and references, the comparison between the coronavirus pandemic and the mobilisation of nations during the Second World War took place globally. For example, the Irish Prime Minister declared 'Never will so many ask so much of so few' (a nod to Sir Winston Churchill) in his acknowledgement of the devotion of healthcare professionals working with patients with COVID-19. Similarly, the governor of New York declared that 'ventilators are to this war what missiles were to World War II'. The president of France, Emmanuel Macron, used the word 'war' multiple times during a televised press conference about measures the country was taking to 'fight' the coronavirus pandemic.[62] One of the remarkable things about the coronavirus pandemic is that it has allowed a much older version of the military metaphor to infiltrate public discourse about healthcare. For much of the twentieth century, the 'enemy' faced by surgeons and other healthcare professionals was more difficult to identify. While disease remained a worthy opponent, increasingly doctors and nurses were fighting against governments, policymakers, patients, administrators, and managers rather than bacteria or viruses. The coronavirus pandemic hurtled the world back in time, to an age where infectious diseases had the capacity to radically alter the global landscape.

As both Kohlt and Bivins acknowledge, these military metaphors served useful functions during the pandemic. They cultivated a sense of belonging, commitment, and duty on behalf of both healthcare professionals and the public, prompted citizens to give generously to charitable causes, and allowed politicians to mitigate criticisms of their efforts. However, framing the coronavirus pandemic as a battle, with healthcare professionals on the 'front line', posed particular challenges to surgeons.[63] One component of the surgical self-image is the 'paradigm of sorting out problems'.[64] Self-efficacy is a vital component of the mental training necessary for surgical performance and uncertainty fits uneasily into a surgeon's personal or professional narrative. When interviewed, one surgeon said, 'For me, I became a surgeon to fix people … So, when someone dies … I put them in a box, marked "I can't fix you anymore." Then I take a deep breath and try and fix the things I can fix.'[65] For some surgeons, this professional 'paradigm' proved particularly challenging in 2020 both because COVID-19 is a difficult disease to treat, and because they felt underprepared to participate in the NHS's pandemic response. For those surgeons who were redeployed to support non-surgical roles – or, in the words of the Royal College of Surgeons of England, 'to extend temporarily the scope of their practice beyond the normal range of their expertise'[66] – the pandemic was a time of specific worries and frustration. In interviews, surgeons spoke of anxieties about risks to their personal health and safety and the slow distribution of adequate personal protective equipment, but also new and particular concerns about whether to operate or not, what counted as an elective or less-urgent intervention, and what if anything they could do to support their colleagues on COVID wards. In June 2020, Health Education England published a podcast that addressed the question of whether healthcare workers should 'run towards the front line' or remain 'on the sidelines'. For many surgeons, COVID-19 prompted new anxieties about what they could do from the healthcare 'sidelines'.[67]

Resilience

Despite the continuing prevalence of medical 'front lines' and 'trenches', the military metaphor that perhaps has been taken up with the most enthusiasm by surgeons is their supposed capacity for resilience. In December 2020, author and businesswoman Arianna Huffington wrote a blog post entitled 'And the Word of the Year Is … Resilience'.[68] Huffington disagreed with Collins Dictionary, Merriam-Webster, and the Oxford English Dictionary over their predictable and pedestrian choices for 'word of the year'. Instead of 'lockdown', 'pandemic', 'quarantine', 'doom scrolling', and 'coronavirus', she picked 'resilience': 'There is a single word that sums up 2020 and does encapsulate, in a deeper sense, the shared experience of billions of people this year … that word is resilience.'[69] She quoted the Oxford English Dictionary definition of the term: 'the capacity to recover quickly from difficulties; toughness. The ability of a substance or object to spring back into shape; elasticity'. She claimed that resilience is

> that quality that allows us to overcome challenges, obstacles, hardship and adversity, instead of being defeated by them. The reason resilience is my word of the year is because, unlike quarantine and social distancing, resilience is the only one that's going to be just as relevant when the pandemic is over. Resilience is the quality that was summoned in us by all the challenges of 2020. And it's also the quality that's going to carry us forward in 2021.[70]

Resilience is a psychological concept, defined as 'that ineffable quality that allows some people to be knocked down by life and come back stronger than ever; the capacity to recover quickly from difficulties, often equated with toughness'.[71] It is a type of emotional armour, a 'plastic shield' comprised of personality traits such as a robust sense of humour and what psychologists call 'stress immunity'.

It entered the lexicon of business and management from the military, and in 2002, Diane Coutu wrote an article for the *Harvard Business Review* entitled 'How Resilience Works'.[72] It did not take long for this language and associated psychological concepts to infiltrate healthcare generally, and surgery specifically. In 2014, the General Medical Council introduced resilience training to the medical school curriculum. Three years later, in a blog post for the Association for Academic Surgery website, Dawn Coleman applied Coutu's account of resilience to surgery.[73] Coleman quoted from Coutu's article, 'more than education, more than experience, [and] more than training, a person's level of resilience will determine who succeeds and who fails. That's true in the cancer ward, it's true in the Olympics, and it's true in the boardroom.' Coleman went on, 'I pose to you, members of the AAS, that it's also true in surgery.'[74]

Today, the idea that surgeons need to be resilient – and that the most successful surgeons are high achievers partly because of their robust 'emotional armour' – is prevalent. Prominent voices in the profession suggest that it is not only something surgeons should possess – and something that should be selected for when recruiting medical students and surgical trainees – but that it is also something that surgeons and other healthcare professionals can learn and develop. There is a widespread view in the medical profession that doctors, and particularly surgeons, should possess an inherent heightened mental robustness to manage the highly stressful nature of their work. In the section of the Royal College of Surgeons of England's website devoted to 'Careers in Surgery', on a page titled 'Skills and Qualities of a Surgeon', 'emotional resilience' has now made the brief shortlist of required attributes for professional success.[75]

In the 2010s, resilience among surgeons and physicians became an expanding area of research and associated with other twenty-first-century wellbeing preoccupations like burnout, stress, and 'moral injury'.[76] Most of the studies conducted into resilience have been undertaken in Australia and the USA. While researchers acknowledge that resilience is 'complex' and 'multifactorial', these studies use and investigate doctors' 'resilience scores', quantitative and supposedly objective measures of personal resilience.[77] These studies also tend to demonstrate that doctors in fact report relatively low resilience, and even surgeons are no more robust than the general population, and indeed might even be less so.[78]

As a result, resilience training is now big business. Professional societies, royal colleges, and individual institutions contract private organisations to provide general or tailored courses designed to 'upskill' surgeons and improve their ability to cope with the emotional turmoil of their jobs. The RCSEd have a page on their website where they write, 'Resilience is now recognised in healthcare as a collection of features that can be learned by individual doctors.' They offer their members a 'simple 10 step Programme' developed for medical staff by the Deans of Yale and ICAHN School of Medicine and have published 'expert tips for Resilience' on their website. These tips include 'try to maintain a positive outlook' and 'find an exercise regimen you'll stick to'. The Medical Protection Society offers free online workshops to its paying members designed to help them 'recognise the signs of burnout' and 'prevent recurrence'.[79] In 2020, Healthcare Conferences UK offered a one-day event devoted to 'enhancing resilience, reducing stress, and supporting the wellbeing of doctors'. Registration cost £438.

In twenty-first-century surgery, therefore, 'resilience' is everywhere. However, this has not always been the case. Indeed, while resilience might have been Arianna Huffington's word of 2020, its deployment in discussions about work and wellbeing is not a product of the coronavirus pandemic. It is, however, a relatively recent phenomenon. As a term and as a concept, it well predates the twenty-first century, but its widespread use, its application to business and management, and its infiltration of the surgical community emerged only after around 2000.[80] The Google Ngram Viewer is an online search engine that charts the frequencies of any set of search terms found in sources printed between 1500 and 2019 in Google's text corpora in English, Chinese, French, German, Hebrew, Italian, Russian, or Spanish. It is, therefore, a blunt instrument and cannot be used to evidence claims about the changing language of surgery or any other profession. It can, however, be used to illustrate them. If you plug 'resilience' into the engine, there was a clear uptick in the use of the word in the late 1990s, rising steeply past 2010.

As indicated by the Ngram chart, and demonstrated by searches through digitised journals, before c. 2000, 'resilience' as a word and notion was barely mentioned in medical and surgical literature, and when it did appear it was used to refer to patients, not practitioners. People with serious illnesses or injuries were the resilient ones, not the men and women who cared for them. Resilience in surgery is, therefore, a historical phenomenon, a response to a specific social, cultural, and political environment that exists now and did not exist before. Indeed, 'resilience' emerged as a topic of discussion just as the emotional landscape of the British hospital was undergoing a profound transformation in the first few years of the twenty-first century.

As demonstrated in Chapter 6, surgeons argued that the shorter sessions of work mandated by the EWTD led to complex rotas and frequent handovers which have made it difficult to maintain continuity of care with implications for patient safety and professional wellbeing alike. Interviewees reflected on an age of long working hours made bearable by the emotional support provided by their colleagues and the compassionate connections they could form with their patients when they were able to maintain a lasting relationship. The early twenty-first century witnessed, therefore, a shifting culture of emotional expression; increased workloads, more frequent hand-overs, staff shortages, and restricted resources that colluded to intensify the stresses and strains of surgical life; and a decline in informal support structures that were not being replaced by formal interventions designed to ameliorate emotional and mental ill health. This was the climate that made the emergence of resilience rhetoric possible. Prevailing understandings of emotional health and the language that dominated discussions about wellbeing in healthcare settings became increasingly individualised rather than collective. As chapters 3, 4, and 5 revealed, the surgical 'collective' was exclusionary and served a specific demographic. However, those included in that community felt as though they were supported by their colleagues and bolstered by a workplace in tune with their needs and requirements. They maintained enough professional autonomy, independence, and identity to protect themselves from the ample stresses and strains of surgical life.

Moreover, key to the emergence of resilience rhetoric is the language's origin in the military, as well as in business and management. It is no coincidence that Coutu's article was published in the *Harvard Business Review* or that Coleman quotes a reference to 'the boardroom' in her advocacy for resilience in surgery.[81] As discussed, the 1980s, 1990s, and early 2000s saw an increasing influence of management consultancy practices, policies, and language on the health service which are problematic in part precisely because of the focus they place on individuals rather than systems.

Resilience training specifically has its origins in the military. The British Army's Mental Resilience Training programme is designed to help soldiers recognise and regulate the signs of stress and help them to prepare for difficult events and circumstances. Similarly, the UK Royal Air Force offers its recruits a 'novel military health and well-being approach' called SPEAR that emphasises key activities: 'participating in Social networks, capitalising on Personal strengths and weaknesses, managing Emotions, enhancing Awareness of psychological symptoms and learning methods to promote Resilience'.[82] Much of the research into resilience has also taken place in military settings. From the early 2000s onwards, healthcare researchers into professional wellbeing and system management began looking to the army, navy, and air force for lessons and inspiration. In 2015, the chair of the General Medical Council, Terence Stephenson, told the House of Commons Health Committee: 'I am struck by how much the military invest in resilience training … they do not wait until they are out in Helmand province; they start at recruitment and training.' He thought this strategy might apply to healthcare: 'That is probably something that we could think about exploring … building in resilience training when people are medical students and young trainees rather than waiting … until you've been reported or had a complaint, and then trying to develop that resilience.'[83]

While seductive, some have challenged the applicability of the military to the medical. Authors of a *BMJ* article argued in 2010, 'Many of the organisations studied are solely military or include military personnel, which brings an acceptance and adherence to routines and procedures.'[84] Moreover, there is limited evidence that the military's resilience training programmes work – even for the soldiers and settings they are designed for. A randomised controlled trial published in *Occupational & Environmental Medicine* in 2019 found 'no evidence that resilience-based training had any specific benefit to the health and well-being of UK military recruits'.[85] While research has found that *feedback* for resilience training for surgeons is generally positive, there has not been similar rigorous testing of such interventions in healthcare settings.[86]

Conclusion

Psychological research into resilience has shifted since the beginning of the twenty-first century. While the first wave of work yielded descriptions of resilience phenomena, along with concepts and methodologies, it focused on individuals. As research and theoretical interests developed, psychologists have largely adopted a more dynamic account of resilience, focused on exchanges between individuals and the many systems in which they are embedded. They attend to resilient organisations or institutions, rather than just resilient individuals. While researchers into resilience in surgery have increasingly acknowledged the important role played by colleagues and employing institutions, mainstream surgical discussion has not been so subtle or sophisticated. Hospitals are now papered with posters that implore staff to 'be optimistic' and 'never give up'. It is unclear where the evidence for these interventions comes from or whether they can even be counted as interventions at all.

There is much to critique about resilience rhetoric in surgery today. It is individualistic, locating responsibility in people rather than policies, and allows proponents to sidestep serious and sustained engagement with the political and systemic contexts in which surgeons now work. It also focuses the collective mind on surgeons' emotional wellbeing rather than patients' experiences of healthcare. However, it is worth remaining alert to those who seek out services to support their own resilience. In a world where professional organisations, providers of surgical education and training, and surgeons themselves have little else available to them to address inadequate working conditions, resilience training and posters imploring practitioners to 'be optimistic!' are a bare-minimum stand-in for well thought-through, evidence-based responses to high turnover, mental illness, and emotional ill health in surgery. In other words, we should take the widespread nature of resilience rhetoric and critiques of that rhetoric as an indication that all is not well in the surgical world and better solutions are needed.

However, there are also risks associated with taking surgeons' assessments of their working conditions at face value. As discussed throughout this book, there are versions of the surgical stereotype that are positive, or at least reflect well on surgeons. In this chapter, I have explored the various iterations of the military metaphor and its repeated deployment to insist on the mental and emotional robustness of surgeons, their heroic tendencies, and their stoicism. In addition, and as explored in chapters 3, 4, and 5, there are also aspects of the surgical myth that serve certain members of the profession – particularly wealthy, white, male practitioners. Nostalgic reflections among surgeons today – when practitioners wax lyrical about the benefits of now long-gone hospital cultures and communities – tend to gloss over the exclusionary nature of those communities and the way they made working life much worse for some, even as they made it much better for others. In addition, the idea that individualistic resilience rhetoric emerged after the supposed collapse of these hospital communities with the introduction of the EWTD in part suggests the validity of that nostalgia. It is simultaneously true that resilience as an idea and term could only have been applied to surgery in this current historical moment – that it is tied up with contemporary wellbeing culture and neoliberal models of workplace mental health protection – and that the 'good old days', when surgeons looked after one another and hospitals were places that fostered a sense of belonging and commitment, were also harmful in their own way.

Notes

1 Jing-Bao Nie et al., 'Healing without Waging War: Beyond Military Metaphors in Medicine and HIV Cure Research', *American Journal of Bioethics*, 16:10 (2016), 3–11, 3.

2 Dhruv Khullar, 'The Trouble with Medicine's Metaphors', *The Atlantic* (7 August 2014), www.theatlantic.com/health/archive/2014/08/the-trouble-with-medicines-metaphors/374982/ (accessed 22 May 2021).

3 Agnes Arnold-Forster, *The Cancer Problem: Malignancy in Nineteenth-Century Britain* (Oxford: Oxford University Press, 2021); Lorenzo Servitje, *Medicine is War: The Martial Metaphor in Victorian Literature and Culture* (Albany, NY: SUNY Press, 2021).

4 Barron H. Lerner, *The Breast Cancer Wars: Hope, Fear and the Pursuit of a Cure in Twentieth-Century America* (New York: Oxford University Press, 2001), 75.

5 Steven Poole, '"Frontline": Is it Misleading to Apply Military Metaphors to Medicine', *The Guardian* (16 April 2020), www.theguardian.com/books/2020/apr/16/frontline-is-it-misleading-to-apply-military-metaphors-to-medicine (accessed 30 May 2021).

6 David Edgerton, *Warfare State: Britain, 1920–1970* (Cambridge: Cambridge University Press, 2006), 1.

7 Ibid.
8 Quoted in Edgerton, *Warfare State*, 6–7.
9 Khullar, 'The Trouble with Medicine's Metaphors'.
10 Susan Sontag, *Illness as Metaphor & AIDS and its Metaphors* (London: Penguin, 2009).
11 Jessica Morris, 'John McCain's Brain Cancer, and Mine', *New York Times* (20 July 2017), www.nytimes.com/2017/07/20/opinion/john-mccain-brain-cancer-glioblastoma.html (accessed 22 May 2021).
12 Agnes Arnold-Forster, 'Metaphors and Malignancy in Senator McCain's Cancer Diagnosis', *Nursing Clio* (31 July 2017), https://nursingclio.org/2017/07/31/metaphors-and-malignancy-in-senator-mccains-cancer-diagnosis/ (accessed 22 May 2021).
13 Barack Obama, Twitter Post (19 July 2017), https://twitter.com/BarackObama/status/887836712822558720?s=20.
14 David Casarett et al., 'Can Metaphors and Analogies Improve Communication with Seriously Ill Patients?', *Journal of Palliative Medicine*, 13:3 (2010), 255–260.
15 Khullar, 'The Trouble with Medicine's Metaphors'.
16 Agnes Arnold-Forster, 'Resilience in Surgery', *British Journal of Surgery*, 107:4 (2020), 332–333.
17 Michael Brown, '"Like a Devoted Army": Medicine, Heroic Masculinity, and the Military Paradigm in Victorian Britain', *Journal of British Studies*, 49:3 (2010), 592–622, 594.
18 Ibid.
19 Ibid.
20 Ibid., 596.
21 Ibid.
22 Ibid., 594.
23 C. Yorke, 'Heroic Conduct of Surgeons in the Crimea', *The Lancet*, 66:1669 (1855), 178.
24 Laura Otis, *Membranes: Metaphors of Invasion in Nineteenth-Century Literature, Science, and Politics* (Baltimore, MD: Johns Hopkins University Press, 2000), 23.
25 Quoted in Otis, *Membranes*, 34.
26 Quoted in Otis, *Membranes*, 23.
27 J. Bland-Sutton, 'A Lecture on the Cancer Problem', *The Lancet*, 169 (1907), 1342.
28 Charles Ryall, 'The Technique of Cancer Operations, with Reference to the Danger of Cancer Infection', *British Medical Journal*, 2:2492 (1908), 1005.
29 P. A. Simpson, 'An Address on Post-Graduate Possibilities', *British Medical Journal*, 2:1400 (1887), 923–928, 927.

30 Frederick Treves, 'Address in Surgery: The Surgeon in The Nineteenth Century', *British Medical Journal*, 2:2066 (1900), 284–289, 285.
31 Brown, '"Like a Devoted Army"', 595.
32 Ibid.
33 Ibid.
34 Michael Brown, 'Surgery and Emotion: The Era Before Anaesthesia', in Thomas Schlich (ed.), *The Palgrave Handbook of the History of Surgery* (London: Palgrave Macmillan, 2017), 327–348.
35 Brown, '"Like a Devoted Army"', 595.
36 This is, of course, a simplified account of the processes by which surgeons came to be trusted by the lay public. As Claire Brock has pointed out, at the end of the nineteenth century female surgeons were still likely to be perceived as inherently 'risky'. Claire Brock, 'Risk, Responsibility and Surgery in the 1890s and Early 1900s', *Medical History*, 57:3 (2013), 317–337. Sally Wilde has also written about the 'culture of innovation' of late Victorian surgery in which both practitioners and patients moved incrementally towards a shared belief in the possibilities of safe surgery: Sally Wilde, 'The Elephants in the Doctor–Patient Relationship: Patients' Clinical Interactions and the Changing Surgical Landscape of the 1890s', *Health and History*, 9:1 (2007), 2–27.
37 'The Military Medical Services', *British Medical Journal*, 1:2818 (1915), 18–20, 19.
38 'A Great Surgeon', *Manchester Guardian* (19 January 1918), 6.
39 'A Surgeon's Heroism', *The Observer* (29 August 1915), 10.
40 'Ninety-Seven Wounds and Doing Well', *Manchester Guardian* (9 October 1914), 8.
41 Ibid.
42 'Terror and "Funk"', *The Observer* (13 December 1914), 9.
43 See Tracey Loughran, *Shell-Shock and Medical Culture in First World War Britain* (Cambridge: Cambridge University Press, 2017).
44 Richard Heindel, 'War and Medicine', *Social Studies*, 32:2 (1931), 78.
45 Norman Colgan, 'New Nerves for Old! War-time Surgery Reveals Fresh Marvels', *Answers*, 109:2814 (1943), 11.
46 British Empire Cancer Campaign, 'Onwards to Victory' (1953); British Empire Cancer Campaign, 'The Modern Crusaders' (1958).
47 Arnold-Forster, *The Cancer Problem*, 190–214.
48 'Cancer Research: Is Progress Too Slow?', *The Lancet*, 288:7453 (1966), 33–34, 33.
49 Wilfred Kark, *A Synopsis of Cancer: Genesis and Biology* (Bristol: John Wright & Sons, 1966), 258–259.
50 Ibid., 262.

51 R. T. Gordon and D. Gordon, 'Neuro-Cardiovascular Surgery: Innovations for the Treatment and Prevention of Cardiovascular Disease', *Medical Hypotheses*, 5 (1979), 915–936, 934–935.

52 Scrutator, 'The Week: A Personal View of Current Medicopolitical Events', *British Medical Journal*, 295 (1987), 1008.

53 Donald Trunkey, 'Report to the Council of the Association of Surgeons of Great Britain and Ireland', *British Medical Journal*, 299 (1989), 31–33, 33.

54 Fiona Godlee, 'A Seven Day NHS: Confrontational Micromanagement Has Turned this Reasonable Idea into a Battleground', *British Medical Journal*, 352 (2016), 1–2, 1.

55 Ibid.

56 Maya Anaokar, 'War. What is it Good For? Metaphors', *LinkedIn* (20 April 2020), www.linkedin.com/pulse/war-what-good-metaphors-maya-anaokar/ (accessed 31 May 2021).

57 Kat Lay, 'The Frontline NHS Staff Battling to Keep Britain Safe During Coronavirus', *The Times* (8 January 2021), www.thetimes.co.uk/article/the-frontline-nhs-staff-battling-to-keep-britain-safe-during-coronavirus-wdn77c8zq (accessed 24 May 2021).

58 British Medical Association, www.bma.org.uk/news-and-opinion/under-fire-on-the-front-line-doctors-share-their-experiences-of-work-during-the-covid-19-crisis (accessed 24 May 2021).

59 Franziska E. Kohlt, '"Over by Christmas": The Impact of War-Metaphors and Other Science-Religion Narratives on Science Communication Environments During the Covid-19 Crisis', *SocArXiv*, preprint (10 November 2020), https://doi.org/10.31235/osf.io/z5s6a.

60 Roberta Bivins, 'Commentary: Serving the Nation, Serving the People: Echoes of War in the Early NHS', *Medical Humanities*, 46 (2020), 154–156, 154.

61 Boris Johnson, 'We Are So Nearly Out of Our Captivity', *Mail on Sunday* (28 November 2020), www.dailymail.co.uk/news/article-8996881/We-just-throw-away-not-freedom-sight-writes-BORIS-JOHNSON.html (accessed 31 May 2021).

62 James J. Kimble, 'The Real Lessons of World War II for Mobilizing Against Covid-19', *Washington Post* (25 March 2020), www.washingtonpost.com/outlook/2020/03/25/real-lesson-world-war-ii-mobilizing-against-covid-19/ (accessed 30 May 2021).

63 Agnes Arnold-Forster, 'Has Covid Put Practitioners Back in Touch with their Reasons for Becoming Healthcare Professionals?', *BMJ Opinion* (23 April 2020), https://blogs.bmj.com/bmj/2020/04/23/agnes-arnold-forster-has-covid-put-practitioners-back-in-touch-with-their-reasons-for-becoming-healthcare-professionals/ (accessed 23 May 2021).

64 Agnes Arnold-Forster, '"A Small Cemetery": Death and Dying in the Contemporary British Operating Theatre', *Medical Humanities*, 46 (2020), 278–287, 283.
65 Interview with male surgeon; interviewed by author, 24 November 2017.
66 Royal College of Surgeons of England, 'Covid-19: Good Practice for Surgeons and Surgical Teams' (31 March 2020), www.rcseng.ac.uk/standards-and-research/standards-and-guidance/good-practice-guides/coronavirus/covid-19-good-practice-for-surgeons-and-surgical-teams/#ptc (accessed 24 May 2021).
67 Health Education England, https://london.hee.nhs.uk/covid-19-hub/online-well-being-resources/podcasts/episode-6 (accessed 23 May 2021).
68 Arianna Huffington, 'And the Word of the Year Is … "Resilience"', *Thrive Global* (4 December 2020), https://thriveglobal.com/stories/arianna-huffington-resilience-word-of-the-year-2020/ (accessed 24 May 2021).
69 Ibid.
70 Ibid.
71 Anon, 'Resilience', *Psychology Today*, www.psychologytoday.com/gb/basics/resilience (accessed 23 May 2021).
72 Diane Coutu, 'How Resilience Works', *Harvard Business Review* (May 2002), https://hbr.org/2002/05/how-resilience-works (accessed 6 May 2021).
73 Dawn Coleman, 'Resiliency in Surgery', *Association for Academic Surgery* (August 2017), www.aasurg.org/blog/resiliency-in-surgery/ (accessed 21 May 2021).
74 Ibid.
75 Royal College of Surgeons of England, 'Skills and Qualities of a Surgeon', www.rcseng.ac.uk/careers-in-surgery/careers-support/skills-and-qualities-of-a-surgeon/ (accessed 31 May 2021).
76 Nicola McKinley et al., 'Resilience, Burnout and Coping Mechanisms in UK Doctors: A Cross-Sectional Study', *BMJ Open*, 10 (2020), 1–8, 1.
77 Ibid., 2.
78 H. Bolderston et al., 'Resilience and Surgeons: Train the Individual or Change the System?', *Royal College of Surgeons Bulletin*, 102:6 (2020), 244–247.
79 Medical Protection, www.medicalprotection.org/uk/articles/building-resilience-and-avoiding-burnout-workshop (accessed 31 May 2021).
80 Mark Jackson, *The Age of Stress: Science and the Search for Stability* (Oxford: Oxford University Press, 2013).

81 Dawn Coleman, 'Resiliency in Surgery', *Association for Academic Surgery* (August 2017), www.aasurg.org/blog/resiliency-in-surgery/ (accessed 21 May 2021).
82 Norman Jones et al., 'Resilience-based Intervention for UK Military Recruits: A Randomised Controlled Trial', *Occupational & Environmental Medicine*, 76:2 (2019), 90–96, 90.
83 House of Commons Health Committee: Accountability Hearing with the GMC (6 January 2015), www.parliamentlive.tv/Main/Player.aspx?meetingId=16853 (accessed 23 May 2021).
84 Charles Vincent, Jonathan Benn, and George B. Hanna, 'High Reliability in Health Care', *British Medical Journal*, 340:7740 (2010), 225–226, 225.
85 Jones et al., 'Resilience-based Intervention for UK Military Recruits', 90.
86 Ibid.

Conclusion: moving myths

In her 2009 review of Gabriel Weston's semi-fictionalised memoir, *Direct Red*, journalist Elizabeth Day commented on the allure of healthcare: 'We are all, to varying degrees, fascinated by the practice of medicine because of its curious combination of dispassionate abstraction and extreme human emotion.'[1] Since the beginning of the twenty-first century, surgeons have increasingly capitalised on this allure by writing and publishing autobiographical accounts of their careers. Just as the post-war period saw an increasing dramatisation of the clinical arena in the form of romantic novels or comic films, the early twenty-first century has witnessed more and more surgeons exposing themselves to scrutiny and supposedly baring their souls for all to see. These memoirs allow us – or so they insist – into the surgeon's mind, and into the surgeon's heart. These are emotional autobiographies; less about the technicalities of operations, or the mundane day-to-day lives of jobbing healthcare practitioners, they are sometimes-philosophical reflections on life and death, and the surgeon's responsibility to navigate a path between.

As this book has shown, the surgical stereotype and its associated myths have proven remarkably enduring. Constructed around 200 years ago, the caricature of the emotionally detached, paternalistic, male, white, socially elite, and professionally committed practitioner was maintained, reinforced, and reconfigured throughout the nineteenth and twentieth centuries. After the Second World War and the foundation of the National Health Service in 1948, the surgeon became more than just a vaunted professional, he was transformed into a star of screen and page. The fictionalising process rendered him into a caricature – best embodied by Sir Lancelot Spratt. This caricature was, however, often questioned, complicated, and rejected by surgeons themselves, as well as by those seeking to represent surgery to a larger, non-specialist audience. Despite these various shades of grey, the surgical stereotype has not only shaped the cultures and communities of modern British surgery, but dictated the demographic profile of the profession, contributed to a tendency towards overwork, and resulted in some uncomfortable metaphors that neither accurately describe surgery, nor ameliorate surgeons' workplace-related distress or dysfunction. As I have argued throughout this book, one of the reasons why the stereotype has proven so enduring is that there are elements of the popular surgical identity that serve the profession and its members. Paternalism and heroism place the surgeon in an elevated position compared not only to his patients, but also to society more broadly. While occasionally accompanied by less flattering representations of old-school practitioners as domineering and indifferent, you can see why surgeons have sometimes enjoyed the social and indeed financial capital this image has conferred. Similarly, notions of exceptionalism and vocation, while harmful in some ways, also helped to solidify surgery's vaunted status in Britain and cultivated respect and admiration.

Despite the many and various continuities this book has identified, the world has changed dramatically since the foundation of the NHS. Social norms have shifted, the rigid hierarchies that dominate healthcare have flexed slightly, and the power imbalances between doctor and patient have levelled somewhat. We live in a more emotionally expressive era, one where mental illness is more openly discussed, and where there are new expectations around wellbeing and its maintenance, particularly in the workplace. British society has also become increasingly diverse, and women and people of colour have more opportunities to participate in the workforce than ever before. While chapters 4 and 5 were relatively damming about surgery's ability to keep pace with some of these gradual and often all-too-slow changes, there has been some success. However, despite these transformations, and in some cases because of them, surgery seems currently to be undergoing something of a crisis. Some practitioners have joined many of their predecessors in lamenting the loss of a sense of vocation and commitment, particularly among trainees, and others decry the decline of patient deference. Professional organisations as well as individuals are being more vocal about inequalities and abuse within surgery, and institutions are – rightly – being held to a higher standard.

There is also a palpable crisis of wellbeing. Whether that is because hospitals are less pleasant places to work now than they have been in the past, or whether it is because professionals demand more from their jobs and their employers is difficult to say. Either way, all does not seem to be well in the world of surgery. There is the unresolved and protracted calamity of recruitment and, along with other members of the clinical workforce, plenty of surgeons are considering leaving the NHS. Multiple studies have demonstrated that medical students have a low opinion of surgeons and that very old, even crass, caricatures not only continue to inform their perceptions of the profession, but they also seem to describe some of their experiences of surgical placements while at university.[2] Sir Lancelot Spratt was a fictional character, but one based in reality. Living and breathing Spratts might now be a rare occurrence on British hospital wards, but he is not yet extinct.

In response, and over the course of the past twenty years, some surgeons – like Gabriel Weston – have taken matters into their own hands and attempted to reconfigure their profession's reputation by penning moving, emotionally rich, and seemingly frank memoirs. This genre of personal writing that exposes the affective vicissitudes of clinical and operative life has since exploded. Beyond autobiographies (which continue to be widely read, bought, and commissioned), first-hand accounts of what it is to be a surgeon populate newspapers, magazines, and social media. These texts are often framed, by both authors and reviewers, as revelatory, 'brutally honest', and frank descriptions of what hospital life is 'really like'. In his relatively brief review of Henry Marsh's *Do No Harm*, Euan Ferguson uses the word 'honest' on three separate occasions.[3] Much like their fictional post-war predecessors, but with added claims to authenticity and accuracy, these memoirs are supposed to allow readers into the operating theatre – to glimpse behind the curtain into an otherwise closed and restricted world.

Fundamental to these memoirs is a theme that has been a central component of the myth of the modern surgeon for the past century and a half: emotional detachment. As discussed in the first two chapters, both real and fictional surgeons had an uneasy relationship with their emotional closeness to their patients. The stereotype indicates complete dispassion, but surgical textbooks, films, fiction, and television series all portrayed more nuanced versions of emotional investment and distance.

As this book has shown, surgeons have always felt things about their work, whether that was grief and dismay at the death of a patient, anxiety and apprehension at an impending operation, or fury and frustration at their hospital's administration. Emotional detachment has, throughout the twentieth century, been much more a norm, expectation, standard, or stereotype than a reality, and you need not spend long reading the words of past surgeons to appreciate that they rarely, if ever, are capable of putting their feelings aside entirely. In addition, and as demonstrated in Chapter 2, that stereotype has been much less consistent or coherent than it sometimes seems. Even in the heady, 'golden age' of surgery in post-war Britain, surgeons insisted on the emotional complexity of their craft. Moreover, if you take a step away from the operating theatre, it is clear that surgeons feel and felt strongly about their own lives, careers, colleagues, places of work, and profession. Widening the lens beyond the doctor–patient relationship has revealed an array of surgical emotions, ranging from friendship to hostility; from joy to frustration.

In the twenty-first century, what was once a 'trickle' of professional memoirs has since 'become something of a flood; the drip something of a serious arterial haemorrhage'. As the writer William Boyd puts it, the surgical profession has suddenly 'found its collective voice', and surgeons 'feel the need to express and explain themselves'.[4] Many of the authors have sought to reframe public perceptions of their supposed emotional detachment. As discussed right at the very beginning of this book, the blurb to the genre's most famous member, Henry Marsh's *Do No Harm*, compels the reader to challenge their assumptions of neurosurgery as a 'precise and exquisite craft, practised by calm and detached surgeons'.[5] These questions carry new potency in the tail-end of Britain's coronavirus crisis, as the nation's healthcare workers' 'heroic' status has been re-emphasised and the inner lives of doctors have been repeatedly exposed and politicised.

Do No Harm also begins with this quotation from the mid-twentieth-century surgeon René Leriche: 'Every surgeon carries within himself a small cemetery, where from time to time he goes to pray – a place of bitterness and regret, where he must look for an explanation for his failures.'[6] Marsh's book is, in some ways, a steady catalogue of the different tombstones he 'carries within himself'. In the first few pages he describes the emotional costs of an operation gone wrong:

> Early the next morning I lay in bed thinking about the young woman I had operated on the previous week. She had a tumour in her spinal cord ... and – although I do not know why, since the operation had seemed to proceed uneventfully – she awoke from the operation paralysed down the right side of her body.[7]

He wrote about his 'grief', about the 'memory of her lying in her hospital bed, with a paralysed arm and leg'.[8] This operation disrupted the normal narrative arc of surgery, and inflected his feelings about the next one he had planned: 'I longed for this next operation, the operation on the pineal tumour, to go well – for there to be a happy ending, for everybody to live happily ever after, so that I could feel at peace with myself once again.'[9] However, he also acknowledged that he knew that his memory of the woman he had inadvertently paralysed would fade, 'would become a scar rather than a painful wound', another case on his 'list of ... disasters', another 'headstone in that cemetery'.[10]

When asked why they thought so many of their colleagues were invested in contributing to a more emotionally enriched public image of surgeons, the practitioners I interviewed offered up one of two reasons: first, that the burden of mental ill health among surgeons was gaining more and more attention and was becoming increasingly untenable; and second, that society more generally was becoming more emotionally expressive, which meant that surgeons – as part of society – were following suit. It is certainly true that the mental and emotional health of surgeons has been subjected to greater care and consideration in recent years. Partly in response to some of the social, cultural, and occupational trends described in Chapter 6, questions around surgical 'wellbeing' are increasingly prevalent. Professionals, policymakers, and researchers now suggest that a degree of emotional openness, awareness, and even 'intelligence' might protect practitioners from the stress, strain, moral injury, or burnout that seem to accompany the surgical career.

As discussed, there is also some evidence to suggest that British society has become more emotionally expressive since the start of the twenty-first century. There is a certain degree of cultural pressure to talk about your feelings, acknowledge trauma and distress publicly, and seek help and support when unhappy, anxious, or depressed. This can be seen in the many media campaigns run by mental health charities designed to encourage people to share their experiences of depression and other mental illnesses. The #TimeToTalk hashtag is everywhere on Twitter, and public figures like Matt Haig have built their brands around this kind of emotional platitude. Many of these campaigns direct particular attention to men in an attempt to encourage them to overcome their socialised tendencies towards silence and emotional repression. As argued in Chapter 4, surgery was and remains an overwhelmingly male-dominated profession and so the intersection between gender and feelings are particularly pertinent. Sociological research suggests that men might have become more emotionally expressive or are practising a 'softer' or 'more emotional' form of masculinity, which could help explain the recent trend in surgical memoirs.[11]

Whatever the reason, twenty-first-century autobiographies written by surgeons attempt to position practitioners as emotionally rich, thoughtful, and reflective. They openly discuss the pain involved in caring for patients – the ones who survive as well as the ones that do not. Together with other forms of personal life-writing – published in both the medical and mainstream press – they cultivate a new image and identity for the contemporary surgeon, one that is not only in touch with their emotions, but with something important and profound to say about the conditions of life and death, the autonomy of individuals, and the responsibilities of the state.

However, while surgeon-writers' and their books' reviewers insist that these memoirs offer a counterweight to the conventional Spratt stereotype, these memoirs not only reconfirm many aspects of the original caricature – even exploiting them for narrative gain – but they also align with tendencies of life-writing more generally. In her analysis of nineteenth-century middle-class men and their autobiographies, Donna Loftus argues that these texts are characterised by a particular narrative of improvement that was employed to articulate claims to success and public recognition. For all their claims to 'honesty', surgeons' memoirs cannot escape their authors' desires to cast themselves and their profession in a positive light. This is by no means specific to surgery, and as M. R. Somers and G. D. Gibson argue, individuals are limited in their ability to craft narratives about themselves. Instead, they must ' "choose" from the repertoire of available representations and stories'.[12] Crucially, too, these memoirs not only repeatedly inscribe individual achievements, but argue for the broader social benefits of their authors' successes.

Indeed, and despite all their best efforts, these memoirs still manage to reflect some elements of a very old surgical stereotype. While they are often emotionally rich testaments to the grief and pain associated with surgery, they also repeatedly reconfirm the fundamental truth and value of professional dispassion. Marsh describes the 'defensive psychological armour'[13] he wore throughout his career, and in an interview published in the *Financial Times* said, 'you certainly don't want to be empathetic'.[14] His friend and fellow surgeon Stephen Westaby similarly insisted on the importance of emotional detachment:

> When I started heart surgery in 1972, at least one in four patients would die, so you had to have a specific type of character to be a heart surgeon. You had to be able to put behind you what happened during the day. If you killed one patient, or two patients, you put it behind you and you came back the next day.[15]

Surgeons have long had an ambivalent relationship with emotions. They occasionally acknowledge that feelings are unavoidable, but they frequently see them as a kind of emotional contaminant, something that interferes in the 'real work' of surgery.

Many surgeons are seduced by their craft's exceptional status. Marsh reflected, 'I thought brain surgery was exquisite – that it represented the highest possible way of using both hand and brain, of combining art and science.'[16] He goes on to discuss how his idea of surgery had shifted over the course of his career – he had become more realistic, more pragmatic, more nihilistic about what surgeons could offer their patients. Nonetheless, it remains true that surgery and surgeons are held in high regard by the public, and as demonstrated by Chapter 3, they at least used to come from affluent and socially elite family backgrounds. Even the most progressive surgeons today are reluctant to relinquish all that regard and respect. Of course, much of that respect is duly earnt – they are specialists with ample and useful expertise. However, and as discussed in Chapter 6, the notion that surgery is an exceptional profession – distinct from other types of labour or alternative jobs – carries both negatives and positives, harms and benefits, for surgeons themselves. Admittedly with some irony, Marsh commented on his anxieties about retirement: 'I will become a member of the underclass of patients – as I was before I became a doctor, no longer one of the elect.'[17]

This double-bind is a perpetual problem for surgeons and it is a theme that runs throughout this book. The surgical identity and the myth of the modern surgeon are both marked by contradictions, simultaneously paternalistic and compassionate; emotionally detached and empathetic; social and profoundly individualistic; elite, esoteric, and plagued by bureaucracy; robust, resilient, but suffering under unique emotional pressures. It is precisely these contradictions that has made the surgical stereotype so enduring. Rather than just a straightforward caricature that quickly became outdated as the world changed around it, it was a flexible and mutable category. As I have argued throughout this book, elements of the surgical stereotype served members of the profession, and particularly those in positions of power within society and the speciality. The myth of the modern surgeon might have caused much harm, but it forms a key part of surgeons' professional identity, both past and present.

Notes

1 Elizabeth Day, 'Incisions, Incisions', *The Guardian* (15 February 2009), www.theguardian.com/books/2009/feb/15/direct-red-a-surgeon-s-story-gabriel-weston (accessed 31 May 2021).

2 Christos Kontovounisios, 'The Impact of Surgical Clinical Placements on Medical Student's Career Preferences', *International Surgery Journal*, 6:3 (2016), 2365–2366.

3 Euan Ferguson, '*Do No Harm: Stories of Life, Death and Brain Surgery* Review – "a bloody splendid book"', *The Guardian* (30 March 2014), www.theguardian.com/books/2014/mar/30/do-no-harm-stories-brain-surgery-review-henry-marsh (accessed 31 May 2021).

4 William Boyd, 'A Matter of Life and Death: William Boyd on the Rise of the Surgeon-Memoir', *The Guardian* (6 May 2017), www.theguardian.com/books/2017/may/06/surgeon-writer-life-hands-william-boyd (accessed 23 May 2021).
5 Henry Marsh, *Do No Harm: Stories of Life, Death and Brain Surgery* (London: Hachette, 2014).
6 Quoted in Marsh, *Do No Harm*, epigraph.
7 Marsh, *Do No Harm*, 4–5.
8 Ibid., 5.
9 Ibid.
10 Ibid.
11 Sam de Boise and Jeff Hearn, 'Are Men Getting More Emotional? Critical Sociological Perspectives on Men, Masculinities and Emotions', *Sociological Review*, 65:4 (2017), 779–796.
12 Margaret R. Somers and Gloria D. Gibson, 'Reclaiming the Epistemological "Other": Narrative and the Social Construction of Identity', in C. Calhoun (ed.), *Social Theory and the Politics of Identity* (Oxford: Blackwell, 1994), 37–99, 73.
13 Henry Marsh, *Admissions: A Life in Brain Surgery* (London: Hachette, 2017), 21.
14 'What Makes a Great Surgeon? Two of Britain's Best Discuss', *Financial Times* (8 September 2017), www.ft.com/content/d53f2422-9314-11e7-a9e6-11d2f0ebb7f0 (accessed 31 May 2021).
15 Ibid.
16 Marsh, *Admissions*, 13.
17 Ibid., 9.

Bibliography

Archival Material

James IV Association of Surgeons Records, The Drs. Barry and Bobbi Coller Rare Book Reading Room, New York Academy of Medicine Library, New York, USA

Belzer, Folkert O., 'Report to the James IV Association of Surgeons', Surgical Traveller for 1977 to England, Poland, the Netherlands, and Sweden.

Colcock, Bentley P., 'Report to the James IV Association of Surgeons', 1964.

Dudley, Hugh, 'Excerpts from Tributes to Sir John Bruce (1905–1975) by the Hon. David A. Balfour, Adam N. Smith and Professor Hugh Dudley'. Word from the James IV Association of Surgeons, Inc., Spring 1976, Box 1, Folder 2, Minutes, etc. 1971, 1975–1982.

Ferguson, Colin C., 'Summary of a Visit to England, Scotland and Ireland as a James IV Surgical Traveller', 1965.

Kennedy, Terence, 'Visit to the USA as James IV Surgical Traveller from Ireland', c. 1964.

Macbeth, R. A., 'Report on the James IV Association of Surgeons Inc. Surgical Travelership to the United Kingdom, Eire, Denmark and Sweden', 1960s.

Minutes of an Interim Meeting of the North American Members, James IV Association of Surgeons, Inc. October 23, 1979.

Minutes of the Meeting of the Board of Directors, James IV Association of Surgeons, Inc., September 9, 1983, 'Discussion and Selection of Candidates for Election to Active Membership'.

Muir, E. G., 'Report on a Visit to the United States and Canada as James IV Travelling Professor', 1961.

Riddell, Victor, 'Visit to India as James IV Surgical Traveller 1963'.

Stephenson, Hugh E., ‘Undergraduate Surgical Teaching in the United Kingdom and Ireland’. Reprinted from *Surgery*, 65 (1964), 321–333.

Tuckwell, Edward G., ‘Report of the First Ian Aird Surgical Traveller, United States and Canada 1963’.

Mills & Boon Special Collections, University of Reading, Reading, UK

‘Biography’, MB AB/1/035a.

Letter from Elizabeth Gilzean to Alan W. Boon, 8 June 1957, MB AB/1/035a.

Letter from Elizabeth Gilzean to Alan W. Boon, 1 October 1957, MB AB/1/035a.

Letter from Elizabeth Gilzean to Alan W. Boon, 5 December 1957, MB AB/1/035a.

Letter from Elizabeth Gilzean to Alan W. Boon, 21 December 1957, MB AB/1/035a.

Letter from Elizabeth Gilzean to Alan W. Boon, 3 June 1958, MB AB/1/035b.

Letter from Alan W. Boon to Elizabeth Gilzean, 1 November 1960, MB AB/1/035d.

Synopsis for *No Time for Love*, MB/AB/1/035b.

The National Archive, London, UK

Comments to Royal Commission on the National Health Service, Professor James Parkhouse, December 1976, BS6/5.

Letter from Dr F. A. Lodge to Dr Summerskill, 8 December 1975, BS6/44.

Letter from Philip Hugh-Jones to Mr de Peyer (The Secretary), 5 January 1976, BS6/211.

Letter from Mr P. Harding to A. Merrison, 21 March 1976, BS6/10.

Letter from Keith A. Mallinson to A. Merrison, 7 May 1976, BS6/12.

Letter from R. D. D. Henderson to A. Merrison, 19 May 1976, BS6/16.

Letter to A. Merrison, 25 May 1976, BS6/59.

Letter from Miss M. Williams to A. Merrison, 26 May 1976, BS6/75.

Letter from Mr Vellacott FRCS to A. Merrison, 29 May 1976, BS6/79.

Letter from Miss E. M. Henslow SRN SCM to A. Merrison, 2 June 1976, BS6/80.

Letter from The Somerset Local Pharmaceutical Committee to Sir Alec Merrison, 22 June 1976, BS6/272.

Wellcome Library, London, UK

History and Origins of the NHS, GC/201/A/1/63.

Published Material

A General Practitioner's Wife, 'Married Quarters', *British Medical Journal*, 1:5538 (1967), 505.

Adler, Paul S., Linda C. Forbes, and Hugh Willmott, 'Critical Management Studies', *Academy of Management Annals*, 1:1 (2007), 119–179.

Ahmed, Sara, *On Being Included: Racism and Diversity in Institutional Life* (Durham, NC: Duke University Press, 2012).

Alam, Eram, 'Cold War Crises: Foreign Medical Graduates Respond to US Doctor Shortages, 1965–1975', *Social History of Medicine*, 33 (2018), 132–151.

Alam, Eram, 'The Care of Foreigners: A History of South Asian Physicians in the United States, 1965–2016' (2016). Publicly Accessible Penn Dissertations. https://repository.upenn.edu/edissertations/2161.

Anaokar, Maya, 'War. What is it Good For? Metaphors', *LinkedIn* (20 April 2020), www.linkedin.com/pulse/war-what-good-metaphors-maya-anaokar/ (accessed 31 May 2021).

Anders, David L., 'Aequanimitas Centennial', *Southern Medical Journal*, 82:11 (1989), 1403–1404.

Anon, '"It is Absurd," Says Dr Anne Gruneberg, "That it should be a Handicap in Obstetrics to have had a Baby"', *The Guardian* (7 April 1980), 8.

Anon, 'A Great Surgeon', *Manchester Guardian* (19 January 1918), 6.

Anon, 'Annual Representative Meeting', *British Medical Journal*, 3:5714 (1970), 41–54.

Anon, 'A Surgeon's Heroism', *The Observer* (29 August 1915), 10.

Anon, 'Annual Representative Meeting, Folkestone, 1973', *British Medical Journal*, 2:5868 (1973), 138–155.

Anon, 'Annual Representative Meeting, Swansea 1965', *British Medical Journal*, 2:5454 (1965), 29–68.

Anon, 'Appeasement 1977 Style', *British Medical Journal*, 2:6103 (1977), 1619–1620.

Anon, 'C. G. Irwin, M.B., F.R.C.S.Ed.', *British Medical Journal*, 2:5156 (1959), 889–890.

Anon, 'Cancer Research: Is Progress Too Slow?', *The Lancet*, 288:7453 (1966), 33–34.

Anon, 'Canvassing for Hospital Appointments', *British Medical Journal*, 2:1194 (1883), 981.

Anon, 'Cecil Joll, M.D., M.S., M.Ch., F.R.C.S.' *British Medical Journal*, 1:4387 (1945), 168.

Anon, 'Clarke "To Act on Doctors' Hours"', *Daily Mail* (10 January 1989).

Anon, 'Gratuitous Medical Practice', *The Lancet*, 2 (1854), 217.

Anon, 'Hospital Junior Staffs', *British Medical Journal*, 1:5343 (1963), 260–261.

Anon, 'Hospital Junior Staffs Group Council', *British Medical Journal*, 2:5217 (1960), 269–271.

Anon, 'Hospital Junior Staffs Group Council', *British Medical Journal*, 1:5240 (1961), 294–297.

Anon, 'Hospital Junior Staffs Group Council', *British Medical Journal*, 2:5425 (1964), 229–231.

Anon, 'I Will Help to Cut These Hospital Hours, says Mellor', *Daily Mail* (3 January 1989).

Anon, 'London Hospitals and Dispensaries', *The Times* (30 January 1869).

Anon, 'Maud Mary Chadburn C.B.E., M.D. Lond.', *The Lancet*, 269:6975 (1957), 938–940.

Anon, 'Medical Notes in Parliament: Objectionable Examples', *British Medical Journal*, 1:5227 (1961), 755–757.

Anon, 'More than Half of UK Female Surgeons have Experience of Workplace Discrimination, Poll Suggests', *British Medical Journal* (2018), www.bmj.com/company/newsroom/more-than-half-of-uk-female-surgeons-have-experience-of-workplace-discrimination-poll-suggests/ (accessed 4 August 2022).

Anon, 'Ninety-Seven Wounds and Doing Well', *Manchester Guardian* (9 October 1914), 8.

Anon, 'Resilience', *Psychology Today*, www.psychologytoday.com/gb/basics/resilience (accessed 23 May 2021).

Anon, 'Sir James Walton, K.C.V.O., M.S., F.R.C.S.', *British Medical Journal*, 2:4940 (1955), 684.

Anon, 'Sleep If and When You Can', *Daily Mail* (7 October 1981).

Anon, 'T. C. Graves, B.Sc., M.D., F.R.C.S., M.R.C.V.S.', *British Medical Journal*, 1:5399 (1964), 1711.

Anon, 'T. L. Clark, M.D., F.R.C.S.Ed.', *British Medical Journal*, 1:5064 (1958), 225–226.

Anon, 'Terror and "Funk"', *The Observer* (13 December 1914), 9.

Anon, 'The Military Medical Services', *British Medical Journal*, 1:2818 (1915), 18–20.

Anon, 'The Orthopaedic Surgeon', *British Medical Journal*, 1:5698 (1970), 748–749.

Anon, 'The Week in Dundee', *British Medical Journal (Clinical Research Edition)*, 287:6385 (1983), 139–155.

Anon, 'Top Surgeons', *British Medical Journal*, 1:5129 (1959), 1100.

Anon, 'Trying to Overcome Racism in the NHS', *British Medical Journal*, 320:7235 (2004), 657.

Anon, 'What Makes a Great Surgeon? Two of Britain's Best Discuss', *Financial Times* (8 September 2017), www.ft.com/content/d53f2422-9314-11e7-a9e6-11d2f0ebb7f0 (accessed 31 May 2021).

Appignanesi, Lisa, 'Happily Ever After', *New Statesman* (13 July 1984), 24.

Arklay Steel, W., 'Charges for Residence', *British Medical Journal*, 2:4890 (1954), 128–129.

Armes Gius, John, *Fundamentals of General Surgery* (Chicago: Year Book Medical Publishers, 1962), 241.

Arnold-Forster, Agnes, '"A Small Cemetery": Death and Dying in the Contemporary British Operating Theatre', *Medical Humanities*, 46 (2020), 278–287.

Arnold-Forster, Agnes, 'Doctors' Wellbeing: Learning from the Past Can Help Improve the Future', *British Medical Journal*, 363 (2018), https://doi.org/10.1136/bmj.k4101 (accessed 15 February 2023).

Arnold-Forster, Agnes, 'Gender and Pain in Nineteenth-Century Cancer Care', *Gender and History*, 32:1 (2020), https://doi.org/10.1111/1468-0424.12468.

Arnold-Forster, Agnes, 'Has Covid Put Practitioners Back in Touch with their Reasons for Becoming Healthcare Professionals?', *BMJ Opinion* (23 April 2020), https://blogs.bmj.com/bmj/2020/04/23/agnes-arnold-forster-has-covid-put-practitioners-back-in-touch-with-their-reasons-for-becoming-healthcare-professionals/ (accessed 23 May 2021).

Arnold-Forster, Agnes, 'Metaphors and Malignancy in Senator McCain's Cancer Diagnosis', *Nursing Clio* (31 July 2017), https://nursingclio.org/2017/07/31/metaphors-and-malignancy-in-senator-mccains-cancer-diagnosis/ (accessed 22 May 2021).

Arnold-Forster, Agnes, 'Resilience in Surgery', *British Journal of Surgery*, 107:4 (2020), 332–333.

Arnold-Forster, Agnes, 'Review of *The Butchering Art: Joseph Lister's Quest to Transform the Grisly World of Victorian Medicine*', *Reviews in History* (2018), https://doi.org/10.14296/RiH/2014/2256 (accessed 25 March 2020).

Arnold-Forster, Agnes, 'Sexism in Surgery: Little has Changed', *BMJ Opinion* (2018), https://bit.ly/3ozkOPL (accessed 20 May 2021).

Arnold-Forster, Agnes, *The Cancer Problem: Malignancy in Nineteenth-Century Britain* (Oxford: Oxford University Press, 2021).

Arnold-Forster, Agnes, 'The Emotional Landscape of the Hospital Residence in Post-war Britain', in Agnes Arnold-Forster and Alison Moulds (eds), *Feelings and Work in Modern History: Emotional Labour and Emotions about Labour* (London: Bloomsbury, 2022), 58–75.

Arnold-Forster, Agnes, 'The Social and Emotional World of Twentieth-Century Anglo-American Surgery: The James IV Association of Surgeons', *Bulletin of the History of Medicine*, 96:1 (2022), 71–101.

Arnold-Forster, Agnes and Michael Brown, 'Healthcare Workers and their Emotions in the Time of Covid-19', *Surgery and Emotion*, www.surgeryandemotion.com/blog/view/emotions-healthcare-workers-and-covid-19 (accessed 31 May 2021).

Arnold-Forster, Agnes, and Alison Moulds, 'Medical Women in Popular Fiction', *BMJ Opinion* (2018), https://blogs.bmj.com/bmj/2018/09/26/agnes-arnold-forster-alison-moulds-medical-women-popular-fiction/ (accessed 20 May 2021).

Arnold-Forster, Agnes, and Sam Schotland, 'Covid-19 Only Exacerbated a Longer Pattern of Health-Care Worker Stress', *Washington Post* (29 April 2021), www.washingtonpost.com/outlook/2021/04/29/covid-19-only-exacerbated-longer-pattern-healthcare-worker-stress/#click=https://t.co/81YIkeqjZX (accessed 20 May 2021).

Arnold-Forster, Agnes, Caitjan Gainty, and Lucas Camino, 'Covid-19 and Health Inequality', *History Workshop Online* (8 June 2020), www.historyworkshop.org.uk/covid-19-and-health-inequality/ (accessed 21 May 2021).

Ashton-James, C. E., J. M. Tybur, V. Grießer, and D. Costa, 'Stereotypes About Surgeon Warmth and Competence: The Role of Surgeon Gender', *PLoS One*, 14 (2019), e0211890.

Aspinall, Peter J., 'Ethnic/Racial Terminology as a Form of Representation: A Critical Review of the Lexicon of Collective and Specific Terms in Use in Britain', *Genealogy*, 4:87 (2020), 1–4.

Atkins, Hedley, *The Surgeon's Craft* (Manchester: Manchester University Press, 1965).

Baily, Hamilton, and R. J. McNeill Love (eds), *Surgery for Nurses* (London: H. K. Lewis, 1946).

Baker, Catherine, 'Beyond the Island Story?: The Opening Ceremony of the London 2012 Olympic Games as Public History', *Rethinking History: The Journal of Theory and Practice*, 19:3 (2015), 409–428.

Baker, Clarice A., 'Married Quarters in Hospital', *British Medical Journal*, 2:5348 (1963), 51.

Banks, Peter, 'Part IV: Decompartmentalizing Art and Science', *CMA Journal*, 119 (1978), 1239.

Bates, Victoria, '"Humanizing" Healthcare Environments: Architecture, Art and Design in Modern Hospitals', *Design for Health*, 2 (2018), 5–19.

Beaumont, Berenice, 'Talking Point: Training and Careers of Women Doctors in the Thames Regions', *British Medical Journal*, 1:6106 (1978), 191–193.

Bedford, Thomas, S. A. Roach, D. G. Harvey, and J. E. Braham, 'First Conference of the British Occupational Hygiene Society', *British Journal of Industrial Medicine*, 11:1 (1954), 49–62.

Begley, Philip, and Sally Sheard, 'McKinsey and the "Tripartite Monster": The Role of Management Consultants in the 1974 NHS Reorganisation', *Medical History*, 63:4 (2019), 390–410.

Bellini, Maria Irene, Yitka Graham, Catherine Hayes, Roxanna Zakeri, Rowan Parks, and Vassilios Papalois, 'A Woman's Place is in Theatre: Women's Perceptions and Experiences of Working in Surgery from the Association of Surgeons of Great Britain and Ireland Women in Surgery Working Group', *BMJ Open*, 9 (2019), 1–8.

Bergen, Leo, 'Surgery and War: The Discussions About the Usefulness of War for Medical Progress', in Thomas Schlich (ed.), *The Palgrave Handbook of the History of Surgery* (London: Palgrave Macmillan, 2017), 389–407.

Berkowitz, Carin, *Charles Bell and the Anatomy of Reform* (Chicago: Chicago University Press, 2015).

Berrey, Ellen, 'Diversity is for White People: The Big Lie Behind a Well-Intended Word', *Salon* (26 October 2015), www.salon.com/2015/10/26/diversity_is_for_white_people_the_big_lie_behind_a_well_intended_word/ (accessed 21 May 2021).

Beveridge, William, *Social Insurance and Allied Services* (London: His Majesty's Stationery Office, 1942).

Biske, Evelyn Mary, 'On Call to a Nation', *British Medical Journal*, 2:5105 (1958), 1162.

Bivins, Roberta, 'Commentary: Serving the Nation, Serving the People: Echoes of War in the Early NHS', *Medical Humanities*, 46 (2020), 154–156.

Bivins, Roberta, *Contagious Communities: Medicine, Migration, and the NHS in Post War Britain* (Oxford: Oxford University Press, 2015).

Bivins, Roberta, 'Picturing Race in the British NHS, 1948–1988', *Twentieth Century British History*, 28:1 (2017), 83–109.

Bland-Sutton, J., 'A Lecture on the Cancer Problem', *The Lancet*, 169 (1907), 1342.

Boddice, Rob, *Humane Professions: The Defence of Experimental Medicine, 1876–1914* (Cambridge: Cambridge University Press, 2021).

Bolderston, H., M. Greville-Harris, K. Thomas, A. Kane, and K. Turner, 'Resilience and Surgeons: Train the Individual or Change the System?', *Royal College of Surgeons Bulletin*, 102:6 (2020), 244–247.

Bonner, T. N., *Becoming a Physician: Medical Education in Great Britain, France, Germany and the United States, 1750–1945* (New York: Johns Hopkins University Press, 1995).

Booth, Robert, 'Residential Homes "Desperate" for PPE, As Two Care Workers Die', *The Guardian* (6 April 2020), www.theguardian.com/society/2020/apr/06/residential-homes-desperate-for-ppe-as-two-care-workers-die (accessed 21 May 2021).

Bornat, Joanna, Parvati Raghuram, and Leroi Henri, '"Without Racism There Would be No Geriatrics": South Asian Overseas-Trained Doctors and the Development of Geriatric Medicine in the UK, 1950–2000', in Laurence Monnais and David Wright (eds), *Doctors Beyond Borders: The Transnational Migration of Physicians in the Twentieth Century* (Toronto: University of Toronto Press, 2016), 185–207.

Bourke, Joanna, 'Pain, Sympathy and the Medical Encounter between the Mid-Eighteenth and the Mid-Twentieth Centuries', *Historical Research*, 85:229 (2012), 430–452.

Bourke, Joanna, 'Some Surgeons may be Psychopaths – But that's No Bad Thing', *Prospect* (21 June 2017), https://prospectmagazine.co.uk/magazine/two-new-books-explore-how-surgeons-must-be-resolute-and-merciless (accessed 18 May 2021).

Bourke, Joanna, *The Story of Pain: From Prayer to Painkillers* (Oxford: Oxford University Press, 2014).

Boyd, Milo, 'NHS Staff can now Refuse to Treat People who are Racist or Sexist Towards Them', *Mirror* (18 February 2020), www.mirror.co.uk/news/uk-news/nhs-staff-now-refuse-treat-21523570) (accessed 21 May 2021).

Boyd, William, 'A Matter of Life and Death: William Boyd on the Rise of the Surgeon-Memoir', *The Guardian* (6 May 2017), www.theguardian.com/books/2017/may/06/surgeon-writer-life-hands-william-boyd (accessed 23 May 2021).

Boym, Svetlana, *The Future of Nostalgia* (New York: Basic, 2001).

British Empire Cancer Campaign, 'Onwards to Victory' (1953).

British Empire Cancer Campaign, 'The Modern Crusaders' (1958).

British Medical Association, *Medicine on Radio and Television* (London: British Medical Association, 1961), 7–8.

Brock, Claire, *British Women Surgeons and their Patients, 1860–1918* (Cambridge: Cambridge University Press, 2017).

Brock, Claire, 'Risk, Responsibility and Surgery in the 1890s and Early 1900s', *Medical History*, 57:3 (2013), 317–337.

Brown, J. D., and K. Walsh-Childers, 'Effects of Media on Personal and Public Health', in J. Bryant and D. Zillman (eds), *Media Effects: Advances in Research* (Hillsdale, NJ: Erlbaum, 1994), 389–415.

Brown, Michael, *Emotions and Surgery in Britain, 1793–1912* (Cambridge: Cambridge University Press, 2022).

Brown, Michael, '"Like a Devoted Army": Medicine, Heroic Masculinity, and the Military Paradigm in Victorian Britain', *Journal of British Studies*, 49:3 (2010), 592–622.

Brown, Michael, 'Medicine, Reform and the "End" of Charity in Early Nineteenth-Century England', *English Historical Review*, 124 (2009), 1353–1388.

Brown, Michael, *Performing Medicine: Medical Culture and Identity in Provincial England, c. 1760–1850* (Manchester: Manchester University Press, 2011).

Brown, Michael, 'Redeeming Mr Sawbone: Compassion and Care in the Cultures of Nineteenth-Century Surgery', *Journal of Compassionate Health Care*, 4:13 (2017), 1–7.

Brown, Michael, 'Robert Liston, the "Fastest Knife in the West End"? Part 1: Historical Myth-Making', *Surgery & Emotion*, http://www.surgeryandemotion.com/blog/view/robert-liston-the-fastest-knife-in-the-west-end-part-1-historical-myth-making (accessed 6 April 2023).

Brown, Michael, 'Surgery and Emotion: The Era Before Anaesthesia', in Thomas Schlich (ed.), *The Palgrave Handbook of the History of Surgery* (London: Palgrave Macmillan, 2017), 327–348.

Bryan, Charles S., '"Aequanimitas" Redux: William Osler on Detached Concern versus Humanistic Empathy', *Perspectives in Biology and Medicine*, 49:3 (2006), 384–392.

Caiach, Sian, 'Training Doctors', *British Medical Journal*, 310:6992 (1995), 1473.

Callard, Felicity, and Des Fitzgerald, *Rethinking Interdisciplinarity across the Social Sciences and Neurosciences* (London: Palgrave Macmillan, 2015).

Campbell Gosling, George, *Payment and Philanthropy in British Healthcare, 1918–48* (Manchester: Manchester University Press, 2017).

Campbell, Tricia, 'You Can't Have Diversity without Inclusion', *British Orthopaedic Association* (15 July 2020), www.boa.ac.uk/resources/knowledge-hub/you-can-t-have-diversity-without-inclusion.html (accessed 21 May 2021).

Canter, Richard, 'Impact of Reduced Working Time on Surgical Training in the United Kingdom and Ireland', *The Surgeon*, 9 (2011), 6–7.

Cantor, A. M., 'Personal View', *British Medical Journal*, 2:6146 (1978), 1224.

Casarett, David, Amy Pickard, Jessica M. Fishman, Stewart C. Alexander, Robert M. Arnold, Kathryn I. Pollak, and James A. Tulsky, 'Can Metaphors and Analogies Improve Communication with Seriously Ill Patients?', *Journal of Palliative Medicine*, 13:3 (2010), 255–260.

Cassell, Joan, 'Doing Gender, Doing Surgery: Women Surgeons in a Man's Profession', *Human Organization*, 56:1 (1997), 47–52.

Chaney, Sarah, 'Dying Scientifically: Sex and Scandal in Victorian Medicine', *The Lancet*, 379:9831 (2012), 2042.

Christopher, Frederick (ed.), *A Textbook of Surgery by American Authors*, 4th edition (Philadelphia and London: W. B. Saunders, 1945).

Clarke, Jackie, 'Closing Time: Deindustrialization and Nostalgia in Contemporary France', *History Workshop Journal*, 79 (2015), 107–125.

Coleman, Dawn, 'Resiliency in Surgery', *Association for Academic Surgery* (August 2017), http://www.aasurg.org/blog/resiliency-in-surgery/ (accessed 21 May 2021).

Colgan, Norman, 'New Nerves for Old! War-time Surgery Reveals Fresh Marvels', *Answers*, 109:2814 (1943), 11.

Commonwealth Immigrants Act (1962), 1–24.

Cook, T., E. Kursumovic, and S. Lennane, 'Exclusive: Deaths of NHS Staff from Covid-19 Analysed', *Health Service Journal* (21 June 2020), www.hsj.co.uk/exclusive-deaths-of-nhs-staff-from-covid-19-analysed/7027471.article (accessed 21 May 2021).

Coombes, Rebecca, 'Press: The Consultant Contract', *British Medical Journal*, 325:7372 (2002), 1120.

Cooper, Cary L., and Roy Payne, *Stress at Work* (London: John Wiley & Sons, 1978).

Coutu, Diane, 'How Resilience Works', *Harvard Business Review* (May 2002), https://hbr.org/2002/05/how-resilience-works (accessed 6 May 2021).

Crebbin, Wendy, Graeme Campbell, David A. Hillis, and David A. Watters, 'Prevalence of Bullying, Discrimination and Sexual Harassment in Surgery in Australia', *Australia and New Zealand Journal of Surgery*, 85 (2015), 905–909.

Creighton, Sarah, 'Reviewed Work(s): The Woman in the Surgeon's Body by Joan Cassell', *British Medical Journal*, 317:7165 (1998), 1088.

Crenshaw, Kimberlé, 'Demarginalizing the Intersection of Race and Sex: A Black Feminist Critique of Antidiscrimination Doctrine, Feminist Theory and Antiracist Politics', *University of Chicago Legal Forum*, 1:8 (1989), 139–167.

Cromwell, 'Married Quarters in Hospital', *British Medical Journal*, 2:5348 (1963), 52.

Cronin, A. J., *The Citadel* (London: Picador, 2019).

Crowe, Sophie, Nicholas Clarke, and Ruairi Brugha, '"You Do Not Cross Them": Hierarchy and Emotion in Doctors' Narratives of Power Relations in Specialist Training', *Social Science and Medicine*, 186 (2017), 70–77.

Crowther, Anne, and Marguerite Dupree, *Medical Lives in the Age of Surgical Revolution* (Cambridge: Cambridge University Press, 2007).

Cummins, Eleanor, 'How Dr Glaucomflecken Overcame Death to Get Internet Laughs', *Medscape* (10 March 2021), www.medscape.com/viewarticle/947199 (accessed 20 May 2021).

Darbyshire, Daniel, and Paul Baker, 'A Systematic Review and Thematic Analysis of Cinema in Medical Education', *Medical Humanities*, 38 (2012), 28–33.

Davis, Fred, 'Nostalgia, Identity and the Current Nostalgia Wave', *Journal of Popular Culture*, 11:2 (1977), 414–424.

Davis, Fred, *Yearning for Yesterday: A Sociology of Nostalgia* (New York: Free Press, 1979).

Davis, Neville, and H. Stephen Pasmore, 'Anxious Patient and Worried Doctor', *British Medical Journal*, 1:5061 (1958), 40.

Day, Elizabeth, 'Incisions, Incisions', *The Guardian* (15 February 2009), www.theguardian.com/books/2009/feb/15/direct-red-a-surgeon-s-story-gabriel-weston (accessed 31 May 2021).

Day, George, 'Personal View', *British Medical Journal*, 3:5611 (1968), 182.

de Boise, Sam, and Jeff Hearn, 'Are Men Getting More Emotional? Critical Sociological Perspectives on Men, Masculinities and Emotions', *Sociological Review*, 65:4 (2017), 779–796.

de Bronkart, Dave, 'From Patient Centred to People Powered: Autonomy on the Rise', *British Medical Journal*, 350 (2015), 1–3.

de Noronha, Leslie, 'Nationalities of Junior Staff', *British Medical Journal*, 2:5269 (1961), 1777–1778.

DelVecchio Good, Mary-Jo, and Byron J. Good, 'Disabling Practitioners: Hazards of Learning to Be a Doctor in American Medical Education', *American Journal of Orthopsychiatry*, 59:2 (1989), 303–309.

Digby, Anne, and Nick Bosanquet, 'Doctors and Patients in an Era of National Health Insurance and Private Practice, 1913–1938', *Economic History Review*, 41 (1988), 74–94.

Dingwall, D. W., 'Special Article: Provision of Married-Quarters for House Officers', *British Medical Journal*, 1:5436 (1963), 1664–1665.

Dobbin, Frank, *Inventing Equal Opportunity* (Princeton, NJ: Princeton University Press, 2011).

Donohoe, Claire L., and H. M. Mohan, 'Pregnancy, Parenthood and Second-Generation Bias: Women in Surgery', *British Journal of Surgery*, 108:1 (2021), 1–2.

Doyle, Barry, and Rosemary Wall, 'What was Healthcare Like before the NHS?', *The Conversation* (3 July 2018), https://theconversation.com/what-was-healthcare-like-before-the-nhs-99055 (accessed 28 April 2020).

Drabble, Margaret, *The Millstone* (London: Weidenfeld & Nicolson, 1965).

Drabble, Margaret, *The Millstone* (London: Penguin, 2016).

Duffy, Mignon, 'Doing the Dirty Work: Gender, Race, and Reproductive Labor in Historical Perspective', *Gender & Society*, 21:3 (2007), 313–336.

Edgerton, David, *Warfare State: Britain, 1920–1070* (Cambridge: Cambridge University Press, 2006).

Edwards, Harold C., *Recent Advances in Surgery*, 3rd edition (London: J. & A. Churchill, 1948).

Edwards, Matthew L., 'On William Osler, Psychiatry, and the Law: Reflections on "Aequanimitas" at 130 Years', *American Journal of Psychiatry Residents' Journal*, 15:1 (2019), 3, https://doi.org/10.1176/appi.ajp-rj.2019.150102.

Elkomy, Shimaa, Graham Cookson, and Simon Jones, 'Cheap and Dirty: The Effect of Contracting Out Cleaning on Efficiency and Effectiveness', *Public Administration Review*, 79:2 (2019), 193–202.

Elston, Mary Ann, 'Medicine: Half our Future Doctors?', in Rosalie Silverstone and Audrey Ward (eds), *Careers of Professional Women* (London: Routledge, 1980), 99–139.

Elston, Mary Ann, *Women and Medicine: The Future* (London: Royal College of Physicians, 2009).

Evans, M. J., 'Sacrificed to an Archaic Training System', *British Medical Journal*, 303:6793 (1991), 65.

Evans, P. Catherine, 'Mr. Cecil A. Joll', *British Medical Journal*, 1:4391 (1945), 314.

Feasey, Rebecca, *Masculinity and Popular Television* (Edinburgh: Edinburgh University Press, 2008).

Feiner, Natasha, 'Pilot Fatigue and the Regulation of Airline Schedules in Post-war Britain', in Mark Jackson and Martin D. Moore (eds), *Balancing the Self: Medicine, Politics, and the Regulation of Health in the Twentieth Century* (Manchester: Manchester University Press, 2020), 190–215.

Ferguson, Euan, 'Do No Harm: Stories of Life, Death and Brain Surgery Review – "a bloody splendid book"', *The Guardian* (30 March 2014), www.theguardian.com/books/2014/mar/30/do-no-harm-stories-brain-surgery-review-henry-marsh (accessed 31 May 2021).

Firth Cozens, Jenny, 'Medicine and the Media', *British Medical Journal (Clinical Research Edition)*, 295:6607 (1987), 1199–1200.

Fitzharris, Lindsey, *The Butchering Art: Joseph Lister's Quest to Transform the Grisly World of Victorian Medicine* (London: Penguin, 2017).

Fletcher, Ian, 'The Price of a Surgeon's Devotion to Work', *Daily Mail* (9 January 1981).

Flyn, Cal, 'NHS Strikes and the Decades of Discontent', *Wellcome Collection Stories* (12 July 2018), https://wellcomecollection.org/articles/WyjRuCcAACvGno__ (accessed 23 May 2021).

Forrester, R. M., 'Married Quarters in Hospital', *British Medical Journal*, 2:5348 (1963), 51.

Forster, Peter, 'Equal Opportunities: Progress so Far', *British Medical Journal*, 304:6827 (1992), 630–632.

Fox, Renée C., *Experiment Perilous: Physicians and Patients Facing the Unknown* (Glencoe, IL: Free Press, 1959).

Fox, Renée C., 'Is There a "New" Medical Student?: A Comparative View of Medical Socialization in the 1950s and the 1970s', in *Essays in Medical Sociology: Journeys into the Field* (New York: John Wiley & Sons, 1979).

Franklin, Benjamin, 'Advice to a Young Tradesman' (21 July 1748), Founders Online, National Archives, https://founders.archives.gov/documents/Franklin/01-03-02-0130 (accessed 28 February 2023).

Gabriel, Yiannis, 'Organisational Nostalgia: Reflections on the Golden Age', in S. Fineman (ed.), *Emotions in Organisations* (London: SAGE, 1993).

Gavrus, Delia, 'Men of Dreams and Men of Action: Neurologists, Neurosurgeons and the Performance of Professional Identity, 1920–1950', *Bulletin of the History of Medicine*, 85:1 (2011), 57–92.

Gerbner, G., and L. Gross, 'Living with Television: The Violence Profile', *Journal of Communication*, 26:2 (1976), 172–199.

Gerbner, G., L. Gross, M. Morgan, and N. Signorielli, 'The Mainstreaming of America: The Violence Profile', *Journal of Communication*, 30:11 (1980), 10–29.

Godlee, Fiona, 'A Seven Day NHS: Confrontational Micromanagement has turned this Reasonable Idea into a Battleground', *British Medical Journal*, 352 (2016), 1–2.

Goffman, Erving, *Asylums: Essays on the Social Situation of Mental Patients and Other Inmates* (New York: Anchor Books, 1961).

Gordon, Richard, *Doctor at Large* (London: Harmondsworth, 1975).

Gordon, Richard, *Doctor in the House* (London: Michael Joseph, 1952).

Gordon, Richard, *Great Medical Disasters* (London: Hutchinson & Co., 1983).

Gordon, R. T., and D. Gordon, 'Neuro-Cardiovascular Surgery: Innovations for the Treatment and Prevention of Cardiovascular Disease', *Medical Hypotheses*, 5 (1979), 915–936.

Gordon-Taylor, G., 'Cecil A. Joll, F.R.C.S', *British Medical Journal*, 1:4389 (1945), 238–239.

Gorsky, Martin, '"Searching for the People in Charge": Appraising the 1983 Griffiths NHS Management Inquiry', *Medical History*, 57:1 (2013), 87–107.

Gorsky, Martin, John Mohan, and Tim Willis, *Mutualism and Health Care: British Hospital Contributory Schemes in the Twentieth Century* (Manchester: Manchester University Press, 2006).

Gunaratnam, Yasmin, *Researching Race and Ethnicity* (London: SAGE, 2003).

Hadley, Tessa, 'The Millstone: The Crucial 1960s Feminist Novel', *The Guardian* (15 May 2015), www.theguardian.com/books/2015/may/15/the-millstone-the-crucial-1960s-feminist-novel (accessed 28 April 2020).

Hagiwara, Nao, Frederick W. Kron, Mark W. Scerbo, and Ginger S. Watson, 'A Call for Grounding Implicit Bias Training in Clinical and Translational Frameworks', *The Lancet*, 2:395 (2020), 1457–1460.

Hailey, Arthur, *The Final Diagnosis* (New York: Doubleday & Co, 1959).

Hale, R., and L. Hudson, 'The Tavistock Study of Young Doctors: Report of the Pilot Phase', *British Journal of Hospital Medicine*, 47:6 (1990), 452–464.

Hallam, Julia, 'Grey's Anatomy: Scalpels, Sex, and Stereotypes', *Medical Humanities*, 35 (2009), 60–61.

Halpern, Jodi, *From Detached Concern to Empathy: Humanizing Medical Practice* (New York: Oxford University Press, 2001).

Hamad, Hannah, 'Contemporary Medical Television and Crisis in the NHS', *Critical Studies in Television: The International Journal of Television Studies*, 11:2 (2016), 136–160.

Hansard, HC Deb 18 April 1975 vol 890 c176W, https://api.parliament.uk/historic-hansard/written-answers/1975/apr/18/manual-workers-average-wage (accessed 19 May 2021).

Hansard, HC Deb 24 March 1976 vol 908 cc190-1W, https://api.parliament.uk/historic-hansard/written-answers/1976/mar/24/doctors-pay (accessed 19 May 2021).

Hardy, Carter, 'Clinical Sympathy: The Important Role of Affectivity in Clinical Practice', *Medicine, Health Care and Philosophy*, 22:4 (2019), 499–513.

Harries, R. L., Vimal J. Gokani, Peter Smitham, and J. Edward F. Fitzgerald, 'Less than Full-Time Training in Surgery: A Cross-Sectional Study Evaluating the Accessibility and Experiences of Flexible Training in the Surgical Trainee Workforce', *BMJ Open*, 6 (2016), e010136.

Harrison, Stephen, 'New Labour, Modernisation and the Medical Labour Process', *Journal of Social Policy*, 31:3 (2002), 465–485.

Hayward, Rhodri, *The Transformation of the Psyche in British Primary Care, 1870–1970* (London: Bloomsbury, 2015).

Health Foundation, The, *Person-Centred Care Made Simple: What Everyone Should Know About Person-Centred Care* (London: The Health Foundation, 2016).

Heindel, Richard, 'War and Medicine', *Social Studies*, 32:2 (1931), 78.

Hendry, N. G. C., J. H. E. Bergin, J. M. Armitt, and A. T. Seaton, 'Differences and Differentials', *British Medical Journal*, 1:5388 (1964), 984–985.

Hession, Michael, 'Married Quarters in Hospital', *British Medical Journal*, 1:5436 (1963), 1475.

Hoffarth, Matthew J., 'The Making of Burnout: From Social Change to Self-Awareness in the Postwar United States, 1970–82', *History of the Human Sciences*, 30:5 (2017), 30–45.

Housden, E. Gerard, 'The Health Service Bill', *British Medical Journal*, 1 (1946), 846–847.

House of Commons Health Committee: Accountability Hearing with the GMC (6 January 2015), www.parliamentlive.tv/Main/Player.aspx?meetingId=16853 (accessed 23 May 2021).

Howard, S. H. F., 'Medicine Broadcast', *British Medical Journal*, 1:5225 (1961), 595.

Howieson, W., and D. Cloke, 'The Hidden Curriculum and its Implications for Surgical Specialties: Preventing the Unspoken Academic and Social Messages Taught to Trainees that Lead to Unwanted Behaviours and Results', *Royal College of Surgeons of England Bulletin*, 101:7 (2019), 282–284.

Huffington, Arianna, 'And the Word of the Year Is … "Resilience"', *Thrive Global* (4 December 2020), https://thriveglobal.com/stories/arianna-huffington-resilience-word-of-the-year-2020/ (accessed 24 May 2021).

Huggins, Mike, 'Sport and the British Upper Classes c.1500–2000: A Historiographic Overview', *Sport in History*, 28 (2008), 364–388.

Hughes, David, 'The Reorganisation of the National Health Service: The Rhetoric and Reality of the Internal Market', *Modern Law Review*, 54:1 (1991), 88–103.

Jackson, Mark, *The Age of Stress: Science and the Search for Stability* (Oxford: Oxford University Press, 2013).

Jacobs, Jason, *Body Trauma TV: The New Hospital Dramas* (London: BFI, 2003).

Jacobs, Jason, 'Hospital Drama', in Glen Creeber (ed.) *The Television Genre Book* (London: BFI, 2002), 23–26.

Janesick, Valerie J., 'Oral History Interviewing: Issues and Possibilities', in Patricia Leavy (ed.), *The Oxford Handbook of Qualitative Research* (Oxford: Oxford University Press, 2014).

Jefferson, Laura, Karen Bloor, and Alan Maynard, 'Women in Medicine: Historical Perspectives and Recent Trends', *British Medical Bulletin*, 114:1 (2015), 5–15.

Johnson, Boris, 'We Are So Nearly Out of Our Captivity', *Mail on Sunday* (28 November 2020), www.dailymail.co.uk/news/article-8996881/We-just-throw-away-not-freedom-sight-writes-BORIS-JOHNSON.html (accessed 31 May 2021).

Johnson, Donald McI., 'A G.P. On His Clinical Training', *British Medical Journal*, 2:4677 (1950), 493–496.

Johnson, P. A., 'Married Quarters', *British Medical Journal*, 1:5538 (1967), 505.

Johnson, Sarah, 'NHS Staff Lay Bare a Bullying Culture', *The Guardian* (26 October 2016), www.theguardian.com/society/2016/oct/26/nhs-staff-bullying-culture-guardian-survey (accessed 20 May 2021).

Jones, Cecily, '"Human Weeds, Not Fit to Breed?": African Caribbean Women and Reproductive Disparities in Britain', *Critical Public Health*, 23:1 (2013), 49–61.

Jones, Norman, Chantelle Whelan, Larissa Harden, Andrea Macfarlane, Howard Burdett, and Neil Greenberg, 'Resilience-Based Intervention for UK Military Recruits: A Randomised Controlled Trial', *Occupational & Environmental Medicine*, 76:2 (2019), 90–96.

Kark, Wilfred, *A Synopsis of Cancer: Genesis and Biology* (Bristol: John Wright & Sons, 1966).

Kelly, Laura, 'Migration and Medical Education: Irish Medical Students at the University of Glasgow, 1859–1900', *Irish Economic and Social History*, 39 (2012), 39–55.

Kernahan, Peter J., 'Surgery Becomes a Specialty: Professional Boundaries and Surgery', in Thomas Schlich (ed.), *The Palgrave Handbook of the History of Surgery* (London: Palgrave Macmillan, 2017), 95–113.

Khullar, Dhruv, 'The Trouble with Medicine's Metaphors', *The Atlantic* (7 August 2014), www.theatlantic.com/health/archive/2014/08/the-trouble-with-medicines-metaphors/374982/ (accessed 22 May 2021).

Khunti, Kamlesh, Ash Routen, Manish Pareek, Shaun Treweek, and Lucinda Platt, 'The Language of Ethnicity', *British Medical Journal*, 371 (2020), m4493.

Kimble, James J., 'The Real Lessons of World War II for Mobilizing Against Covid-19', *Washington Post* (25 March 2020), www.washingtonpost.com/outlook/2020/03/25/real-lesson-world-war-ii-mobilizing-against-covid-19/ (accessed 30 May 2021).

King, Janet W. C., and Stephen J. Wigmore, 'How Surgeons Should Behave on Social Media', *Surgery*, 38:10 (2020), 623–626.

Kirby, Jill, *Feeling the Strain: A Cultural History of Stress in Twentieth-century Britain* (Manchester: Manchester University Press, 2019).

Klein, Rudolf, *The New Politics of the NHS: From Creation to Reinvention* (London: Radcliffe, 2013).

Kohlt, Franziska E., '"Over by Christmas": The Impact of War-Metaphors and Other Science-Religion Narratives on Science Communication Environments During the Covid-19 Crisis', *SocArXiv*, preprint (10 November 2020), https://doi.org/ 10.31235/osf.io/z5s6a.

Kontovounisios, Christos, 'The Impact of Surgical Clinical Placements on Medical Student's Career Preferences', *International Journal of Surgery*, 6:3 (2016), 2365–2366.

Kotsis, Sandra V., and Kevin C. Chung, 'Application of See One, Do One, Teach One Concept in Surgical Training', *Plastic Reconstructive Surgery*, 131:5 (2013), 1194–1201.

Lagunes Cordoba, Emmeline, Suzanne Shale, Rachel Clare Evans, and Derek Tracy, 'Time to Get Serious about Distributed Leadership: Lessons to Learn for Promoting Leadership Development for Non-Consultant Career Grade Doctors in the UK', *BMJ Leader*, http://dx.doi.org/ 10.1136/leader-2020-000395 (accessed 21 May 2021).

Lakeman, Geoffrey, 'Spoons OK for Ops, Say Bosses', *Daily Mirror* (21 February 2003), 28.

Lambert, Trevor W., Fay Smith, and Michael J. Goldacre, 'Combining Parenthood with a Medical Career: Questionnaire Survey of the UK Medical Graduates of 2002 Covering Some Influences and Experiences', *BMJ Open*, 7:8 (2017), 1–8.

Langhamer, Claire, 'Feelings, Women and Work in the Long 1950s', *Women's History Review*, 26:1 (2016), 77–92.

Langhamer, Claire, 'Who the Hell are Ordinary People? Ordinariness as a Category of Historical Analysis', *Transactions of the Royal Historical Society*, 28 (2018), 175–195.

Lawrence, Christopher, 'Democratic, Divine and Heroic: The History and Historiography of Surgery', in Christopher Lawrence (ed.), *Medical Theory, Surgical Practice: Essays in the History of Surgery* (London: Routledge, 1992).

Lawrence, Christopher (ed.), *Medical Theory, Surgical Practice: Studies in the History of Surgery* (London: Routledge, 1992).

Lawrie, Jean, 'Training our Specialists', *The Lancet*, 289:7484 (1967), 74.

Lay, Kat, 'The Frontline NHS Staff Battling to Keep Britain Safe During Coronavirus', *The Times* (8 January 2021), www.thetimes.co.uk/article/the-frontline-nhs-staff-battling-to-keep-britain-safe-during-coronavirus-wdn77c8zq (accessed 24 May 2021).

Lederer, Susan E., 'Surgery and Popular Culture: Situating the Surgeon and the Surgical Experience in Popular Media', in Thomas Schlich (ed.), *The Palgrave Handbook of the History of Surgery* (London: Palgrave Macmillan, 2017), 349–367.

Lerner, Barron H., *The Breast Cancer Wars: Hope, Fear and the Pursuit of a Cure in Twentieth-Century America* (New York: Oxford University Press, 2001).

Lewis, Jane, 'Myrdal, Klein, *Women's Two Roles* and Postwar Feminism 1945–1960', in Harold L. Smith (ed.), *British Feminism in the Twentieth Century* (Aldershot: Edward Elgar, 1990), 167–168.

Lewis, Natalie J., Charlotte E. Rees, J. Nicky Hudson, and Alan Bleakley, 'Emotional Intelligence Medical Education: Measuring the Unmeasurable?', *Advances in Health Sciences Education*, 10:4 (2005), 339–355.

Lewis, Richard, 'Personal View', *British Medical Journal (Clinical Research Edition)*, 284:6332 (1982), 1867.

Lief, Harold I., and Renée C. Fox, 'Training for "Detached Concern" in Medical Students', in Harold I. Lief, Victor F. Lief, and Nina R. Lief (eds), *The Psychological Basis of Medical Practice* (New York: Harper & Row, 1963), 12–35.

Lindsay, Rachel, 'Love Unspoken', *Woman's Own* (18 March 1954).

Linklater, Eric, 'Prometheus and To-Morrow', *British Medical Journal*, 2 (1955), 1517–1520.

Loftus Dale, H. W., 'Cecil Joll. M.Ch., F.R.C.S.', *British Medical Journal*, 1:4388 (1945), 202–203.

Long, Vicky, and Victoria Brown. 'Conceptualizing Work-Related Mental Distress in the British Coalfields (c.1900–1950)', *Palgrave Communications*, 4 (2018), 1–10.

Lothian-McLean, Moya, 'How to Become an Orthopaedic Surgeon, By the Woman who was First in her Field', *Stylist*, https://bit.ly/3f8NADV (accessed 21 May 2021).

Loughran, Tracey, *Shell-Shock and Medical Culture in First World War Britain* (Cambridge: Cambridge University Press, 2017).

Lupton, Deborah, 'Grey's Anatomy is Unrealistic, But it Might Make Junior Doctors More Compassionate', *The Conversation* (19 February 2018), https://theconversation.com/greys-anatomy-is-unrealistic-but-it-might-make-junior-doctors-more-compassionate-92040 (accessed 20 May 2021).

Lussier, Kira, 'What the History of Diversity Training Reveals About its Future', *The Conversation* (7 September 2020), https://theconversation.com/what-the-history-of-diversity-training-reveals-about-its-future-143984 (accessed 21 May 2021).

Luu, Shelly, Priyanka Patel, Laurent St-Martin, Annie So Leung, Glenn Regehr, M. Lucas Murnaghan, et al., 'Waking up the Next Morning: Surgeons' Emotional Reactions to Adverse Events', *Medical Education*, 46 (2012), 1179–1188.

Macaulay, Duncan, 'Nationalities of Junior Staff', *British Medical Journal*, 2:5269 (1961), 1777–1778.

Macbeth, Ronald. 'Married Quarters in Hospital', *British Medical Journal*, 1:5346 (1963), 1674.

Madhok, Rajan, 'Foreword', in Emma L. Jones and Stephanie J. Snow, *Against the Odds: Black and Minority Ethnic Clinicians and Manchester, 1948 to 2009* (Manchester: Manchester NHS Primary Care Trust, in association with the Centre for the History of Science, Technology and Medicine, University of Manchester, 2010).

Marsh, Henry, *Admissions: A Life in Brain Surgery* (London: Hachette, 2017).

Marsh, Henry, *Do No Harm: Stories of Life, Death and Brain Surgery* (London: Hachette, 2014).

Marsh, Henry, 'The Great War's Miracle Worker', *New Statesman*, 13 July 2022, https://www.newstatesman.com/culture/books/2022/07/the-facemaker-review-lindsey-fitzharris-great-war (accessed 7 April 2023).

Matemavi, Praise, *Passion and Purpose: Black Female Surgeons* (Deleon Springs, FL: A 2 Z Press, 2020).

McAleer, James, 'Love, Romance, and the National Health Service', in Clare V. J. Griffiths, James J. Nott, and William Whyte (eds), *Classes, Cultures, and Politics: Essays on British History for Ross McKibbin* (Oxford: Oxford University Press, 2011), 173–191.

McCarthy, Helen, *Double Lives: A History of Working Motherhood in Modern Britain* (London: Bloomsbury, 2020).

McDonald, Ruth, Justin Waring, and Stephen Harrison, 'At the Cutting Edge? Modernization and Nostalgia in a Hospital Operating Theatre Department', *Sociology*, 40:6 (2006), 1097–1115.

McKeigue, P. M., J. D. Richards, and P. Richards, 'Effects of Discrimination by Sex and Race on the Early Careers of British Medical Graduates During 1981–7', *British Medical Journal*, 301 (1990), 961–964.

McKibbin, Ross, 'Politics and the Medical Hero: A. J. Cronin's "The Citadel"', *English Historical Review*, 123:502 (2008), 651–678.

McKinley, Nicola, R. Scott McCain, Liam Convie, Mike Clarke, Martin Dempster, William Jeffrey Campbell, and Stephen James Kirk, 'Resilience, Burnout and Coping Mechanisms in UK Doctors: A Cross-Sectional Study', *BMJ Open*, 10 (2020), 1–8.

Menon, Rajgopalan, 'The NHS Owes Doctors Who Trained Abroad an Apology for Racism', *British Medical Journal*, 361 (2018), https://doi.org/10.1136/bmj.k2360.

Merrison, Alec, *Royal Commission on the National Health Service: Report* (London, 1979).

Miller, Jessica, 'Passionate Virtue: Conceptions of Medical Professionalism in Popular Romance Fiction', *Literature and Medicine*, 33:1 (2015), 70–90.

Milner, Adrienne, and Sandra Jumbe, 'Using the Right Words to Address Racial Disparities in COVID-19', *The Lancet*, 5 (2020), e419–e420.

Ministry of Health: Consultative Council on Medical and Allied Services, *Interim Report on the Future Provision of Medical and Allied Services* (London, 1920), http://www.nhshistory.net/Dawson%20report.html (accessed 28 April 2021).

Moberly, Tom, 'A Fifth of England's Surgeons are Women', *British Medical Journal*, 363 (2018), 209.

Mold, Alex, 'Making the Patient-Consumer in Margaret Thatcher's Britain', *Historical Journal*, 54:2 (2011), 509–528.

Morris, Jessica, 'John McCain's Brain Cancer, and Mine', *New York Times* (20 July 2017), www.nytimes.com/2017/07/20/opinion/john-mccain-brain-cancer-glioblastoma.html (accessed 22 May 2021).

Moulds, Alison, *Medical Identities and Print Culture, 1830s–1910s* (London: Palgrave Macmillan, 2021).

Moulds, Alison, 'Medical Women: Perspectives from the Victorian Medical Profession', *Royal College of Surgeons Bulletin* (2017), 255–257.

Mullally, Sasha, and David Wright, 'Connecting to Canada: Experiences of the South Asian Medical Diaspora during the 1960s and 1970s', in Laurence Monnais and David Wright (eds) *Doctors Beyond Borders: The Transnational Migration of Physicians in the Twentieth Century* (Toronto: University of Toronto Press, 2016), 230–256.

Murray, J. F., 'Improving the Hospital Service', *British Medical Journal*, 1:6008 (1976), 507–508.

National Health Service Reorganisation Act (1973), www.legislation.gov.uk/ukpga/1973/32/enacted.

Newby, Malcolm, 'Nursing at the Movies', *Nursing Standard*, 3:32 (1989), 13.

NHS Voices of Covid-19, 'Women, Work and the NHS: Balance for Better', www.nhs70.org.uk/story/women-work-and-nhs-balance-better (accessed 20 May 2021).

Nickson, Hilda, *Surgeons in Love* (London: Mills & Boon, 1962).

Nie, Jing-Bao, Adam Gilbertson, Malcolm de Roubaix, Ciara Staunton, Anton van Niekerk, Joseph D. Tucker, and Stuart Rennie, 'Healing without Waging War: Beyond Military Metaphors in Medicine and HIV Cure Research', *American Journal of Bioethics*, 16:10 (2016), 3–11.

Norredam, Marie, and Dag Album, 'Prestige and its Significance for Medical Specialities and Diseases', *Scandinavian Journal of Public Health*, 35:6 (2007), 655–668.

O'Farrell, P. T., 'British Medical Association One Hundred and Twentieth Annual Meeting, Dublin, 1952 President's Address: Topics, Thoughts, and Tendencies', *British Medical Journal*, 2 (1952), 53–57.

Obama, Barack, Twitter Post (19 July 2017), https://twitter.com/BarackObama/status/887836712822558720?s=20.

Osler, William, *Aequanimitas: With Other Addresses to Medical Students, Nurses and Practitioners of Medicine* (Philadelphia: P. Blakiston, 1922).

Otis, Laura, *Membranes: Metaphors of Invasion in Nineteenth-Century Literature, Science, and Politics* (Baltimore, MD: Johns Hopkins University Press, 2000).

Ottley, C. M., 'Emergency Ward 10', *British Medical Journal*, 1:5174 (1960), 728.

Ovens, Gerald H. C., *An Approach to Clinical Surgery* (London: J. & A. Churchill, 1953).

Oxtoby, Kathy, 'Love on the Wards: Relationships between Doctors', *British Medical Journal*, 351 (2015).

Paget, Derek, *No Other Way to Tell It: Docudrama on Film and Television* (Manchester: Manchester University Press, 2011).

Patey, David H. (ed.), *An Introduction to Surgery* (London: Lloyd-Luke Ltd., 1958).

Payne, Lynda, *With Words and Knives: Learning Medical Dispassion in Early Modern England* (Burlington, VT: Ashgate, 2007).

Pernick, Martin S., 'More than Illustrations: Early Twentieth-Century Health Films as Contributors to the Histories of Medicine and of Motion Pictures', in Leslie J. Reagan, Nancy Tomes, and Paula A. Treichler (eds), *Medicine's Moving Pictures: Medicine, Health, and Bodies in American Film and Television* (Rochester, NY: University of Rochester Press, 2007), 19–35.

Peters, William, 'A New Heart for Pamela', *Woman's Own* (16 December 1954).

Pfau, Michael, Lawrence J. Mullen, and Kirsten Garrow, 'The Influence of Television Viewing on Public Perceptions of Physicians', *Journal of Broadcasting & Electronic Media*, 39:4 (1995), 441–458.

Phillips, E. A., Tony Nimeh, Julie Braga, and Lori B. Lerner, 'Does a Surgical Career Affect a Woman's Childbearing and Fertility? A Report on Pregnancy and Fertility Trends Among Female Surgeons', *Journal of the American College of Surgery*, 219 (2014), 944–950.

Pitchford, Mark, *The Conservative Party and the Extreme Right 1945–1975* (Manchester: Manchester University Press, 2011).

Poole, Steven, '"Frontline": Is it Misleading to Apply Military Metaphors to Medicine', *The Guardian* (16 April 2020), www.theguardian.com/books/2020/apr/16/frontline-is-it-misleading-to-apply-military-metaphors-to-medicine (accessed 30 May 2021).

Prentice, Rachel, *Bodies in Formation: An Ethnography of Anatomy and Surgical Education* (Durham, NC: Duke University Press, 2012).

Press Association, 'Medical Students "Humiliated by Senior Doctors"', *The Guardian* (1 October 2004), www.theguardian.com/education/2004/oct/01/highereducation.uk1 (accessed 19 May 2021).

Pressley, Hilda, *Staff Nurses in Love* (London: Mills & Boon, 1962).

Razai, Mohammad S., Hadyn K. N. Kankam, Azeem Majeed, Aneez Esmail, and David R. Williams, 'Mitigating Ethnic Disparities in Covid-19 and Beyond', *British Medical Journal*, 372 (2021), 1–14.

Reagan, Leslie J., Nancy Tomes, and Paula A. Treichler, 'Introduction: Medicine, Health, and Bodies in American Film and Television', in Leslie J. Reagan, Nancy Tomes, and Paula A. Treichler (eds), *Medicine's Moving Pictures: Medicine, Health, and Bodies in American Film and Television* (Rochester, NY: University of Rochester Press, 2007), 1–16.

Reddy, William, *The Navigation of Feeling: A Framework for the History of Emotions* (Cambridge: Cambridge University Press, 2001).

Redhead, Grace, '"A British Problem Affecting British People": Sickle Cell Anaemia, Medical Activism and Race in the National Health Service, 1975–1993', *Twentieth Century British History*, 32:2 (2021), 189–211.

Redman, N. R., J. P. Toby, and J. B. Peniket, 'Hospital Junior Doctors: Survey at Northampton General Hospital', *British Medical Journal*, 3:5669 (1969), 522–525.

Reed, Graham, 'Hospital Doctors Need a New Career Structure', *British Medical Journal*, 330:7504 (2005), 1397.

Reid, Iona, 'Patients' Preference for Male or Female Breast Surgeons: Questionnaire Study', *British Medical Journal*, 317:7165 (1998), 1051–1060.

Richards, Tessa, 'The Overseas Doctors Training Scheme: Failing Expectations', *British Medical Journal*, 308:6944 (1994), 1627–1631.

Rimmer, Abi, 'The Firm: Does it Hold the Answers to Teamworking and Morale?', *BMJ*, 365 (2019), l4104.

Rimmer, Abi, 'Working Time Restrictions May Have Increased Tensions Between Trainees and Consultants, Studies Find', *British Medical Journal*, 348 (2014).

Rivett, Geoffrey, '1998–2007: Labour's Decade', Nuffield Trust, www.nuffieldtrust.org.uk/chapter/1998-2007-labour-s-decade (accessed 22 May 2021).

Rivett, Geoffrey, *From Cradle to Grave: Fifty Years of the NHS* (London: King's Fund, 1998).

Roberts, Shirley, 'Sophia Louisa Jex-Blake (1840–1912)', *Oxford Dictionary of National Biography*, www.oxforddnb.com/view/10.1093/ref:odnb/9780198614128.001.0001/odnb-9780198614128-e-34189 (accessed 20 May. 2021).

Rosenstein, Alan H., and Michelle O'Daniel, 'A Survey of the Impact of Disruptive Behaviors and Communication Defects on Patient Safety', *Joint Commission Journal on Quality and Patient Safety*, 34:8 (2008), 464–471.

Rosenwein, Barbara H., 'Worrying about Emotions in History', *American Historical Review*, 107:3 (2002), 821–845.

Rosner, L., *Medical Education in the Age of Improvement: Edinburgh Students and Apprentices, 1760–1826* (Edinburgh: Edinburgh University Press, 1991).

Royal College of Physicians, 'Helen Marion Macpherson Mackay', https://history.rcplondon.ac.uk/inspiring-physicians/helen-marion-macpherson-mackay (accessed 20 May 2021).

Royal College of Surgeons, 'Statistics', www.rcseng.ac.uk/careers-in-surgery/women-in-surgery/statistics/ (accessed 20 May 2021).

Royal College of Surgeons of England, 'Black Surgeons Past and Present' (27 October 2020), www.rcseng.ac.uk/news-and-events/news/archive/black-surgeons-past-present/ (accessed 21 May 2021).

Royal College of Surgeons of England, 'Covid-19: Good Practice for Surgeons and Surgical Teams' (31 March 2020), www.rcseng.ac.uk/standards-and-research/standards-and-guidance/good-practice-guides/coronavirus/covid-19-good-practice-for-surgeons-and-surgical-teams/#ptc (accessed 24 May 2021).

Royal College of Surgeons of England, 'Joll, Cecil Augustus (1885–1945)', *Plarr's Lives of the Fellows* (23 July 2013).

Royal College of Surgeons of England, 'Skills and Qualities of a Surgeon', www.rcseng.ac.uk/careers-in-surgery/careers-support/skills-and-qualities-of-a-surgeon/ (accessed 31 May 2021).

Royal College of Surgeons of England, 'The Royal College: Our Professional Home. An Independent Review on Diversity and Inclusion for the Royal College of Surgeons of England. An Exciting Call for Radical Change' (March 2021).

Rudman, L. A., and P. Glick, 'Feminized Management and Backlash toward Agentic Women: The Hidden Costs to Women of a Kinder, Gentler Image of Middle Managers', *Journal of Personal and Social Psychology*, 77:1004 (1999).

Ryall, Charles, 'The Technique of Cancer Operations, with Reference to the Danger of Cancer Infection', *British Medical Journal*, 2:2492 (1908), 1005.

Sanerkin, N. G., 'Hospital Junior Staff', *British Medical Journal*, 2:5514 (1966), 646.

Saunders, Jack, 'Emotions, Social Practices and the Changing Composition of Class, Race and Gender in the NHS, 1970–79', *History Workshop Journal*, 88 (2019), 204–229.

Saunders, Jack, 'The Junior Doctors' Strike: What's Really New About it?', *The Guardian* (6 January 2016), www.theguardian.com/science/the-h-word/2016/jan/06/nhs-junior-doctors-strike-whats-really-new-about-it (accessed 22 May 2021).

Saunders, Jack, 'When do Doctors' Strikes End? A Perspective from 1975', *People's History of the NHS* (8 February 2016), https://peopleshistorynhs.org/when-do-doctors-strikes-end-a-perspective-from-1975/ (accessed 22 May 2021).

Scanlon, Lesley, 'White Coats, Handmaidens and Warrior Chiefs: The Role of Filmic Representations in Becoming a Professional', in Lesley Scanlon (ed.), *"Becoming" a Professional: An Interdisciplinary Analysis of Professional Learning* (New York: Springer, 2011), 109–127.

Schlich, Thomas, 'Degrees of Control: The Spread of Operative Fracture Care with Metal Implants. A Comparative Perspective of Switzerland, East Germany, and the USA, 1950s–1990s', in Jenny Stanton (ed.), *Innovations in Health and Medicine: Diffusion and Resistance in the Twentieth Century* (London: Routledge, 2002), 106–125.

Schlich, Thomas, 'Introduction: What is Special about the History of Surgery', in Thomas Schlich (ed.), *The Palgrave Handbook of the History of Surgery*, (London: Palgrave Macmillan, 2017), 1–24.

Schlich, Thomas, '"One and the Same the World Over": The International Culture of Surgical Exchange in an Age of Globalization, 1870–1914', *Journal of the History of Medicine and Allied Sciences*, 71 (2016), 247–270.

Schlich, Thomas, *Surgery, Science and Industry: A Revolution in Fracture Care, 1950–1990s* (Basingstoke: Palgrave, 2002).

Schlich, Thomas (ed.), *The Palgrave Handbook of the History of Surgery* (London: Palgrave Macmillan, 2017).

Schlich, Thomas, and Christopher Crennner (eds), *Technological Change in Modern Surgery: Historical Perspectives on Innovation* (Rochester, NY: University of Rochester Press, 2017).

Schofield, Camilla, *Enoch Powell and the Making of Postcolonial Britain* (Cambridge: Cambridge University Press, 2013).

Schwarz, Bill, *The White Man's World* (Oxford: Oxford University Press, 2013).

Schulz, Amy J., and Leigh Mullings (eds), *Gender, Race, Class, and Health: Intersectional Approaches* (San Francisco: Jossey-Bass, 2006).

Scrutator, 'The Week: A Personal View of Current Medicopolitical Events', *British Medical Journal*, 295 (1987), 1008.

Seaton, Andrew, 'Against the 'Sacred Cow': NHS Opposition and the Fellowship for Freedom in Medicine, 1948–72', *Twentieth Century British History*, 26 (2015), 424–449.

Secretary of State for Health, 'The New NHS: Modern. Dependable' (Department of Health and Social Care, 1997), https://assets.publishing.service.gov.uk/government/uploads/system/uploads/attachment_data/file/266003/newnhs.pdf.

Segal, Francesca, 'Who Said Romance was Dead?', *The Observer* (27 January 2008), www.theguardian.com/books/2008/jan/27/fiction.features1 (accessed 18 May 2021).

Servitje, Lorenzo, *Medicine is War: The Martial Metaphor in Victorian Literature and Culture* (Albany, NY: SUNY Press, 2021).

Sex Discrimination Act (1975), www.legislation.gov.uk/ukpga/1975/65/pdfs/ukpga_19750065_en.pdf (accessed 20 May 2021), 1–81.

Shah, Jyoti, 'Knife, Life, and Wife: Old Stereotypes Persist in Surgery', *Health Service Journal* (1 December 2015), www.hsj.co.uk/women-leaders-network/knife-life-and-wife-old-stereotypes-persist-in-surgery/7000785.article (accessed 13 May 2020).

Sharma, Malika, and Shail Rawal, 'Intersections of Race and Gender in Surgical Training', *JAMA Surgery*, 156:5 (2021), 498.

Shepherd, John, 'Married Quarters', *British Medical Journal*, 1:5538 (1967), 505.

Simpson, Julian M., *Migrant Architects of the NHS: South Asian Doctors and the Reinvention of British General Practice (1940s–1980s)* (Manchester: Manchester University Press, 2018).

Simpson, Julian M., Stephanie J. Snow, and Aneez Esmail, 'Providing "Special" Types of Labour and Exerting Agency: How Migrant Doctors Have Shaped the UK's National Health Service', in Laurence Monnais and David Wright (eds), *Doctors Beyond Borders: The Transnational Migration of Physicians in the Twentieth Century* (Toronto: University of Toronto Press, 2016), 208–229.

Simpson, P. A., 'An Address on Post-Graduate Possibilities', *British Medical Journal*, 2:1400 (1887), 923–928.

Sinclair, Simon, *Making Doctors: An Institutional Apprenticeship* (London: Routledge, 2020).

Smith, Allen C., and Sherryl Kleinman, 'Managing Emotions in Medical School: Students' Contacts with the Living and the Dead', *Social Psychology Quarterly*, 52:1 (1989), 56–69.

Smith, Nicola P., Evelyn H. Dykes, George S. Youngson, and Paul D. Losty, 'Is the Grass Greener? A Survey of Female Pediatric Surgeons in the United Kingdom', *Journal of Pediatric Surgery*, 41:11 (2006), 1879–1881.

Snow, Stephanie, and Emma Jones, 'Immigration and the National Health Service: Putting History to the Forefront', *History & Policy* (8 March 2011), www.historyandpolicy.org/policy-papers/papers/immigration-and-the-national-health-service-putting-history-to-the-forefron (accessed 21 May 2021).

Sokol, Daniel K., 'How to Be a Cool Headed Clinician', *British Medical Journal*, 344 (2012), e3980.

Somers, Margaret R., and Gloria D. Gibson, 'Reclaiming the Epistemological "Other": Narrative and the Social Construction of Identity', in C. Calhoun (ed.), *Social Theory and the Politics of Identity* (Oxford: Blackwell, 1994), 37–99.

Sontag, Susan, *Illness as Metaphor & AIDS and its Metaphors* (London: Penguin, 2009).

Spencer, John, 'Some Activity But Still Not Much Action on Patient and Public Engagement', *Medical Education*, 50 (2016), 3–23.

St Clair Strange, F. G., *The History of the ABC Club of Travelling Fellows* (London: British Editorial Society of Bone and Joint Surgery, 1998).

Stahel, Philip F., *Blood, Sweat & Tears: Becoming a Better Surgeon* (Shrewsbury: TFM, 2016).

Stanley, Peter, *For Fear of Pain: British Surgery, 1790–1850* (Amsterdam: Rodopi, 2003).

Stearns, Peter N., *American Cool: Constructing a Twentieth-Century Emotional Style* (New York: New York University Press, 1994).

Stein, Leonard I., 'The Doctor–Nurse Game', *American Journal of Nursing*, 68:1 (1968), 101–105.

Stidolph, Neville, 'Training of Surgeons', *British Medical Journal*, 4:5627 (1968), 379–383.

Stobbs, N., and E. Ward, 'Do Modern-Day Surgeons Break the Stereotype and Show Emotional Intelligence in their Leadership?', *Bulletin of the Royal College of Surgeons of England*, 96 (2013), 5–8.

Strangleman, Tim, 'The Nostalgia of Organisations and the Organisation of Nostalgia: Past and Present in the Contemporary Railway Industry', *Sociology*, 33:4 (1999), 725–746.

Strangleman, Tim, and Ian Roberts, 'Looking Through the Window of Opportunity: The Cultural Cleansing of Workplace Identity', *Sociology*, 33:1 (1999), 47–67.

Strauman, Elena C., and Bethany C. Goodier, 'The Doctor(s) in House: An Analysis of the Evolution of the Television Doctor-Hero', *Journal of Medical Humanities*, 32:1 (2011), 31–46.

Tan, Ashley, 'Racism on the Frontline: Britain's Asian Healthcare Workers', *Al Jazeera* (27 April 2021), www.aljazeera.com/features/2021/4/27/under-fire-on-the-frontline-britains-asian-healthcare-workers (accessed 21 May 2021).

Taylor, J. G., 'Encouraging Recruits to Medicine', *British Medical Journal*, 2:5752 (1971), 51.

Teo, Hsu-Ming, 'The Romance of White Nations: Imperialism, Popular Culture, and National Histories', in Antoinette Burton (ed.), *After the Imperial Turn: Thinking With and Through the Nation* (Chapel Hill, NC: Duke University Press, 2003), 279–292.

Thomson, Mathew, 'Representations of the National Health Service in the Arts and Popular Culture', in Jennifer Crane and Jane Hand (eds), *Posters, Protests, and Prescriptions: Cultural Histories of the National Health Service in Britain* (Manchester: Manchester University Press, 2022), 231–254.

Timm, Anja, 'The Demise of the Firm: What is Happening to Apprenticeship Learning?', https://bit.ly/2Sb4mZL (accessed 19 May 2021).

Tincknell, Estella, 'The Nation's Matron: Hattie Jacques and British Post-war Popular Culture', *Journal of British Cinema and Television*, 12:1 (2015), 6–24.

Toft, Anthony, 'Has Humanity Disappeared from the NHS?', *British Medical Journal*, 320:7247 (2000), 1483.

Tokarz, J. Pat, William Bremer, and Ken Peters, *Beyond Survival: The Challenge of the Impaired Student* (American Medical Association: Workgroup on Physician Well-Being, Resident Physicians Section, 1979).

Treves, Frederick, 'Address in Surgery: The Surgeon in The Nineteenth Century', *British Medical Journal*, 2:2066 (1900), 284–289.

Trueland, Jennifer, 'And You Thought Surgery was Hard…', British Medical Association (11 June 2021), www.bma.org.uk/news-and-opinion/and-you-thought-surgery-was-hard (accessed 4 August 2022).

Trunkey, Donald, 'Report to the Council of the Association of Surgeons of Great Britain and Ireland', *British Medical Journal*, 299 (1989), 31–33.

Tsouroufli, Maria, Mustafa Özbilgin, and Merryn Smith, 'Gendered Forms of Othering in UK Hospital Medicine: Nostalgia as Resistance Against the Modern Doctor', *Equality, Diversity and Inclusion: An International Journal*, 30:6 (2011), 489–509.

Tune, G. S., 'Sleep and Wakefulness in a Group of Shift Workers', *British Journal of Industrial Medicine*, 26 (1969), 54–58.

Turow, John, *Playing Doctor: Television, Storytelling, and Medical Power* (Ann Arbor: University of Michigan Press, 2010).

Tweedie, J. H., A. Milosevic, and D. Shuttleworth, 'Facilities for Junior Doctors in New Hospitals', *British Medical Journal*, 2:6150 (1978), 1503.

Underman, Kelly, and Laura E. Hirshfield, 'Detached Concern?: Emotional Socialization in Twenty-First Century Medical Education', *Social Science & Medicine*, 160 (2016), 94–101.

University of Sussex, National Union of Students, 'That's What She Said: Women Students' Experiences of "Lad Culture" in Higher Education', http://sro.sussex.ac.uk/id/eprint/49011/1/That's_what_she_said_full_report_Final_web.pdf (accessed 20 May 2021).

Vigna, Xavier, Michelle Zancarini-Fournel, and Sian Reynolds, 'Gender History and Labour History', *Clio. Women, Gender, History*, 38 (2013), 176–203.

Vincent, Charles, Jonathan Benn, and George B. Hanna, 'High Reliability in Health Care', *British Medical Journal*, 340:7740 (2010), 225–226.

Vinson, Alexandra H., and Kelly Underman, 'Clinical Empathy as Emotional Labor in Medical Work', *Social Science & Medicine*, 251 (2020), 112904.

Waddington, Keir, 'Mayhem and Medical Students: Image, Conduct and Control in the Victorian and Edwardian London Teaching Hospital', *Social History of Medicine*, 15:1 (2002), 45–64.

Webster, Charles, *The Health Services Since the War, Volume II. Government and Health Care: The National Health Service 1958–79* (London: Stationery Office, 1996).

Webster, Charles, *The National Health Service: A Political History* (Oxford: Oxford University Press, 2002).

Webster, Wendy, *Englishness and Empire 19939–1965* (Oxford: Oxford University Press, 2005).

Whitfield, A. G. W., 'Women Medical Graduates of the University of Birmingham 1959–63', *British Medical Journal*, 3:5661 (1969), 44–46.

Wild, J. R. L., H. J. M. Ferguson, F. D. McDermott, S. T. Hornby, and V. J. Gokani, 'Undermining and Bullying in Surgical Training: A Review and Recommendations by the Association of Surgeons in Training', *International Journal of Surgery*, 23:1 (2015), S5–S9.

Wilde, Sally, 'The Elephants in the Doctor–Patient Relationship: Patients' Clinical Interactions and the Changing Surgical Landscape of the 1890s', *Health and History*, 9:1 (2007), 2–27.

Wilde, Sally, 'Truth, Trust, and Confidence in Surgery, 1890–1910: Patient Autonomy, Communication, and Consent', *Bulletin of the History of Medicine*, 83:2 (2009), 302–330.

Willett, L. L., Melissa F. Wellons, Jason R. Hartig, Lindsey Roenigk, Mukta Panda, Angela T. Dearinger, et al., 'Do Women Residents Delay Childbearing due to Perceived Career Threats?', *Academic Medicine*, 85 (2010), 640–646.

Wittkower, Eric D., and Kerr L. White, 'Bedside Manners', *British Medical Journal*, 1:4876 (1954), 1432–1434.

Woods, Hannah Rose, *Rule, Nostalgia: A Backwards History of Britain* (London: Ebury, 2022).

Yorke, C., 'Heroic Conduct of Surgeons in the Crimea', *The Lancet*, 66:1669 (1855), 178.

Younge, Gary, 'In these Bleak Times, Imagine a World Where you can Thrive', *The Guardian* (10 January 2020), www.theguardian.com/commentisfree/2020/jan/10/bleak-times-thrive-last-column-guardian (accessed 21 May 2021).

Websites

British Library, 'Oral Histories of Medicine and Health Professionals', www.bl.uk/collection-guides/oral-histories-of-medicine-and-health-professionals (accessed 14 August 2018).

British Medical Association, www.bma.org.uk/news-and-opinion/under-fire-on-the-front-line-doctors-share-their-experiences-of-work-during-the-covid-19-crisis (accessed 24 May 2021).

#HammerItOut, https://twitter.com/hammeritoutuk (accessed 20 May 2021).

Health Education England, https://london.hee.nhs.uk/covid-19-hub/online-well-being-resources/podcasts/episode-6 (accessed 23 May 2021).

KevinMD.com, www.kevinmd.com/blog/2016/03/doctors-marry-doctors-challenges-face.html (accessed 20 May 2021).

Measuring Worth.com, https://measuringworth.com/datasets/ukearncpi/ (accessed 30 November 2020).

Medical Protection, www.medicalprotection.org/uk/articles/building-resilience-and-avoiding-burnout-workshop (accessed 31 May 2021).

Royal College of Surgeons of Edinburgh, www.rcsed.ac.uk/professional-support-development-resources/anti-bullying-and-undermining-campaign (accessed 20 May 2021).

Surgery and Emotion, www.surgeryandemotion.com (accessed 31 May 2021).

Television Heaven, https://televisionheaven.co.uk/reviews/emergency-ward-10 (accessed 18 May 2021).

UK Government, www.ethnicity-facts-figures.service.gov.uk/workforce-and-business/workforce-diversity/nhs-workforce/latest (accessed 21 March 2021).

Index